METROPOLITAN MATERNITY:
MATERNAL AND INFANT WELFARE
SERVICES IN EARLY TWENTIETH
CENTURY LONDON

THE WELLCOME INSTITUTE SERIES IN THE HISTORY OF MEDICINE

Forthcoming Titles

Warm Climates and Western Medicine
Edited by David Arnold

Marshall Hall: 1790–1857: Science and Medicine in
Early Victorian Society
Diana Manuel

The Correspondence of James Jurin (1684–1750):
Physician and Secretary of the Royal Society
Andrea Rusnock

History of Cardiology
P. Fleming

Fantasy Surgery
Ann Dally

Operative Chymist:: A Biography of Thomas N. R. Morson
Anthony F. P. Morson

Academic enquiries regarding the series should be addressed
to the editors W. F. Bynum and Roy Porter at
the Wellcome Institute for the History of Medicine,
183 Euston Road, London NW1 2BE, UK

METROPOLITAN MATERNITY:
MATERNAL AND INFANT WELFARE
SERVICES IN EARLY TWENTIETH
CENTURY LONDON

Lara V. Marks

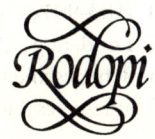

Amsterdam - Atlanta, GA 1996

First published in 1996
by Editions Rodopi B. V., Amsterdam – Atlanta, GA 1996.

© 1996 Lara V. Marks

Design and Typesetting by Christine Buckley, the Wellcome Trust.
Printed and bound in The Netherlands by Editions Rodopi B. V.,
Amsterdam – Atlanta, GA 1996.

British Library Cataloguing in Publication Data
A catalogue record for this book is available from the British Library
ISBN 90-5183-901-4 (Bound)

Marks, Lara V.
Metropolitan Maternity: Maternal and Infant Welfare Services in
Early Twentieth Century London – Amsterdam – Atlanta, GA:
Rodopi. – ill.
(Clio Medica 36/The Wellcome Institute Series in the
History of Medicine)

CIP-GEGEVENS KONINKLIJKE BIBLIOTHEEK, DEN HAAG

Front cover: from a pamphlet published to accompany an
exhibition organized by Woolwich Borough Council in 1928.
Health Week focused on the range of health facilities
available in the borough, healthy living and eating.
Courtesy of London Borough of Greenwich: Local History Library.

Met index, lit. opg.
ISBN 90-5183-901-4 (geb)
Trefw.: Kraamverpleging; Londen; geschiedenis; 20e eeuw;
zuigelingenzorg; Londen; geschiedenis; 20e eeuw
Consultatiebureaus; Londen; geschiedenis; 20e eeuw

© Editions Rodopi B. V. Amsterdam – Atlanta, GA 1996
Printed in The Netherlands

This book is dedicated to David Widgery

Contents

Acknowledgements

This book started as a project on the historical geography of the welfare state and has had a long and varied history. Much of this book was inspired by the troubled times we are now experiencing with the National Health Service and the Welfare State. It is dedicated to David Widgery, whom I only met once and sadly on what turned out to be the last day of his life. His work and commitment, however, have provided me with great insight into the problems of poverty and ill health and the need at all costs to provide a comprehensive and humane health service.

In writing the book I have had the warmth and support of many, to whom it is hard to express enough gratitude. Throughout the process of thinking and writing my mother, father, and brother have proved a vital source of encouragement and patience. Special thanks also go to Humaira Ahmed, Meg Arnot, Cathy Crawford, Sandra den Otter, Irvine Loudon, Hilary Marland, Liz Peretz, Helen Nicholls, Hilary Sapire, Anne Summers and Maridowa Williams, many of whom not only offered the crucial support of friendship but also a critical eye to the manuscript while in its preparation. Much appreciation also goes to Sally Alexander, Bill Bynum, Mary Dobson, Iris Dove, David Edgerton, Lesley Hall, Anne Hardy, Enid Henessey, Lisa Hilder, Ludmilla Jordanova, Jane Lewis, Ornella Moscucci, Naomi Pfeffer, Dorothy Porter, Roy Porter, Ruth Richardson, Richard Smith, Pat Thane, Mathew Thomson, Cornelie Usborne, Signild Vallgarda, Andrew Warwick, Charles Webster, Dan Weinbren, Jerry White and Susan Williams for all their academic advice and constant encouragement during various stages of completing the book. This book would also never have begun or been completed without the help of Roger Lee, John Mohan, Gillian Rose and Humphrey Southall. In addition to this I owe a great deal of gratitude to John Imrie, who not only typed the majority of the original manuscript, but also provided an important critical and challenging eye. Many thanks are also due to Edward Oliver for producing such clear and illustrative maps, and to Linda Neri for her assistance in gathering archive data. Much support was also given to me by the academic and secretarial staff in the Geography Department at Queen Mary and Westfield College, the Health Promotion Sciences Unit at the London School of Hygiene and Tropical Medicine, and the Centre for the History of Science,

Technology and Medicine at Imperial College. Special acknowledgement is also due to the Leverhulme Trust for funding the project. Warm appreciation also goes to all the people I interviewed for the research, whose memories brought the project alive and added a rich texture to my work.

Research for the book was made immeasurably easier by the knowledge and kindness of the staff at the Bodleian Library, the British Library, the British Library of Political and Social Science, Camden Local History Library, the Contemporary Medical Archives Centre at the Wellcome Institute for the History of Medicine, the Francis Countway Library, the Fawcett Library, the Greater London Record Office, the Greenwich Local History Library, Kensington Local History Library, the London School of Hygiene and Tropical Medicine, the Public Record Office, the National Museum of Labour History, St Bartholomew's Hospital Archives, Sophia Smith Collection at Smith College, The London Hospital Archives and the Tower Hamlets Local History Library and Archive. I am also grateful to all these libraries and archives for granting me permission to publish their sources.

I am thankful to Greenwich Health Authority, the Family Welfare Association, the Whittington Hospital, and Tower Hamlets Health Authority for granting me permission to use various records relating to the following hospitals and organizations: British Hospital for Mothers and Babies, Charity Organization Society and the City of London Maternity Hospital.

List of Figures

Appendices

List of Tables

List of Tables

xix

List of Abbreviations

Am. Hist. Rev.	*American Historical Review*
Ann. Epidemiol.	*Annals of Epidemiology*
AJA	Anglo Jewish Archives
A/R	*Annual Report*
BL	British Library
BLPES	British Library of Political and Economic Sciences
BMB	British Hospital for Mothers and Babies
Br. J. Obstet. & Gynaecol.	*British Journal of Obstetrics and Gynaecology*
Br. Med. J.	*British Medical Journal*
Bull. Hist. Med.	*Bulletin of the History of Medicine*
Ch.	Chapter
CLMH	City of London Maternity Hospital
CMB	Central Midwives Board
CMAC	Contemporary Medical Archives Centre, Wellcome Institute
COS	Charity Organization Society
Econ. Hist. Rev.	*Economic History Review*
Edn	Edition
EEMH	East End Maternity Home
ELA	*East London Advertiser*
ELNS	East London Nursing Society
ELO	*East London Observer*
Epidemiol. Rev.	*Epidemiological Review*
Eur. J. Popul.	*European Journal of Population*
Fem. Stud.	*Feminist Studies*
Gender and Hist.	*Gender and History*
GLH	Greenwich Local History Library
GLRO	Greater London Record Office
HCSW	Hampstead Council for Social Welfare
HLHL	Hampstead Local History Library
Hist.	*History*
Hist. J.	*Historical Journal*
Hist. Workshop J.	*History Workshop Journal*
IMR	Infant Mortality Rate
IWC	Infant Welfare Centre
Instit. Br. Geog. Trans.	*Institute of British Geographers Transactions*
Intro.	Introduction
JBG	Jewish Board of Guardians
JC	*Jewish Chronicle*
JMH	Jewish Maternity Home
JWB	Jewish Welfare Board Archive

J. Biosoc. Sci.	*Journal of Biosocial Science*
J. Br. Stud.	*Journal of British Studies*
J. Contemp. Hist.	*Journal of Contemporary History*
J. Eur. Econ. Hist	*Journal of European Economic History*
J. Hist. Geog.	*Journal of Historical Geography*
J. Hist. Med.	*Journal of the History of Medicine*
J. Interdisc. Hist.	*Journal of Interdisciplinary History*
J. Publ. Health	*Journal of Public Health*
J. Roy. Stat. Soc.	*Journal of the Royal Statistical Society*
J. Sanitary Institute	*Journal of the Sanitary Institute*
J. Soc. Hist.	*Journal of Social History*
J. Soc. Pol.	*Journal of Social Policy*
J. Stat. Soc.	*Journal of the Statistical Society*
KLHL	Kensington Local History Library
LGB	Local Government Board
LCC	London County Council
LH	London Hospital Archive
MS	Manuscript
MCW	Maternal and Child Welfare
Med. Hist.	*Medical History*
Med. Offr.	*Medical Officer*
MH	Ministry of Health
MP	Member of Parliament
MMR	Maternal Mortality Rate
MOH	Medical Officer of Health
Mocatta	Mocatta Library, University College, London University
NCVO	National Council for Voluntary Organizations
NKWWC	North Kensington Women's Welfare Centre
NNMR	Neonatal Mortality Rate
Oral Hist.	*Oral History*
Popul. Stud.	*Population Studies*
PP	Parliamentary Papers
P & P	*Past and Present*
PNNMR	Post-neonatal Mortality Rate
PRO	Public Record Office
Publ. Health	*Public Health*
Repr.	Reprint
R. C.	*Royal Commission on*
RMC	Royal Maternity Charity
St Barts	St Bartholomew's Hospital Archive
SA	Salvation Army Archive
SAMH	Salvation Army's Mothers Hospital
Ser.	Series
SRHS	Sick Room Helps Society
Soc. Hist.	*Social History*

List of Abbreviations

Soc. Hist. Med.	Social History of Medicine
Soc. Serv. Rev.	Social Services Review
SS	Sophia Smith Collection, Smith College
THL	Tower Hamlets Local History Library
Trans. Obstet. Soc.	Transactions of the Obstetrical Society of London
Twentieth Cent. Br. Hist.	Twentieth Century British History
Unpub.	Unpublished
Vict. Stud.	Victorian Studies
Vol.	Volume
WDA	Westminster Diocese Archive, Catholic Church

Introduction

London has always been at the heart of the social and economic fabric of British life and empire. Its dominance in international financial markets and its focus as the centre of the national transport system have always promoted its powers beyond its geographical boundaries. London has also been a key site for the initiation and implementation of legislation. Not only did the city host Parliament, but also, from 1888, the London County Council, which served as a model for other local government administrations within Britain, and was the largest municipal authority in the world in the late nineteenth and early twentieth centuries. The metropolis is also the headquarters for many of the professions, and a home for much of the country's intellectual élite.

To see London as an organic and unified entity is to miss its variety and complexity. In reality London might more accurately be described as a mosaic of communities within a geographical region, each jostling for recognition and power. London has always had a disproportionately large number of middle- and upper-class residents. The image of London as the city which had streets paved with gold lured many working-class residents, many of whom found employment in the city's large service sector.[1] As a port, London has also attracted many groups of immigrants, such as the Huguenots, the Irish and East European Jews. The class and ethnic composition of London has probably never been homogeneous. Each of the groups who came to settle in the great metropolis tended to settle in distinct areas, forming communities in themselves with their own agendas and social and religious needs.

In addition to the different classes and immigrant groups, London hosted multiple government bodies, each with their own jurisdiction and purpose. The most centralized regional body in the late nineteenth century was the London County Council, which was the capital's first democratic metropolitan authority. Modelled on its predecessor the Metropolitan Board of Works, the aim of the London County Council was to coordinate and initiate public services within and for London as a whole, including drainage, buildings, the fire service, housing, parks, recreational spaces, education and the transport system. In 1930 Poor Law Infirmaries also passed into the London County Council's hands.

1

On a more local level were the 28 local authorities, also known as borough councils, created by the Local Government Act of 1899. Built upon the basis of existing vestries and other countervailing authorities, these borough councils were originally set up under the Conservative ministry of Lord Salisbury in the late nineteenth century as a measure to check the power of the London County Council and the Progressive Party that dominated its administration. Both the London County Council and the borough councils were given very similar powers, which did not always make for easy relationships and could lead to overlapping services.[2] Like the London County Council, the borough councils were expected to take responsibility for sanitation, health, housing and other public services. Within each borough, these local authorities had enormous autonomy in determining expenditure levels and the types of services provided. Alongside the borough councils, were the Boards of Guardians who administered the various forms of parish relief: including care for the elderly, the unemployed, unmarried mothers, orphans and the sick poor.

All these authorities were answerable to a different electorate, each of which had its own visions and demands. As the regional institution, the London County Council represented the whole of London. The borough councils and Boards of Guardians were governed largely by more local needs and demands, determined by the particular socio-economic conditions, class composition, and political affiliations of each district.

London's significance stretches beyond its diverse population and unique institutional structures. London suffered particularly acute social and economic problems, having witnessed more rapid and greater growth than the rest of Britain during the nineteenth century, bringing along with it evils such as overcrowding, poor sanitation, and social and economic dislocation. Such problems were not confined to London alone, but as the capital of the nation and the heart of the Empire they were treated with special gravity. Indeed, London had a distinct place in many of the political and social debates concerning the physical, military and economic strength of the nation in the early twentieth century.[3]

During the South African War (1899–1902)[4] between 29 and 32 per cent of men recruited to the war effort had failed to pass the fitness test to join the army, revealing the appalling level of ill health among the male population.[5] The gravity of the problem was highlighted by the Royal Commission on Physical Deterioration, whose report was published in 1904. Many medical experts and

2

social reformers had given evidence to the commission and had indicated that a large proportion of the male working-class population were small in stature, malnourished, physically weak, had decayed teeth and poor eyesight, and were often suffering from tuberculosis and venereal disease.[6] Similar revelations of poor health were revealed among recruits for the First World War (1914–18).

The physical incapacity of many within the population was deeply disturbing to many politicians and social reformers concerned about the increasing military and industrial competition Britain was facing from America and Germany in these years. Compounding their anxiety was also the prediction of population decline in the light of a falling birth rate. Nor were their fears eased by the high rates of infant mortality during these years. Indeed, unlike other forms of mortality which underwent a sharp drop from the 1870s, infant mortality remained high, and even rose in the late 1890s and early twentieth century.[7] Some idea of the concern this caused can be seen from a statement made in 1915 by Henry Ashby, a medical expert on infant mortality. He declared,

> A high rate of infant mortality implies not only a wastage of life, but also a large number of our fellow citizens are living under wretched conditions, deprived of most of the advantages which alone can make life bright and happy.[8]

Ashby's assertion highlights the link that medical experts and social reformers were making between health and the environment in the early twentieth century. Growing urbanization, poor housing, inadequate diets and squalid living conditions were just some of the factors cited as the reason for the increasing ill health of the British population.[9] For many politicians and health reformers one solution to the prevailing ill health among the population was the provision of good health care services by the state, which would raise health standards among the population and enable individuals to realize their full potential as citizens, particularly as soldiers and workers.

Starting at a time of great debate in the wake of the South African War and ending just before the outbreak of the Second World War, *Metropolitan Maternity* covers a period in which the debate over the future and the welfare of the nation was particularly fraught. This book explores the call for state provision of health care in these years and shows that many of the services arose amid as much conflict as the health policies being pursued today. Women and infants became the most important priority group during this period.[10] These years were crucial for legislation on maternal and infant health services,

3

including the first regulation of midwives in 1902, the introduction of the Maternity Benefit in 1913, the Maternal and Child Welfare Act of 1918, and the Public Health Act and Midwives Act of 1936 which brought in a comprehensive state midwifery service for the first time. These measures were not without their irony: aimed at ensuring the survival of infants and the future generation, many of the children nurtured under them were later maimed or killed either in the First World War or the Second World War. Driven partly by military concerns, these measures, therefore, had a double-edge to their outcome.

Maternal and infant health services provide an invaluable insight into early state health and welfare developments in Britain and the foundations on which they were built. The establishment of these services are particularly interesting in the light of the changes that are going on in the health service today, and the increasing turn away from state provision. To many who regarded the Welfare State and National Health Service as an irreversible feature of British society which arose from the consensus policy which emerged during the Second World War and an inevitable consequence of the progress of modernization and medicine, recent changes have come as a surprise. Yet, as *Metropolitan Maternity* shows, state provision of health services has always been a matter of contest. The establishment of the Welfare State and the National Health Service was not predetermined, nor was the form each institution took. Each arose from particular needs and within a specific context.

Many historians have viewed British state welfare provision either as a manipulative reform imposed by the wealthier classes from above in order to quell discontent from below, or by contrast, as the cumulative result of the increasing political mobilization and power of the underprivileged to secure social and economic benefits available to the wealthier members of society.[11] Such approaches, however, are often simplistic and polarized. As Baldwin has argued in his comparative history of welfare states in Europe,

> Most examinations of the social bases of welfare reform narrate a scenario pitting upper and lower, rich and poor, middle and working class in combat for redistributive advantage. Workers and society's disinherited sought solidarity. The bourgeoisie and other well-positioned groups, in turn, resisted any such designs on their pockets. The outcome of this dichotomized contest over redistribution depended on the respective strengths of these polar actors. A strong, self-confident bourgeoisie was able to turn back ambitions for solidaristic reform. Conversely a sufficiently powerful labour movement might overcome such obstacles.[12]

4

Instead, as Baldwin suggests, and as this book takes as its premise, the development of the British Welfare State arose from conflicts between different classes and interest-groups rooted in particular historical, national and local situations, and which altered over time. In depicting the history of the Welfare State either as the triumph for the forces above or below, historians have tended to concentrate either on the history of government institutions and professions, or on the importance of the labour movement.[13]

In recent years historians have begun to modify their view of the creation of the British Welfare State to one which is more nuanced and more focused on what was going on at the local rather than the national level.[14] Following in this tradition, *Metropolitan Maternity* shows that decisions on welfare taken nationally interacted and were intrinsically informed by those made at a local level. This was vital to the formation of the British Welfare State, not only in terms of expenditure but also in policy formation and the general acceptance of services by those they were intended to serve.

Focusing on London, the book explores the process by which national and local ideas intersected and diverged in the shaping of health and welfare provision. In the book I concentrate on the initiatives from local voluntary groups, from political pressure groups, and labour organizations, as well as the efforts of individual women themselves. While these groups were greatly affected by the policies taken at the centre, their concerns and interests were influenced by a range of popular interests and influences which differed from those on a national level and can only be understood within a local context.[15] Most of these groups were acting from a local perspective, but when taken together, their collective efforts can be seen to have been a vital force in determining both the extent and the type of services provided.

By focusing on grassroot movements and organizations I aim to demonstrate the diversity of groups that were involved in the provision of services and the wide variety of services they established. As we shall see the care they helped provide extended beyond the remit of the hospital and other formal institutions which have all too often been the focus of much of the literature on the history of health services. I also hope to illuminate some of the experiences individuals had in using the services. Their voices and demands had a profound influence on the facilities provided, a factor which is all too often overlooked by historians concentrating on the centralized administrative developments of these years.

London is an especially rich area for undertaking a study of health care provision. As the capital of Britain and as home to the nation's parliament and the most centralized local government, it was a crucial site for generating health care and welfare policies, many of them forming the basis for national measures. Just before the Second World War almost a quarter of the national expenditure on centralized health care was spent in London.[16] London was also unique in the high number of its specialized voluntary hospitals.[17] The abundance of hospitals within London is particularly interesting in the light of recent studies of other British urban areas which have linked the rise of hospitals closely with the social, political and economic strife stirred by industrialization.[18] Yet London never experienced the same intensity of industrialization as elsewhere. One of the reasons for the large concentration of specialized hospitals in London lies in the dominant presence of the medical profession as well as the large number of wealthy patients who were able to pay for their services within the city.

As this book shows, maternal and infant welfare services were also far more comprehensive and far-reaching in London than elsewhere. Yet, within London such provision was highly variable, reflecting the great diversity of socio-economic conditions within each of its boroughs and the degree of autonomy local authorities had within the metropolis. The four boroughs of Hampstead, Kensington, Stepney and Woolwich were chosen to show the differing levels of living and health standards within London as a whole. In Stepney and Woolwich the overwhelming proportion of residents were working class, but in Stepney most were involved in the casual labour market while the majority in Woolwich tended to be skilled artisans. Stepney, with its densely packed population and poor housing also contrasts with Woolwich which was one of the least densely populated areas of London. Hampstead and Kensington were renowned for their prosperity, but they included areas of severe deprivation. Of these two boroughs poverty was greatest in Kensington. It tended to be concentrated in the north of the borough where overcrowding, poor housing and sanitation were comparable to those found in Stepney.

While such variations in socio-economic conditions were important in determining the levels of mortality found in each borough, as Chapter 3 reveals, no simple and direct relationship seems to have existed between the social deprivation and mortality patterns of each area. Stepney, which was the poorest of the four boroughs, experienced remarkably lower rates of maternal mortality than the other three. This disparity can partly be accounted for by the good charitable maternity care that was available in Stepney through its large number of voluntary teaching hospitals. The importance of this care can be seen by the fact that Stepney was one of the few places where maternal mortality fell in the early twentieth century. No such fall occurred in the other boroughs, or indeed nationally. Mothers in Hampstead, who had the financial means to purchase the expertise of a general practitioner or private midwife, were less likely to receive strict antiseptic care which governed the charitable provision afforded to poorer women in Stepney.

None the less, while it would seem that medical care outweighed the importance of social and economic factors in determining levels of maternal mortality, this was not so in the case of infant mortality. Of the four boroughs, Stepney and Kensington had the highest rates of infant mortality, reflecting the overcrowding and poor housing of many of their residents. Hampstead and Woolwich, by contrast, had significantly lower rates of infant mortality. The contrast in infant mortality patterns is particularly striking between the richer borough of Kensington and the poorer borough of Woolwich, indicating that social and economic conditions were not the only determinants of infant mortality. Remarkably Stepney and Woolwich, which were the poorest of the boroughs and had more municipal commitment to funding maternal and infant welfare services, experienced a greater reduction in their infant mortality rates than Hampstead or Kensington.

It would therefore seem that while socio-economic conditions played an important role in determining the levels of mortality in each borough, some of the negative effects of deprivation can be outweighed by the good provision of medical and welfare services. As Chapters 4 to 6 make clear, however, what provisions were made and the degree to which services reached those in most need, was highly dependent on the political outlook and social relations within each area. Hampstead and Kensington, which were politically more conservative than the two other boroughs, provided far fewer municipal maternal and infant welfare services and were much more reliant on the voluntary sector for provision of such care. Stepney and Woolwich, by contrast, appear to have made more provision for their residents, partly reflecting the greater political commitment of these two councils.

While politics and policies influenced the comprehensiveness and quality of the services provided in each borough, the degree to which these services were used varied greatly and was dependent on the expectations and perceptions of those they were intended to serve. What these demands were and the extent to which they were satisfied is the subject of Chapters 7 and 8. The success of maternal and infant welfare services was not only determined by the efficiency

and type of care provided, but also by the attitude of the professionals towards those they catered for and the outlook of mothers
themselves. In these chapters we will see that the early twentieth
century not only witnessed a growth in the provision of maternal
and child welfare services and an extension in the type of care
provided, but also a shift in the expectations surrounding the provision and uptake of such facilities. By the 1930s many of the
services provided for mothers and children had been transformed
from the philanthropic and patronizing enterprises which had dominated much of the provision at the turn of the century, and had
become more democratic and inclusive of the mothers they were
intended to serve.

Such a change in the orientation of maternal and child welfare
services reflected the growing campaign in the 1920s and 1930s for
citizen participation in civic life, as well as the extension of suffrage
to women. Newly won rights to vote and to stand for parliament
highlight only the surface of the ways in which women were increasing their participation within society. Women's entry into the work-
force in unprecedentedly large numbers during the First World War,
and into new areas of employment after the War, had resulted in a
growing confidence among many women.[19] Smaller families, shorter
working days, higher wages for those in work and the rise in the
general standard of living, all contributed to a new sense of being a
woman in the inter-war years.

The appearance of cropped hair, the wearing of increasingly short
dresses, plus the growing number of women smokers, all show the
growing assertiveness and changing consciousness of women during this
period. As Alexander has shown, women's expectations and demands
were also changing as a result of women's strengthened activities within
trade unions, education, local government and feminist groups. The
growth in advertising and of the cinema in these years, also played on
women's fantasies and desires, enabling them to 'imagine an end to
domestic drudgery and chronic want'.[20] Advertising billboards and cin-
emas projecting offers of streamlined kitchens, effective cleaning
equipment, cheap and pretty clothes and make-up, even if difficult to
purchase in reality, gave many women a vision of an easier and more
fulfilling life than they had ever dreamed possible before.[21]

Women's growing assertiveness in these years was not confined to
their increasingly important role in the work-place and the outside
world. The heightened awareness of the nation's health and the need
for good infant health placed a new emphasis on women's roles as
mothers. As John Burns, President of the Local Government Board,

put it to the first National Conference on Infant Mortality in 1906:

> At the bottom of infant mortality, high or low, is good or bad motherhood. Give us good motherhood, and good pre-natal conditions, and I have no despair for the future of this or any other country.[22]

While limited in scope and in provision, increasing state recognition of motherhood gave many mothers a new sense of pride and awareness. The value attached to motherhood was not only seen in the growing provision of maternal and infant services in these years, but also in the boom in literature on motherhood and childcare.[23]

The new stress upon the importance of motherhood came with its own difficulties. As Alexander has pointed out, a mother's self worth and respect within a neighbourhood depended greatly on being able to maintain the health of her children. Outward signs of cleanliness were all important in this effort. Thus clean and tidy hair and dress were seen as marks of good mothering. 'The child's fall from grace was a reproach to the mother's capabilities, a sign to the neighbours or street that she had been momentarily defeated in the battle against bugs, infection, and ill-health.' A mother's pride was thus greatly invested in that of the appearance of her children. This was not always easy to achieve given the bad housing and scarcity of amenities in these years.[24]

Starting with women's view of motherhood, this book explores how the increasing focus on the nation's health and good mothering affected women's experience of motherhood in the early twentieth century. Concentrating on those mothers who were living in one of the most urbanized parts of Britain, *Metropolitan Maternity* examines the special features of the city that both hindered and helped women in carrying out their tasks of motherhood and securing the survival of their infants while continuing to preserve their own health.[25]

Notes

1. D. Feldman and G. Stedman Jones (eds), *Metropolis London: Histories and Representations since 1800* (London: 1989), intro.; J. White, 'Old Worlds for New', unpub. MS, Chs 2 and 3.
2. For more information on the history and structure of the LCC and the borough councils see essays in A. Saint (ed.), *Politics and the People of London: The LCC 1889–1965* (London: 1989); S. Pennybacker, '"The Millenium by Return of Post:" Reconsidering London Progressivism, 1889–1907', in Feldman & Stedman Jones, *op. cit.* (note 1); R. Porter, *London: A Social History* (London: 1994), Chs 10, 11, 14.

3. Feldman & Stedman Jones, *op. cit.* (note 1), White, *op. cit.* (note 1), Porter, *op. cit.* (note 2).
4. Also commonly known as the Boer War.
5. *Report of the Interdepartmental Committee on Physical Deterioration,* PP 1904, XXXII (Cd. 2175 and Cd. 2210), Minutes of Evidence, Appendix. See particularly evidence of Major General H. C. Bourrett, Q163, p.157.
6. *Ibid.*
7. Such attitudes were not unique to Britain. Apprehension was also apparent in other European countries during these years, the most notable being France which had experienced one of the earliest and sharpest declines in population and the birth rate. This anxiety had led France into providing some of the earliest state funded maternity care. For more information see M. M. Huss, 'Pronatalism and the Popular Ideology of the Child in Wartime France: The Evidence of the Picture Postcard', in R. Wall and J. Winter (eds), *The Upheaval of War: Family, Work and Welfare in Europe, 1914–1918* (Cambridge: 1988); R. G. Fuchs, 'Preserving the Future of France: Aid to the Poor and Pregnant in 19th Century Paris', in P. Mandler (ed.), *The Uses of Charity: The Poor on Relief in the Nineteenth Century Metropolis* (Philadelphia: 1990).
8. H. J. Ashby, *Infant Mortality* (Cambridge: 1915), 1.
9. Similar explanations were apparent in the *Report of the Inter-departmental Committee, op. cit.* (note 5).
10. For a pioneering article on maternal and infant health services see A. Davin, 'Imperialism and Motherhood', *Hist. Workshop J.*, 5 (1978), 9–66.
11. An interesting summary of different historical approaches to the welfare state and critiques of these theories can be found in P. Abrams, *Historical Sociology* (Somerset: 1982), 9–16.
12. P. Baldwin, *The Politics of Social Solidarity: Class Bases of the European Welfare State 1875–1975* (Cambridge: 1990; 1992), 11.
13. Some examples of this are D. M. Fox, *Health Policies and Health Politics: The British and American Experiences 1911–1965* (Princeton, NJ.: 1986); D. Fraser, *The Evolution of the British Welfare State* (London: 1984); F. Honigsbaum, *Health, Happiness and Security: The Creation of the National Health Service* (London: 1989); R. Klein, *The Politics of the National Health Service* (London: 1983); W. J. Mommsen (ed.), *The Emergence of the Welfare State in Britain and Germany, 1850–1950* (London: 1981); P. Thane, *The Foundations of the Welfare State* (London: 1982); C. Webster, *Problems of Healthcare: The British National Health Service Before 1957* (London: 1988). See also *Twentieth Century British History,* 1/2 (1990) for some critiques on the literature on the history of the welfare state and health services, particularly the essays R. Lowe, 'The Second World War and the Foundations of the Welfare State'; C. Webster, 'Conflict and Consensus: Explaining the

British Health Service'; M. Freeden, 'The Stranger at the Feast: Ideology and Public Policy in Twentieth Century Britain'; and G. Finlayson, 'A Moving Frontier: Voluntarism and the State in British Social Welfare, 1911–1949', *Twentieth Cent. Br. Hist*, 1/1 (1990), 183–206; See also J. Lewis, *What Price Community Medicine? The Philosophy, Practice and Politics of Public Health Since 1919* (Brighton: 1986); and *eadem, Women in Social Action in Victorian and Edwardian England* (London: 1991).

14. For some interesting work which highlights this approach in the context of MCW, see E. P. Peretz, 'Local Authority Maternal and Child Welfare Services in England and Wales, 1919–1939: A Comparative Study', unpub. Ph.D., Middlesex University, 1992; M. Lodge, 'Aspects of Infant Welfare in Coventry 1900–40', in B. Lancaster and T. Mason (eds), *Life and Labour in a Twentieth Century City: The Experience of Coventry* (Coventry: 1986); and J. Mark-Lawson, M. Savage and A. Warde, 'Gender and Local Politics: Struggles over Welfare Policies, 1918–1919', in The Lancaster Regionalism Group, *Localities, Class and Gender* (London: 1985).

15. This is a point made by P. Saunders in his research on more recent tensions between local and central government in his article 'Rethinking Local Politics', in M. Boddy and C. Fudge (eds), *Local Socialism? Labour Councils and New Left Alternatives* (London: 1984), 24, 32, 45. See also R. Miliband, *The State in Capitalist Society* (London: 1973), 49, and J. Dearlove, *The Reorganization of British Local Government* (Cambridge: 1979), 244.

16. R. Lee, 'Uneven Zenith: Towards a Geography of the High Period of Municipal Medicine in England and Wales', *J. Hist. Geog.*, 14/3 (1988) 260–80, 268.

17. For a more complete discussion of the unique features of London hospitals see F. K. Prochaska, *Philanthropy and the Hospitals of London: The King's Fund 1897–1900* (Oxford: 1992).

18. An interesting example of this can be seen in J. V. Pickstone, *Medicine and Industrial Society: A History of Hospital Development in Manchester and its Region* (Manchester: 1985).

19. While many women were pushed out of work in the immediate aftermath of the War with the return of the troops, new opportunities were developing for women in office and shop work, and in the new and expanding industries, such as glass, chemicals, light metals, commerce, the manufacture of food and drink which were particularly strong in Greater London. See S. Alexander, 'Becoming a Woman in London in the 1920s and 30s', in S. Alexander, *Becoming a Woman and Other Essays in 19th and 20th Century Feminist History* (London: 1994), 205–6.

20. *Ibid.*, 205.

21. *Ibid.*

22. Cited in Davin, *op. cit.* (note 10), 28.

23. C. Urwin and E. Sharland, 'From Bodies to Minds in Childcare Literature: Advice to Parents in Inter-war Britain', in R. Cooter (ed.), *In the Name of the Child: Health and Welfare, 1880–1940* (London: 1992).

24. Alexander, *op. cit.* (note 19), 217.

25. An exploration of working-class mothers in London for an earlier period appears in E. Ross, *Love and Toil: Motherhood in Outcast London, 1870–1918* (Oxford: 1994).

1

Serving the Needs of Mothers and the State

This woman is 32 and has had six children all under nine. She pays
15s. rent out of the housekeeping money of 45s. .... She had albuminuria before the birth of the last baby and now suffers from high
blood pressure, giddiness and indigestion. The Health Visitor writes
'Her food is quite insufficient owing to the claims of the family and
the giddiness is probably due to want of food. She has very bad
teeth but has not the time or the money for hospital. She is a very
conscientious mother.' The woman states that she has 'no time for
dinner on Monday'.[1]

Drawn from a national investigation in the late 1930s, the experience
of this woman from Woolwich illustrates the widespread ill health
many women were enduring across the nation in these years. Based
on an inquiry into the health of 1,250 working-class women, this
study revealed that such mothers tended to suffer the worst health in
the population. Household drudgery, constant childbearing, and lack
of resources and leisure time, and inadequate access to adequate
medical attention made the fight for good health an uphill battle for
many of these women. They tended to be the most poorly fed and
clothed within the family unit and in society as a whole. Of the 1,250
working-class women analysed, 31.2 per cent were found to be
suffering very grave health problems and 22.3 per cent had 'indifferent
health'. Anaemia, headaches, constipation with or without haemorrhoids, rheumatism, gynaecological disorders, toothache, and vari-
cose veins were common complaints among these women.[2]

Many social reformers and feminist campaigners not only saw such
poor health as tragic for the individual mother, but dangerous to the
well-being of the whole nation.[3] Much of their attitude was intricately
tied to the widespread concern about the overall health of the British

nation that had dominated the social and political discourse since the late nineteenth century. At the heart of this discourse was the perceived physical and military degeneration of the British Empire.[4]

Much of the debate in these years centred on the health and fitness of men, as they were the ones on whom politicians and social reformers placed the responsibility for the economic productivity and military defence of the nation. As the future citizens of Britain and her empire, however, the spotlight was also turned on the health and welfare of infants. This view was succinctly put by one medical expert, who argued,

> By seeing to it that our infant mortality falls below that of other nations, we shall not only tend to keep our numbers up, but increase more rapidly than other nations, and, by the care we shall then exercise, the number of damaged or unhealthy children will be less. Carelessness in connection with infant life is a sure sign of degeneracy in any country.[5]

Mothers, as the reproducers and carers of infants, were also accorded a special prominence in the debates of these years. They were viewed as pivotal to the survival of the infant, and hence the future generation. As a leading doctor and health official, George Newman, argued,

> The infant depends for its life not upon the State or the municipality, nor yet upon this or that system of creche, or artificial milk feeding, so much as upon the health, the intelligence, the devotion, and the maternal instinct of the mother. So that if we would solve this great national problem it would appear that we must first begin with the mother.[6]

Indeed, good mothering was seen as the answer to many of the problems associated with the birth decline and high rates of infant mortality.[7] This attitude was revealed most forcefully in an address by John Burns at the first National Conference on Infant Mortality in 1906, when he declared

> First concentrate on the mother. What the mother is the children are. The stream is no purer than the source. Let us glorify, dignify, purify motherhood by every means in our power.... In every aspect of this subject let us have good mothering; that is at the bottom of happy, healthy children.[8]

Mothers were thus not only perceived as serving the needs of their family, but also those of the nation as a whole and as such were regarded as an important national resource. To what degree the state should help mothers in the attainment of this goal, however, was open to question. As I will show in this chapter and those that follow, this depended greatly not only on the values attached to mothers and their needs, but also on the wider debates taking place in these years over state intervention and the provision of welfare and health services, and citizenship.

Mothers' Voices

While motherhood was a central theme in many of the social and political discourses and policies in the early twentieth century, the voices of the women themselves were rarely acknowledged. Women were not only disregarded by politicians and medical experts in these years, but until recently many historians writing on the development of the welfare state have also ignored their views.[9] Similarly, where historians have uncovered women's voices, it has usually been among those who were the key organizers and campaigners of welfare provision in these years. These tended to be the more middle-class women who had greater strength and power to articulate their needs. Working-class women, however, who were the very ones towards whom much of the maternity and child welfare services of the early twentieth century were directed, are often left out of the picture.[10] Yet the attitudes and behaviour of these mothers were crucial to the success of the facilities provided. Their perceptions and needs as mothers not only had a critical impact on the degree to which they accepted or rejected the material and medical support given, but also in shaping the provision made.

Part of the neglect in representing the voice of the working-class mother stems from the absence of evidence remaining from the women themselves. One way of capturing the voice of the mothers is through oral interviews. The collection of such material, however, is limited by the scarcity of people who can recall the services of these years and whose memories have not been coloured by the passage of time.[11] None the less, while little remains from the mothers themselves, their voices have not been totally lost. Some of their feelings and experiences can be found in questionnaires left from an abortion survey undertaken in 1936–7. This was an investigation mounted by the Joint Council of Midwifery, together with the National Council of Women, the National Birthday Trust Fund, and the Central Midwives Board. While abortion is not the focus of this book, this survey provides an unusually rich source for the working-class women's lives and attitudes in these years. The aim of this survey was to study the incidence of abortion in different areas with a view to combating the high number of consequent maternal deaths (from abortion). A total 3,300 questionnaires were distributed by the Joint Council of Midwives to 19 local authorities in England, Wales and Scotland, and a number of hospitals.[12] This material covered two of the boroughs examined in this book: Kensington and Stepney.

Some of the richest information comes from North Kensington where the survey was conducted under the direction of Dr Fenton. Overall the investigation included a standard questionnaire, which was filled out by a health worker on behalf of the women interviewed.[13] Most of the participants interviewed were working-class women who had attended a municipal clinic or hospital on account of a failed abortion. By contrast, those interviewed in North Kensington by Dr Fenton and his team, had not necessarily experienced an abortion and were being questioned on account of their attendance at an antenatal clinic. This difference in background made the nature of the questions asked of them, and their replies different from those women interviewed elsewhere.

Together with a number of oral interviews I conducted with women in the four London boroughs (Hampstead, Kensington, Woolwich and Stepney) studied in this book, the abortion survey provides an invaluable insight into the perceptions women had of their roles as mothers in these years, as well as the difficulties they faced, and the degree to which maternal and child welfare services provided for their needs. Such material, however, is not without problems. The study by the Joint Council of Midwives did not, for instance, cover those women who procured successful abortions, nor, as in the case of women interviewed in North Kensington, those who had skilfully mastered contraception. Similarly, it did not include those women who visited a private doctor or clinic.[14] Answers to the questions were also not free of bias. The illegality of abortion in these years, for instance, may have induced many women to hide their true feelings when quizzed about any issues connected with abortion. Despite these difficulties, the survey provides some of the richest testimonies we have from working-class women for this period. Each woman was not only asked questions about abortion, but also details about her economic status and occupation as well as that of her husband; her housing conditions; her reproductive history and overall standard of health, the number of live births, miscarriages and stillbirths she had had, and of the babies born alive how many had survived the first year of life. The causes, methods, and results of abortion were also noted, and, in the survey conducted by Dr Fenton in Kensington, the method of contraception.

Mothers' Perceptions of Motherhood

What is clear from both the survey as well as other sources is that motherhood was a much prized ambition for most women in these years.[15] Women interviewed in the North Kensington antenatal clinics, for instance, all stressed the importance of motherhood. As one woman recalled before she gave birth to several children she used 'to sit and dream of having a baby'.[16] Another declared '[I] always longed for a child more than anything else since I was 10 years old'.[17] Indeed, for many of the mothers in North Kensington, motherhood was something they had long desired. Some saw motherhood as a national duty. One newly married woman, for instance, claimed, 'It is a woman's life work to have babies and bring them up in a healthy home.' This woman planned to have three children in total, and was determined not to be persuaded otherwise.

> We are not going to have an only child – they are spoiled and selfish. We want 3. I tell my husband that if the doctor says I have had a bad confinement and should not have another child he is not to pay any attention – even if I ask myself, it is for my permanent happiness to have another baby and I want him to keep to our present plans.[18]

For a number of these women the pleasure of a baby represented a means of dispelling their loneliness. As one first-time pregnant woman claimed, 'This baby will give me something to live for.'[19] Another, who had given birth to five children already but had lost her fifth child, desperately wanted another, declaring, 'I know people say we can't afford it but it was so lonely in the house without my baby I felt I must have another or I shall go mad.'[20]

None the less, for many motherhood was not a joy that came without cost. Even before a child was born, many women were concerned about the pain they would experience in childbirth as well as the very real threat of death.[21] The majority of mothers in North Kensington also feared the financial anxiety a child would impose.[22] Many commented that while they would like to have a large family, it was economically impossible, and a number of them stated it was not fair to bring children into poverty.[23] One woman succinctly summed up this view when she said 'We love children, but how can you support a family on the dole?'[24] A number of recently married couples, aware of the financial burden of having children, intended to save up some money before having children. This view was not confined to the women in Kensington. Mrs P. O. from East London, who had her first child during the Second World

17

War, stated 'You see, I didn't want to have a child, ... because we wanted to get on our feet ... we wanted, naturally to save up a bit of money.'[25] While Mrs P. O. succeeded in preventing pregnancy by using pessaries, many others were less fortunate.

Having another child was not only seen as another mouth to feed, but also adding to the cramped housing conditions many families lived in. As one mother with two children in North Kensington expressed it, 'My nerves are all on edge – the children are too much on top of us in one or two rooms.'[26] Bad housing conditions were not unique to North Kensington. One woman Mrs A., who lived in Kilburn (the poorer area of Hampstead), who bore and reared five children in the 1930s and 1940s with a weekly income of £2, of which 15s. was spent on rent, remembered the struggle she had rearing them in the one room she lived in. Not only was it impossible to live with three children in the small space of one room, but it had no running water and the toilet was three floors down. Clearly these conditions made the task of daily life a great struggle. Although she had wanted the first three children, she recalled

> I was very mad about the last two, I can tell you.... I thought three was enough and I lived at the top of the house in Cambridge Gardens, you couldn't ... couldn't leave your pram down, you had to take it up, upstairs and then you had to take your coal up in buckets because, you know there was nothing there. We shared a toilet with about 16 people, I think, we had no bathroom....[27]

For one mother in North Kensington who had four children and lived in two rooms, the physical conditions of overcrowding were worsened by the threat of authority, as she stated, 'We can't go on having babies so quickly – the sanitary man will be after us because of the overcrowding.' She also added 'I don't feel strong enough either to have another baby for 2 or 3 years anyway.'[28] Indeed, for many women, the prospect of another child was physically exhausting. As one woman with four children in North Kensington admitted, 'I'm never really well – I've no energy; I should like to sit down all the time', while another declared 'I have no desire left in me either for [my] husband or for more children.'[29]

Despite the hardships women faced, many of them seemed resigned to their fate. As Mrs A. from Kilburn, stated 'you got no help at all with the baby, you just had to get on with it.'[30] Miss T. G. who grew up in East London also recalled 'Mother had no time to think about her health. It was considered a woman's lot to be ill in her life, so it was dismissed and no one cared tuppence about it.'[31]

18

The determination of women to make the best of things was told over and over again. This was clear in the case of one woman in North Kensington who lived with five children in four rooms, on a weekly family income of £2 8s. Her husband 'never had much of a job', which meant that in order to make ends meet she was forced to undertake casual daily domestic work as well as rent out one room. While she and her husband practised coitus interruptus, she had become pregnant with a sixth child. However, despite the difficulties this pregnancy imposed, she, like many others, refused to have an abortion. As she stated, 'I've always made the best of it.'[32] Another woman who had eight children and who also opposed abortion, underlined the sacrifice she was willing to undergo for the sake of her children, arguing, 'I don't think one has any rights to risk one's health when there are children. I shouldn't have dared to take anything for the sake of the children I had to help support. I couldn't risk leaving them.'[33] Similarly one woman who had given birth to 13 children, ten of whom survived, firmly opposed abortion and birth control, arguing 'I believe in Providence and I have always been able to find a crust when it had been needed.... I let the child come as they are sent.'[34] Dr Oxley also noted such attitudes among women he worked with in East London. As he commented,

> My long experience of married women of the working classes in the East End of London has made me certain that their ruling passion is to serve their husband and children and no fear of death or thought of self preservation will deter them doing their best for them.[35]

In highlighting the determination of these women what is most striking is their reluctance to undertake an abortion even when facing the impossibilities of caring for yet another child. Many feared abortion would damage their own health or that of the unborn child.[36] Indeed, many of them were terrified that an abortion would lead to their own deaths,[37] a conclusion which was reinforced not only by the stories they picked up from newspapers and from tales told to them by their mothers and other female relatives, but also by the fact that many women in these years did indeed die from abortions.[38] Some of their reticence towards abortion might also have arisen from the illegality of abortion in this period which made them reluctant to express their true feelings. This reticence was observed by Norman and Vera Himes in 1929 at the North Kensington Women's Welfare Centre, where they noted that staff at the clinic were reluctant to ask their patients for information on abortion, because 'induction of abortion is not a fact which women readily admit, at least to strangers'.[39] The degree to which a stigma was attached to abortion can be seen through the experience of Mrs A. A. from East London, who remembered even in the 1940s how upset she felt when she lost her baby through a miscarriage and overheard a doctor in hospital saying that she had attempted an abortion. She recalled,

> I was sure that he had said abortion, and to me that was a dirty, filthy word, and I said 'Doctor, I did not abort my child, I wanted my child, otherwise I would never have gone in for it.' And the lady doctor that was with him ... calmed me down, she said, 'Mrs ..., don't get upset, he didn't mean it the way you've taken it.'[40]

None the less, it is clear that some women, because of their desperate circumstances chose to risk an abortion even when they knew of the hazards they faced. One woman in North Kensington stated that while she had previously placed great value on motherhood and could not understand how a woman would risk an abortion, admitted that in her present circumstances she could now consider such action. She had borne four children and was struggling on an income of 39s. 6d. a week, at least a third of which was paid on rent for two rooms. In addition to the difficult living conditions, she and her husband were in poor health, making the possibility of yet another child too 'dreadful' to contemplate.[41] Another woman who had three children, one of whom was deaf and dumb, declared that despite the hazards of abortion, 'I think I should have taken pills all the same if I had been pregnant again. With so little money you get so desperate.'[42]

While many women who sought an abortion did so for financial reasons, an abortion could be expensive. Doctors could charge as much as 100 guineas. In 1936 the cost of an abortion, if performed by an unqualified abortionist, could be as much as £2 10s. to £3. Those who bought abortifacient pills were expected to pay 12s. 6d.[43] These costs were considerable given that the average family income was not more than £2. Regardless of the expense, for many women abortion represented the only answer to an insoluble problem.

At a time when contraception was severely limited many women saw abortion as the cheapest and most accessible means of controlling their fertility. Indeed, despite the stigma attached to abortion, many women believed that it was perfectly natural if performed early on in the pregnancy, usually up to three months.[44] One woman in North Kensington who induced an abortion for herself stressed that she did it 'always very early'. Every month she would take large doses of aperient before her period and continued to do this until she menstruated, and believed that this always ensured she was 'never more than a day late'.[45] Another woman who took gin and hot salts to abort her child said that her mother had told her there was 'no danger after that'.[46] The frequency with which women resorted to abortion as a means of contraception was also noted by medical experts. As Dr Oxley noted, 'it is common knowledge that very large numbers of married women are prone, if they miss one or two periods, to take strong aperients or to use a strong soap and water douche "to bring themselves on"'.[47] Women attending the North Kensington Women's Welfare Centre, particularly those already with families of four or more children, were also found to use abortion as a means of birth control.[48] Many women who approached the Centre often confused the contraceptive help offered with abortion, and came specifically to ask for an abortion, which they were refused.[49]

Yet while many women saw abortion as a natural means of fertility control and had no regrets about the decision to undertake an abortion in the face of the other hardships they experienced, for others it was clearly a traumatic experience. The dilemmas they faced are most clearly highlighted in the case of one woman in North Kensington who was pestered to have sexual intercourse 'several times every day' with her husband who was sick with tuberculosis. While she tried to use contraception, his continual demands meant that she did not 'always get time to put the cap in' and she inevitably became pregnant. In desperation she tried abortion, but this was clearly a very painful event for her. As she stated,

> I must have been mad last time. It seemed so dreadful having another when my husband was so ill, but he would have killed me if he knew what I had done. I tried pills first, but they didn't work. When I was 6 months pregnant I knew it was my last chance. I bought some slippery elm bark took a piece and shut my eyes while I pushed it up. The room looked like a slaughter house after. I never told anyone. I was taken to hospital and had inflammation for 7 weeks. I would never dream of doing such a thing again. I was sorry directly I had done it.[50]

A harrowing experience was also related by another woman from North Kensington. While she already had one child which she had planned, her second pregnancy was unwanted, chiefly because of restricted accommodation and the fear of unemployment on the part of her husband. They had tried coitus interruptus and quinine pessaries to prevent pregnancy, but this had failed. In the sixth week of her pregnancy she aborted her child:

21

I was desperate. I thought my husband would lose his job. A neighbour told me how she used a syringe and I went and got one. I held the end against the neck of the womb. As the water went in I felt awful: I was afraid I was going to die. I laid down on the floor. It came away that night. I was ill for 2 years afterwards. My nerves were all anyhow and I was weak and irritable. I had floodings at the periods on and off. My husband didn't know I did anything. I would never dream of taking pills now. I realise how dangerous it is.[51]

As we can see these two women had deliberately not informed their husbands of their abortions. While one or two women were actively encouraged by their husbands to have an abortion, the majority of the respondents in Kensington and elsewhere indicated that they kept their attempts at abortion secret from their husbands. Much of this was governed by the nature of married relationships. Indeed, the widespread secrecy of these women's attempts at abortion indicate the unequal power between husbands and wives during these years.[52] For many women undertaking an abortion was a means of asserting some degree of control, and often resulted from their inability to persuade their husbands to use contraception.[53] Within this context, therefore, the responsibility of motherhood was seen as resting solely on women's shoulders. Some women were not only unable to share their attempts at abortion, but often could not persuade their husbands of the importance of birth control. As one woman who had nine children and another on the way stated, 'My husband is the harum and scarum type – he'd never be careful – he asks me what we married for. He's so convinced that any kind of birth control spoils things; he says that he is sure he would feel anything I wore.'[54] One husband refused to allow his wife to use soluble pessaries because they 'would repel him'.[55] Another woman who already had six children and was about to give birth to another, tried birth control but found it ineffective against her husband's sexual demands which she had to face 'every night and sometimes in the morning too'. She admitted 'I get so tired. I'm afraid I encourage him to drink because I notice then he quietens down.'[56]

To sum up the above evidence, it would seem that while motherhood was for many women a genuine pleasure as well as a heavy responsibility, the financial anxieties and living conditions often made their tasks as mothers difficult to fulfil. Clearly for many women, their problems as mothers could not be remedied by good maternity and infant welfare provision alone. As can be seen from their financial desperation and overcrowded conditions, a more general improvement was required in housing and living conditions alongside the expansion of maternal and child welfare services. Many of their difficulties were also not helped by the nature of many married relationships in these years, as many were living in a perpetual fear of the sexual advances of their husbands and the consequences that this would bring. These anxieties were made worse where there was no support or help from the husband as well as the scarcity of resources to help them control their fertility.[57] What is apparent in many of the women's testimonies from these years is the continual contradiction many of them faced between marital sex and motherhood. On the one hand mothers were expected to satisfy their husbands' sexual appetites, but this often meant the appearance of another child, making the task of caring for other children that much greater. In satisfying the needs of both their husbands and children, mothers also frequently found it difficult to satisfy their own sexual and emotional desires.

Many of the difficulties these women faced not only had a bearing on the ways in which they experienced motherhood and carried out their tasks as mothers, but also for the ways in which they interacted in wider society and sought help for easing their situation. Indeed, it had important repercussions not only for their perceptions of themselves and their needs, but for the ways in which they felt they could call on others to support them. As we shall see, this had a vital bearing on the ways in which they perceived the maternal and child welfare facilities provided and the degree to which they used them. Women's own perceptions of motherhood, and their own needs influenced the use they made of maternal and child welfare services.

Communal Versus Individual Responsibility in the Provision of Welfare

What aid was available to mothers was dependent on issues beyond their perceptions of their own roles. Many of the services provided for mothers and their infants were shaped by concerns over the degree to which the state and other agencies should respond to mothers and help them to fulfil their role as mothers. Such questions were bound up with the wider debates over the importance of individual and collective responsibility in the provision of services that had been taking place since the previous century.

For much of the early nineteenth century the doctrines of utilitarianism had dominated social and political discourse. This dogma portrayed the individual as an atomistic self-governing agent juxtaposed to a minimal state. By the end of the nineteenth century, however, increasing emphasis began to be placed on communal organizations rather than the individual. Demands grew for increased state intervention.[58] Many politicians and social reformers were anxious about social and economic dislocation during this period. Large-scale immigration, increasing urbanization, economic depressions and the growing militancy of British workers were all seen as manifestations of the same problem. Such difficulties were felt more acutely in the face of the increasing economic and military competition Britain was beginning to feel from Germany and the United States in these years.

From the 1890s to the outbreak of the First World War the call for greater state intervention took on a renewed sense of urgency. The South African War and the poor health which had been exposed among those recruited to fight in the campaign heightened fears about the nation's future military and economic strength. At the turn of the century, revelations of extensive poverty among the nation's working class by Charles Booth and Seebohm Rowntree added to this anxiety. For many social reformers and progressive statesmen, such poverty not only undermined their beliefs in the progress of industrialization and capitalism, but was seen as a grave threat to the very survival of the British nation. No longer could Britain and her empire be left to the whims of the *laissez-faire* policies pursued in the nineteenth century. Only increased state intervention could rectify the conditions of poverty and the other perceived evils of industrialization. By the Edwardian years, therefore, increasing emphasis began to be placed on the importance of collective or state action, and began to be used as a rallying cry for those seeking to prevent the social disintegration thought to be occurring as a result of urbanization and industrialization.[59]

Welfare measures implemented by the state, such as the provision of a School Medical Service (1907), Old Age Pensions (1908) and National Insurance (1911), indicated the growing move towards state intervention and collective responsibilities in areas previously conceived of as the concern of individuals. Under this legislation individuals continued to be seen as self-governing agents who had a responsibility for their own health and that of their family, but the provision of welfare was increasingly being seen as something which was a joint responsibility between the individual and the state. Indeed, citizens were no longer merely regarded solely as individuals who had to take care of themselves, but were seen as having certain rights which entitled them to expect the state to protect and provide for them. This expectation was reinforced during the First World War, when fit individuals were expected to shed their blood for the sake of their country, and also to finance the war effort through higher taxation. Such taxation hit the working class as hard as the middle class. By 1919/20 there were six times more tax-payers than had been the case in 1914.[60] Growing state intervention in the financial and social lives of citizens made it increasingly impossible to deny state responsibility for the lives of its citizens. The drive towards collective state action was not confined to the years of the war. The inter-war years witnessed an unprecedented rise in government expenditure on social, economic and environmental services.[61]

The growth in state intervention in these areas coincided, and was partly reinforced, by new concepts of citizenship and rights emerging as a result of the extension of the franchise in these years. In 1918 property qualifications were finally abolished as a prerquisite for the male vote, and women were allowed to vote for the first time.[62] This legislation not only brought in new voters, but enlarged the idea of who was considered a citizen and who had a right to participate and share in the full social, economic and political heritage of society.[63]

While state measures in these years indicate a growing shift towards the acceptance of state responsibility for the health and welfare of citizens and increased the number of facilities funded by central government, the individual was still given a special responsibility. It could be argued that by the early twentieth century more emphasis was being placed on the responsibility of the individual for the maintenance of good health than had been witnessed in the previous century. Paradoxically, much of the medical and state intervention during the nineteenth century tended to focus on combating infectious disease and to improve the physical environment.[64] By the early twentieth century the emphasis had changed to one which focused much more on the individual. Part of this shift in emphasis can be linked to the changing conception of health, which was increasingly tied to the physical fitness and health of individuals and had less to do with sickness. Thus, the burden of health was placed on individuals, rather than the environment or other social and economic variables.[65] Maternal and child health services in these years were aimed at drilling mothers in proper infant care and nutrition, placing the onus upon each individual mother.[66]

Individuals were not only burdened with the special responsibility of the maintenance of their own health, but also with protecting and helping others. Indeed, individuals were seen as a critical component to the health and welfare services in these years, particularly in the initiation and running of voluntary provision. The overall structure of the British state itself aided the process. For much of the nineteenth century British state institutions superficially appeared to be unobtrusive. Behind this facade, however, a system of highly centralized control was effected through a complex network of local government and voluntary institutions working in collaboration with the central state. The state kept a tight reign on these different bodies, but much of its power was based on the initiative of local government institutions and of voluntary organizations to superintend, finance and initiate most education and welfare services.[67] While the state was increasing its control, it did so within a framework which was greatly dependent on local areas and their particular social, economic and political networks of power. Similarly, it did so under conditions which enabled individual citizens to participate extensively in its administration and policy making through voluntary bodies. The welfare of the country could still be seen as the responsibility of the individual and the voluntary sector.[68]

Within this context the state and the individual were each given clearly defined functions. The weight given to each, however, varied across the political spectrum and was subject to bitter contest. 'Conservative' campaigners[69] were advocates of cooperation between the voluntary and state sector, seeing voluntary bodies as key initiators of social service.[70] Voluntary work was seen as a crucial extension of the state. Lord Snell, a supporter of the Charity Organization Society, wrote,

> The [Borough] Council can provide meals or milk for necessitous school children. It cannot inquire why the children are hungry. It cannot re-establish the family in health and security. For this humane and essential work the voluntary assistance worker is required. The Council and the State can provide many services for the people, but they cannot ensure that these services are used. Unless the voluntary worker is there to bring all these advantages into the home, fewer parents would benefit and a great many children would go without.[71]

For Lord Snell and many others involved in charitable work, voluntary agencies were the chief providers of welfare provision, and state provision only covered those areas neglected by them.[72] Voluntary workers were crucial not merely for the initiation and provision of the services that the state could not offer; they were also the best arbiters of such provision because they had the greatest familiarity with the local conditions and needs. They were also considered a vital force in maintaining the humane approach in welfare provision.[73] Voluntary effort was seen as less interfering and more respectful of family privacy than state intervention.[74]

An opposite view was put forward by supporters of the Labour Party. Many within the Labour Party recognized that voluntary agencies, when sensitive to local needs, could be as supportive as state institutions. None the less, they argued that state provision would offer a more comprehensive and systematic service than the voluntary sector, and was the only means by which benefits and services could be provided as a matter of right. Similarly they challenged the idea that voluntary workers provided a more human touch to services, arguing that many charitable services were paternalistic in their orientation and unsympathetic to the needs of the poor. They believed state services provided greater scope for the poor to be heard, which was to be achieved through the representation of local communities on local government bodies, particularly through the election of Labour councillors.[75] Accordingly they campaigned for greater participation on the part of citizens either through voting or by standing in elections for positions on borough councils and other local government bodies. This attitude was highlighted in 1922 when the Woolwich Labour Party called on its electorate to assist the party 'to make the world a brighter place to live in. First join the Party yourself and then become a missionary to bring others into our ranks.'[76] They saw this method as the means by which elective local authorities would be made responsible and accountable to its citizens and prevent state services becoming too intrusive and bureaucratic.[77]

State Intervention and the Ambiguities of Motherhood

While the boundaries between individual and state responsibility were being renegotiated in these years, they were based on particular constructs of gender. Such notions of gender had important implications for the different ways in which men and women experienced the growth in state intervention. As the potential soldiers and workers of the nation, men were accorded a different status from women.

This difference in status was most clearly seen in the varying levels of state sponsored medical provision available to men and women. Under the National Insurance Act of 1911, men were provided with medical attention from a panel doctor, paid for by the state. Such provision was limited to men in regular employment and did not extend to their families. Partly inspired out of a concern for men's health so that they could continue to be a productive and industrious member of society, the legislation provided for a curative form of health care. By contrast the provision made for women and children, most noticeably the services provided under the Maternal and Child Welfare Act of 1918, stressed preventative rather than

27

curative care. Such varying levels of medical provision for men and women show the very different priorities that the state accorded to men and women's health. Not seen as workers themselves, the health of women was dismissed as unimportant to the future of the nation. Yet, as we have seen above, women suffered some of the worst health. For them medical treatment rather than prevention was what was needed. Where women's health was given priority was in child-bearing, and this can be seen in the provision of maternity benefits introduced in 1913.

Maternity benefits not only stressed the image of women as mothers, but also as the dependents of their husbands. Significantly, maternity benefits were initially paid to women via their husbands and not in their own right. The payment was also limited to the wives of husbands who were in regular employment and made continual contributions to the state. The maternity benefit was thus conceived of as a benefit for workers' wives and not one which was concerned with the 'private' sphere of social reproduction which entitled women to have the benefit in their own right in the way that men were able to claim as workers under the National Insurance Act. Single women were also not eligible for maternity benefits, reinforcing the notion that motherhood was to be kept strictly within the bonds of marriage.

Much of the discrimination surrounding maternity benefits enhanced the view that women were not citizens in their own right, and reflected, as well as reinforced, wider conceptions about the role of men and women within marriage and the family. Within this context a woman's role was seen to be primarily that of wife and mother and she was to depend on her husband for her economic sustenance. The insistence on a family wage in these years, which enforced higher wages for men on the basis that they were expected to economically support the family, reinforced this notion. Women were not seen as being entitled to earning the same wages as their male counterparts. Similarly, women could not get state support in their own right.[78] This was not only apparent from the regulations surrounding maternity benefits, but also in other forms of welfare provision. Because they were not in full outside employment most mothers were unable to claim social insurance and unemployment benefits, and even when employed were not entitled to the full assistance accorded to men.[79] Nor were many able to claim medical insurance on their own behalf from Friendly Societies.

Yet to see mothers as victims is to ignore the other advantages that they had in these years. Growing state provision of maternal and child welfare services emerged at a time when other forms of state welfare and health care provision were still relatively scarce. Mothers and their infants therefore appear to have been accorded a status not given to other citizens within society. The importance attached to services for mothers and their children is particularly striking when we consider the relative absence of help for other vulnerable groups in society such as the elderly, the chronically sick and the physically or mentally disabled. In 1921, for instance, £9.8 million pounds was being spent on community care in all urban areas, of which £7.7 million was allotted to maternal and child welfare services. While in later years the proportion of the budget spent on maternal and child welfare reduced, it still remained a sizeable sum. By 1937 expenditure on community care provision had increased to £29.5 million, of which just under half (£17.4 million) was accorded to maternal and child welfare services.[80] Thus, while motherhood relegated women to a specific role within society which stressed their reliance on men and discriminated against their independence, it also gave them certain advantages over other members of society.

The disadvantages and the advantages that mothers had in the early twentieth century reflects the ambiguities surrounding the meaning and value of motherhood. While seen as an important asset to the nation in producing future citizens, mothers were believed to have responsibilities for which the state could not always be expected to provide. One physician, Saleeby, highlighted the contradictory nature of the responsibility of the state towards women. Calling for more educational schemes on mothercraft, he categorically maintained, however, that only mothers, and not the state, could solve problems of infant mortality and the decline of the nation: 'There is no State womb, there are no State breasts, there is no real substitute for the beautiful reality of the individual motherhood.'[81] While pinning the responsibility of infant health on mothers, such calls did not necessarily guarantee rights to mothers in the way of provision.

Others, however, were less ambiguous in their advocacy of state support for mothers. The Fabian socialist, Sidney Webb, for instance, called on the state to offer more economic incentives to mothers not only in caring for infants, but also to undertake other occupations commonly associated with the 'feminine' role of mothering, such as school teaching. He believed that

> Once the production of healthy, moral, and intelligent citizens is
> revered as a social service and made the subject of deliberate praise
> and encouragement on the part of the Government it will, we may
> be sure, attract the best and most patriotic of the citizens.[82]

Many women campaigning for more state aid for mothers through groups such as the Women's Co-operative Guild and the women's section in the Labour Party expressed similar arguments. In 1912 a letter published in the Women's Column of *The Pioneer* (newspaper of the Woolwich Labour Party) argued that working mothers would only be able to improve their health and that of their children by demanding a national medical service and better housing.[83]

Some of the most interesting terminology around motherhood was inspired by the military concerns of these years. Thus, the fate of mothers was frequently likened to that of soldiers. Like soldiers, mothers were seen as 'heroines', who, instead of staking their lives on the battlefield, risked them in childbirth and in the home.[84] This cry was not only taken up by politicians but also by mothers who used it as a means for advancing welfare and medical provision for themselves.[85] Such images were particularly strong in a series of letters published by the Women's Co-operative Guild in 1915 as part of a campaign to increase the number of maternity and infant welfare services. As one woman wrote in 1915, 'The child is the asset of the nation, and the mother the backbone.' Rather than seeing this as the total responsibility of mothers, she and others called on the state to do more to help mothers. As this mother stated, 'I think the nation should help to feed and keep that mother, and so help to strengthen the nation by giving birth to strong boys and girls.'[86]

The importance of motherhood was not only conceptualized in a military, or in biological idioms. Women, because of their different roles from men and their experiences as wives and mothers, were seen as having an important part to play in the social well-being of the nation as well as its biological future.[87] A clear example of this appeared in an article by Lady Chance in a local Kensington newspaper which justified the importance of women's suffrage because of women's unique insight into the social problems of the day, such as infant mortality. As she declared,

> The tables of birth and death statistics – those bewildering columns of small-print – are to many men just so many rows of figures like any others, signifying no doubt great national loss and waste; but to women they mean not so much the useless sacrifice of many lives and much economic loss, as the most pitiful human tragedies involved in the individual suffering of each one of the hundreds of thousands of women concerned. Never let it be said that women are indifferent to these things. They are the things that lie at the root of the demand of women for a voice in the ordering of the world they have to live in.

She went on to argue that women had a special part to play in combating bad housing and defective sanitation, the evils commonly associated with poor health. Indeed, she asserted

> The part that women are taking all over the world in helping combat these new and ancient evils ... is striking evidence that women are rapidly and consciously fitting themselves for the responsibilities and duties – not only the privileges – of full citizenship. Everywhere today, where women have been already admitted to this full share of responsibility, they are showing increased activity in those departments of public life which especially affect themselves and their children.[88]

In this context Chance challenged the gender distinctions between the public and private spheres as expressed in the sexual divisions of labour. For her the warmth and emotional bonds embodied in motherhood were important influences in the male public domain of politics and business.[89] Such arguments were reiterated by many other women in these years, including those involved in the Labour Party and the Women's Co-operative Guild and even those further to the right of the political spectrum. For many women the fulfilment of social mothering was attained by their work within the philanthropic world as well as in the expanding professions opening up to women in social welfare services.[90]

Conclusion

From this it would seem that motherhood and the values placed upon it varied from those who were mothers themselves to those who viewed it as playing an important role in the future survival of the state. For mothers, motherhood could bring both joy as well as many difficulties. How they experienced motherhood was greatly dependent not only on their social and economic circumstances and their relationship with their husbands, but also on the types of support they could expect to find in the outside world.

What kind of communal help they could find, however, was highly variable. While motherhood was playing an increasingly important role within the debates around communal responsibility and the nation's future in these years, there was an uneasy relationship between what was conceived as the responsibility of the state and the individual mother. This tension is seen most clearly in the context of the state provision of maternal and child welfare services in the early twentieth century, which were not made mandatory and were far from comprehensive. Similarly, while state funding of maternity and infant welfare services increased greatly during this period, the policies pursued still emphasized the prime responsibility of mothers in the care of their infants and the family and had little conception of mothers being individuals in their own right. None the less, as we shall see, such a view of motherhood, was not static and changed greatly over the years.

Notes

1. M. Spring Rice, *Working-Class Wives: Their Health and Conditions* (London: 1939, repr. 1981), 160.
2. For more information on the medical complaints revealed by the investigation see Spring Rice, *op. cit.* (note 1). Similarly poor health was reported among those women attending birth control clinics. Of those visiting the North Kensington Women's Welfare Centre in the inter-war years, for instance, 50 per cent required treatment for post-natal ailments and were found to have very poor general health. M. Spring Rice, 'The Poor Health of Working Women', *The Eugenics Review,* 32/2 (1940), 50–4, 51. The Marie Stopes clinic reported similar findings. Among the first 10,000 of its patients, 1,321 were found to have a slit cervix, 335 a serious prolapse of the uterus, and 1,508 an internal deformation. N. Pfeffer, *The Stork and the Syringe: A Political History of Reproductive Medicine* (Cambridge: 1993), 84–5, 95.
3. This is most eloquently expressed in Spring Rice, *op. cit.* (note 2), 50.
4. For more information on this see my introduction.
5. H. T. Ashby, *Infant Mortality* (Cambridge: 1915), 6.
6. G. Newman, *The Health of the State,* P. Alden (ed.) , (London: 1907), 123–4.
7. Many have argued that stressing the need for good mothering was a cheaper option than the state providing for more extensive social and medical services. This is most strongly argued by J. Lewis, *The Politics of Motherhood: Child and Maternal Welfare in England, 1900–1939* (London: 1980); A. Davin, 'Imperialism and Motherhood', *Hist. Workshop J.,* 5 (1978), 9–66; C. Dyhouse, 'Working-Class Mothers and Infant Mortality in England, 1895–1914', *J. Soc. Hist.,* 12 (1979), 248–67; and H. Marland, 'A Pioneer in Infant Welfare: The Huddersfield Scheme 1903–1920', *Soc. Hist. Med.* 6/1 (1993), 25–50. One historian who refutes this is D. Dwork, *War is Good for Babies and Other Young Children: A History of the Infant and Child Welfare Movement, 1898–1918* (London: 1987), 216–20.
8. John Burns, MP, 13 June 1906, cited in Newman, *The Health of the State,* 123. John Burns was a socialist engineer. In 1906 he was President of the Local Government Board. S. Alexander, *Becoming a Woman and Other Essays in 19th and 20th Century Feminist History* (London: 1994), 150.
9. Exceptions to this can be seen in a collection of articles in G. Bock and P. Thane (eds), *Maternity and Gender Policies: Women and the*

Rise of European Welfare States 1880–1950, (London: 1991); V. Fildes, L. Marks and H. Marland (eds), *Women and Children First. International Maternal and Infant Welfare 1800–1950* (London: 1992); and S. Koven and S. Michel (eds), *Mothers of a New World: Maternalist Politics and Origins of Welfare States* (London: 1993).

10. See Chs 5 and 6 for the degree to which maternal and child welfare services targeted the working-class mother.

11. Similarly, as Peretz has argued, 'a handful of interviews with men and women in their eighties cannot unveil how many clinic haters, Virol takers, or home confinements there were'. E. P. Peretz, 'Local Authority Maternal and Child Welfare Services in England and Wales, 1919–1939: A Comparative Study', unpub. Ph.D., Middlesex University, 1992, 156. For more information on the difficulties of memory and oral history see P. Thompson, *The Voice of the Past: Oral History* (Oxford: 1988). See also S. J. Pitt, 'Midwifery and Medicine: Gendered Knowledge in the Practice of Delivery', unpub. paper presented to the Conference 'Nursing, Women's History and the Politics of Welfare', Nottingham University, 21–24 July 1993.

12. The hospitals included those run by the LCC such as the Mile End Hospital in the Borough of Stepney and St Mary Abbot's in the Borough of Kensington.

13. L. Carnac Rivett, 'The Report of the Abortion Committee of the Joint Council of Midwives,' *The Journal of the Royal Institute of the Public Health and Hygiene,* 4/11 (November 1941), 263–70. All the questionnaires from the survey in Kensington and for other parts of the country are contained in the National Birthday Trust papers kept at the Contemporary Medical Archives Centre, Wellcome Institute for the History of Medicine. For Dr Fenton's forms see particularly SA/NBTF/S.93 Box 171. All following citations for Dr Fenton's forms will just contain the box number and case number.

14. For more information on the survey carried out in Kensington by Dr J. Fenton see his 'Report on Contraception and Abortion' and V. Russell, 'Report of an Investigation into the Question of Contraception and Abortion', a confidential report for the Royal Borough of Kensington, October 1937.

15. This was also clearly demonstrated by the letters of working women written to the Women's Co-operative Guild and published in 1915. Originally written in response to an appeal by the Women's Co-operative Guild to improve maternal and infant welfare services, many of these letters testify to the great courage and sacrifices many women were willing to undergo in order to carry out what they saw as their role in society. These letters are generally written by women who were more literate and educated working-class women than those targeted by the abortion survey. None the less, their views are remarkably similar to those expressed in the survey over 15 years later. M. Llewellyn Davies (ed.), *Maternity: Letters from Working*

Women (London: 1915; repr. 1978).

16. Box 171, Dr Fenton's forms, case no. 239.
17. *Ibid.*, case no. 240. See also case nos 316 and 492.
18. *Ibid.*, case no. 447. Aged 22, this woman was married to a man ten years her senior. She had originally been a domestic servant, and her husband was a valet and general help. The family income was £2 a week, out of which 11s. 6d. was paid for rent for a tenement dwelling with 2 rooms.
19. *Ibid.*, case no. 297. This woman had been unwell since marrying and had had very bad nerves but felt much better once she became pregnant. Her husband was a railway porter bringing home £2 10s. a week. Out of this 15s. 2d. was spent on rent.
20. *Ibid.*, case no. 415. This woman was married to a labourer and the family income was £2 12s., 9s. of which was spent on rent for two rooms. See also case no. 332.
21. *Ibid.*, case nos 348 and 400. The first case was Jewish and was married to a grocer's manager. Their accommodation was free. The second case was of a 23-year-old married to a 27-year-old casual baker's roundsman. She had been a laundry worker, but took up daily housework once she married. The family income was £2 15s.
22. *Ibid.*, case nos 31, 314.
23. *Ibid.*, case nos 58, 336, 418, 436, 429, 449, 456, 457. See also Box 173, case no. 2712 (477), and St Mary Abbott's Hospital forms, case nos 1915, 2012.
24. Box 171, Dr Fenton's forms, case no. 421.
25. Mrs P. O., interviewed by G. MacFarlane, London, 26 May 1992, transcript, 8.
26. For this woman the only answer lay in birth control, even though as a Roman Catholic she had been taught it was wrong. Box 171, Dr Fenton's forms, case no. 37. See also case no. 456 for worries about finding accommodation with big family.
27. Mrs A. B., interviewed by L. Marks, London, 8 June 1992, transcript, 13.
28. Box 171, Dr Fenton's forms, case no. 38. See also box 174, case no. 2341 (180).
29. Box 171, Dr Fenton's forms, case nos 314, 251 and 260.
30. Mrs A. B., interviewed by L. Marks, transcript, 10.
31. Mrs T. G., interviewed by L. Marks, London, 22 January 1988, transcript, 3.
32. Box 171, Dr Fenton's forms, case no. 59. See also case nos 245 and 387.
33. *Ibid.*, case no. 422. See also case no. 494.
34. *Ibid.*, case no. 67. See also case no. 390.
35. Dr W. H. Oxley letter to Secretary of the Interdepartmental Committee on Abortion, 10 October 1937, 1–2 (PRO file forms: HO326/29). For more information on Dr Oxley see Ch. 2.
36. Dr Fenton's forms, box 171, case nos 243, 387, 403, 404, and box

174, case no. 2698 (381).

37. Box 171, Dr Fenton's forms, case nos 84 and 421.

38. *Ibid.,* case nos 85, 356, 360 and 460.

39. N. and V. Himes, 'A Study of the First Thousand Cases to Visit an English Birth Control Clinic', unpub. MS. *c.*1929, 12, (Francis A. Countway Library of Medicine, Boston, MA, N. Himes Collection BMS C77 [Box 83 fo. 883]). For more information on the North Kensington Women's Welfare Centre see Chs 4, 7 and 8.

40. Mrs A. A., interviewed by G. MacFarlane, London, 26 May 1992, transcript, 15.

41. Box 171, Dr Fenton's forms, case no. 471.

42. *Ibid.,* case no. 78.

43. Box 174, Dr Fenton's forms, case nos 2681 and 2350 (211).

44. B. Brookes, *Abortion in England, 1900–1967,* (London: 1988), 2–7. Such attitudes were also widespread in Germany. See C. Usborne, '"Pregnancy is the Woman's Active Service". Pronatalism in Germany during the First World War', in R. Wall and J. Winter (eds), *The Upheaval of War: Family, Work and Welfare in Europe, 1914–1918* (Cambridge: 1988), 404–5.

45. Box 174, Dr Fenton's forms, case no. 2696 (374).

46. *Ibid.,* case no. 2305 (111).

47. Instead of condemning such practice Oxley argued, 'We have no means of estimating the prevalence of this practice with exactitude, nor, if we had, of stopping it. I am not sure that it is an evil. My experience is that it is almost entirely free from danger, and women who resort to it have good social reasons for not wanting another child present.' Dr W. H. F. Oxley, 'Notes on the Abortion Enquiry', n.d (CMAC, file: NBTF/s2/1[10]).

48. H. Wright, *Memorandum for the Interdepartmental Committee on Abortion* (1938) 1 (PRO file: HO 326/29).

49. Himes, *op. cit.* (note 39), 24.

50. Box 173, Dr Fenton's forms, case no. 2699.

51. *Ibid.,* case no. 2702.

52. For an interesting study of this dynamic in the German context see Usborne, *op. cit.* (note 44), 401–3.

53. For one woman the refusal to undertake an abortion was in fact the means of control. As she argued, 'You go through all that risk and then get pregnant again the month after. I know perfectly well that if I started doing that my husband would stop being careful and I should spend my time bringing on miscarriages'. Box 171, Dr Fenton's forms, case no. 197. This woman was married to a labourer whose income was £2 5s. She herself undertook casual laundry work. Their rent was 7s.10d. for two rooms.

54. Box 171, Dr Fenton's forms, case no. 84. This woman's family income was £2 5s., of which 13s. 6d. was paid in rent for four rooms.

55. Box 174, Dr Fenton's forms, case no. 2698 (381).

56. Box 171, Dr Fenton's forms, case no. 192.

57. For an interesting exploration of the changes in the nature of marital relationships, particularly in relation to the increase in contraception see A. Giddens, *The Transformation of Intimacy: Sexuality, Love and Eroticism in Modern Societies* (London: 1992).

58. For more information on this shift see D. Nicholls, *The Pluralist State* (London: 1975); A. Vincent and R. Plant, *Philosophy, Politics and Citizenship* (Oxford: 1984), 2–4; D. Sutton, 'Liberalism, State Collectivism and Social Relations of Citizenship', in M. Langan and B. Schwarz (eds), *Crises in the British State 1880–1930* (London: 1985); S. Collini, *Liberalism and Sociology. L.T. Hobhouse and Political Argument in England, 1880–1945* (Cambridge: 1979); P. Q. Hirst, *The Pluralist Theory of the State: Selected Writings of G. D. H Cole, J. N. Figgis and H. J. Laski* (London: 1989); M. Freeden, *Liberalism Divided* (Oxford: 1986); S. Den Otter, *Society and Things Social: British Idealists and Social Explanation, 1880–1914* (Oxford: 1995), Ch. 5.

59. A. Fried and R. Elman (eds), *Charles Booth's London* (London: 1969), intro.; G. Stedman Jones, *Outcast London* (London: 1971, 2nd edn, 1984), intro.

60. In 1915 income tax was directed for the first time towards working men earning more than £2 10s. a week. Tax additions to tea and tobacco, and the abolition of the halfpenny postage stamp and six-penny telegram also increased the tax burden of the poor. A. Marwick, *The Deluge: British Society and the First World War* (New York: 1965), 40, 129, 303.

61. Between 1921 and 1931 the proportion of the national income being spent on welfare (social security, health and education) rose from just over 6 per cent to over 10 per cent, the largest proportion being spent on social security. J. Hills, *The Future of Welfare: A Guide to the Debate* (London: 1993), 8–9; R. Lee, 'Uneven Zenith: Towards a Geography of the High Period in Municipal Medicine in England and Wales', *J. Hist. Geog.*, 14/3 (1988), 260–80.

62. Initially only women over the age of 30 were granted the vote. This was lowered to 21 in 1929.

63. T. H. Marshall, *Citizenship and Social Class* (London: 1950), 11.

64. F. B. Smith, *The People's Health, 1830–1910* (London: 1979); and A. S. Wohl, *Endangered Lives: Public Health in Victorian England* (London: 1983).

65. This argument is made most forcefully in J. Lewis, *What Price Community Medicine? The Philosophy, Practice and Politics of Public Health Since 1919* (Brighton: 1986).

66. See Lewis, *op. cit.* (note 7), Davin, *op. cit.* (note 7), Dyhouse, *op. cit.* (note 7), 248–67.

67. P. Thane, 'Women in the British Labour Party and the Construction of State Welfare, 1906–39', in Koven & Michel, *op. cit.* (note 9),

357–61; *eadem*, 'Government and Society in England and Wales 1750–1914', in F. M. L. Thompson (ed.), *Cambridge Social History of Britain: Vol 3: Social Agencies and Institutions* (Cambridge: 1990), 1–61; and *eadem*, *Foundations of the Welfare State* (London: 1982), 196. See also J. V. Pickstone, *Medicine and Industrial Society: A History of Hospital Development in Manchester and its Region* (Manchester: 1985), 6.

68. Thane, 'Women in the Labour Party', 357–61; G. Finlayson, 'A Moving Frontier: Voluntarism and the State in British Social Welfare 1911–1949', *Twentieth Cent. Br. Hist.*, 1/2 (1990), 183–206, and *idem, Citizen, State, and Social Welfare in Britain 1830–1990* (Oxford: 1994).

69. Included among these 'conservative councillors' was Hancock Nunn who started the first Council for Social Welfare in Hampstead in 1907 (a break-away from the Charity Organization Society). His views were similar to those also involved in organizing the Guilds of Help (launched originally in Bradford in 1904). For more information on the development of these organizations see M. J. Moore, 'Social Work and Social Welfare: The Organization of Philanthropic Resources in Britain, 1900–1914', *J. Br. Stud.*, 16 (1977), 85–104.

70. HCSW, *A/R* (1917), 36 (GLRO file: A/FWA/B2/47); *Hampstead and Highgate Advertiser*, 25 October 1919, 5.

71. Lord Snell, 'Voluntary Assistance in the Modern State', *Charity Organization Society Quarterly* (January 1939), 1–2.

72. *Hampstead and Highgate Advertiser*, 12 February 1921. See also P. Thane, 'Visions of Gender in the Making of the Welfare State: The Case of Women in the British Labour Party and Social Policy, 1906–45', in Bock & Thane, *op. cit.* (note 9), 102.

73. For a good analysis of the attitude of voluntarism and its relationship to state provision see F. Prochaska, *Philanthropy and the Hospitals of London: The King's Fund, 1897–1900* (Oxford: 1992); and Finlayson, 'A Moving Frontier' and *Citizen, State, and Social Welfare* (note 68).

74. J. Lewis, *Women and Social Action in Victorian and Edwardian England* (Hants: 1991).

75. *The Labour Woman*, December 1918, 89; Thane, *op. cit.* (note 72), 98, 101. Thane's chapter provides an interesting discussion on the vision formulated by Labour Party members, especially women, of state provision of welfare services, particularly for maternal and infant welfare.

76. *The Pioneer*, 8 April 1921.

77. Thane, *op. cit.* (note 72), 101. The importance of civic participation in local government was particularly strong in Woolwich and was greatly promoted by the Woolwich Labour Party. For more information on this see D. Weinbren, '"The Peace Arsenal" Scheme: The Campaign for Non-munitions Work at the Royal Ordnance Factory, Woolwich after the First World War', unpub. Ph.D., Thames

Polytechnic, 1990, 162, 165–7. Similar calls about the importance of local institutions in giving people greater representation and power in determining the provision of services is being made by many on the left today. For more discussion on this see H. Glennerster, A. Power and T. Travers, 'A New Era for Social Policy: A New Enlightenment or a New Leviathan?', *J. Soc. Pol.*, 20/3 (1993), 389–414; S. J. Smith, 'Society, Space, and Citizenship: A Human Geography for the "New Times"', *Trans. Inst. Br. Geog.*, 14 (1989), 144–56; and A. J. Kearns, 'Active Citizenship and Urban Governance', *Instit. Br. Geog. Trans., New Ser.*, 17 (1992), 20–34, 20–1.

78. This contrasts the maternity benefits paid in Australia which were made straight to the mothers themselves and were not dependent on the contributions made by men. They were also unusual in that they provided for single as well as married women. Yet while such benefits were more universal than those paid in Britain, they were confined to white women and not extended to Aborigines or any other women of black colour. M. Lake, 'A Revolution in the Family: The Challenge and Contradictions of Maternal Citizenship in Australia', in Koven & Michel, *op. cit.* (note 9). For a provocative account of the history of the role of gender and the formation of social policy, particularly around family allowances see S. Pedersen, *Family, Dependence, and the Origins of the Welfare State, Britain and France, 1914–1945* (Cambridge: 1993). See also J. Macnicol, *Family Allowances* (London: 1981).

79. Working women paid eight-ninths of the male contribution to national insurance and received only four-fifths of the benefit. Part of this stemmed from the dominance of the notion of the family wage which assumed that men would take care of their wives. C. Kenner, 'The Politics of Married Working Class Women's Health Care in Britain, 1918–39', unpub. M.Phil., Sussex, 1979, 27. See also Pfeffer, *op. cit.* (note 2), 95.

80. Lee, *op. cit.* (note 21), table 4, 269.

81. C. W. Saleeby, (Eugenicist physician), 'The Human Mother', in *Report of the Proceedings of the Second National Conference on Infantile Mortality'* (London: 1908).

82. Sidney Webb, *The Times,* 6 October 1906, cited in Newman, *The Health of the State,* 108. For more description on the Fabian approach to motherhood see Pfeffer, *op. cit.* (note 2), 7–9.

83. *The Pioneer,* 26 April 1912.

84. Ashby, *op. cit.* (note 5), 5. Comparable arguments were being made elsewhere. See for instance what was going on in Germany, Usborne, *op. cit.* (note 44).

85. Similar moves were made by women in Australia, see Lake, *op. cit.* (note 78).

86. Llewellyn Davies, *op. cit.* (note 15), letter no. 122, 154.

87. Embedded in this concept was the idea of serving the community for

the public good. See for instance the comments made by the Progressive and Municipal Reform women candidates in Kensington council elections in 1909. *Kensington News and West London Times,* 21 May 1909, 5; 22 October 1909, 5.

88. *Kensington News and West London Times,* 17 July 1914, 2. No information remains on who Lady Chance was.

89. This was not only promoted by feminists in England. For an interesting discussion of this within both the English and German context see S. Koven, 'Borderlands: Women, Voluntary Action, and Child Welfare in Britain, 1840–1914', and C. Schasse, 'Social Mothers: The Bourgeois Women's Movement and German Welfare-State Formation, 1890–1929', both Chs in Koven & Michel, *op. cit.* (note 9).

90. P. Hollis, *Ladies Elect: Women in English Local Government, 1865–1914* (Oxford: 1987), 1–29; A. Summers, 'A Home from Home – Women's Philanthropic Work in the 19th Century', in S. Burman (ed.), *Fit Work for Women* (London: 1979); F. Prochaska, *Women and Philanthropy in 19th Century England* (London: 1980); Lewis, *op. cit.* (note 74).

2

London: 'A Mosaic of Communities'

This chapter examines the diverse socio-economic conditions within the boroughs of Hampstead, Kensington, Stepney and Woolwich. As I will show such conditions had important repercussions for the type of resources, the social relations, and the politics of each area. All the boroughs were part of London and as such could be considered integral to the sense of a community bounded by the metropolis. None the less, each borough had their own sense of civic pride and solidarity. It is unclear, however, how far residents and politicians within each borough identified with the borough and its geographical boundaries as a 'local community' rather than just a political administrative unit. Similarly, different levels of prosperity, poverty and overcrowding were not only apparent between these four boroughs, but also within the boroughs themselves, particularly in Kensington where the divide between the rich and the poor was most striking. Such a diversity of circumstances generated contrasting experiences of living conditions and health standards among the residents in these boroughs, as well as very different ways in which the day-to-day basis of an area fostered a sense of togetherness. As following chapters will show, these differences, both in the social and economic conditions of each area and their politics, were crucial in determining the level of commitment each area was willing to make towards maternal and child welfare provision, and influential in the differing standards of health found among mothers and infants in each area.

Socio-Economic Conditions and Class Composition

Described as 'one of the largest and most prosperous of the well-to-do residential suburbs of London', by Charles Booth in 1900, Hampstead had the lowest level of poverty of the four boroughs and in London as

40

a whole in both 1889 and 1929 (Table 2.1). By contrast Stepney was one of the poorest areas in London. According to Llewellyn Smith's survey in 1929, Stepney occupied 'fifth place in the percentage of persons living in poverty', and was only slightly better off than the very poor neighbouring boroughs of Shoreditch, Bethnal Green, and Poplar.[1] Kensington and Woolwich fell somewhere in between the extremes of Hampstead and Stepney, and compared more closely to the average for London as a whole. Such differentiations in the levels of poverty found in each borough partly reflected the occupational and socio-economic base of each borough. When judged according to class composition, Hampstead and Kensington were more closely aligned to each other than to the two other boroughs. As we can see from Table 2.2 while Woolwich and Stepney were predominantly working class, a much larger proportion of the residents in Hampstead and Kensington were middle class.

Table 2.1: Percentage of population living in poverty according to the surveys conducted by Booth in 1889, and Llewellyn Smith in 1929

District	% of poverty; Booth's Survey 1889	% of poverty; Llewellyn Smith's Street Survey 1929
Hampstead	13.5	1.4
Kensington	27.1	7.9
Stepney	35.7	15.5
Woolwich	28.7	8.8
Whole of London (average)	30.7	8.7

Sources: C. Booth (ed.), *Life and Labour of the People in London* (London: 1902–3). First series, *Poverty*, Vol. 1, Tables of Sections and Classes, Tables VII, IX–XIV; H. Llewellyn Smith, *The New Survey of London: The Eastern Area*, (London: 1932), 3, 347, 353, 365, and *The New Survey of London: The Western Area* (London: 1934), 88.

Table 2.2: Percentage of working- and middle-class residents in four London boroughs according to *The New Survey of London*, 1929

Borough	% Middle-class	% Working-class
Hampstead	51.7	48.3
Kensington	37.2	62.8
Stepney	14.3	85.7
Woolwich	20.5	79.5
Whole of London	28	72

Source: H. Llewellyn Smith, *The New Survey of London*, Vols 3 & 4 (London: 1929).

In the case of Hampstead most of the residents were business or professional men, merchants, authors, journalists, musicians, scientists or other professionals.[2] A small number of aristocrats also lived in the area. From the eighteenth century artists' colonies, literary associations, progressive intellectuals and politicians' circles had dominated the social character of the neighbourhood.[3] Like Hampstead, Kensington was also one of the most desirable addresses in London. From the mid-nineteenth century Kensington had been a gathering place for royalty and lesser nobility, attracting not only gentlemen of leisure, but also middle-class professionals, successful tradesmen, and some notable intellectuals such as John Stuart Mill and Sir John Simon.[4] In the first three decades of the twentieth century commerce (shopkeepers and their assistants), clerical work and the professions (including teachers and nurses) dominated the occupations of those resident in Hampstead and Kensington.[5] Figures 2.1 and 2.2 show what proportion of the male workforce these professions constituted in the two boroughs.

Figure 2.1: Percentage of men occupied in different trades in Hampstead, 1931

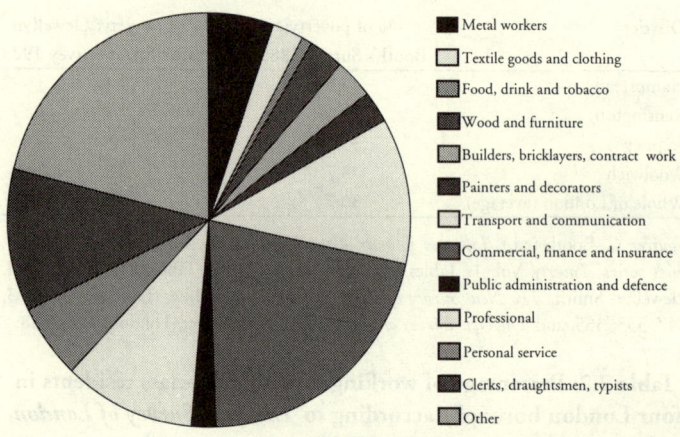

- ■ Metal workers
- □ Textile goods and clothing
- ▨ Food, drink and tobacco
- ■ Wood and furniture
- ▨ Builders, bricklayers, contract work
- ■ Painters and decorators
- □ Transport and communication
- ▨ Commercial, finance and insurance
- ■ Public administration and defence
- □ Professional
- ■ Personal service
- ■ Clerks, draughtsmen, typists
- ▨ Other

Source: Census for England and Wales (London: 1931)

Upper- and middle-class residents were not the only ones dwelling within Hampstead and Kensington. Both these areas, particularly Kensington, housed a sizeable working-class population. Very few workers in these boroughs laboured in the industrial sector, reflecting the relative absence of significant productive industries in the areas. The one exception was the Potteries in the western part of Kensington in the nineteenth century. Many of the poor living in

Hampstead and Kensington were chiefly employed in occupations serving the richer residents of the borough.[6] According to the censuses of 1901 to 1931 most of the male working class in Hampstead and Kensington were employed in building, local transport, retailing, clothing and repair work, and personal service.

Figure 2.2: Percentage of men occupied in different trades in Kensington, 1931

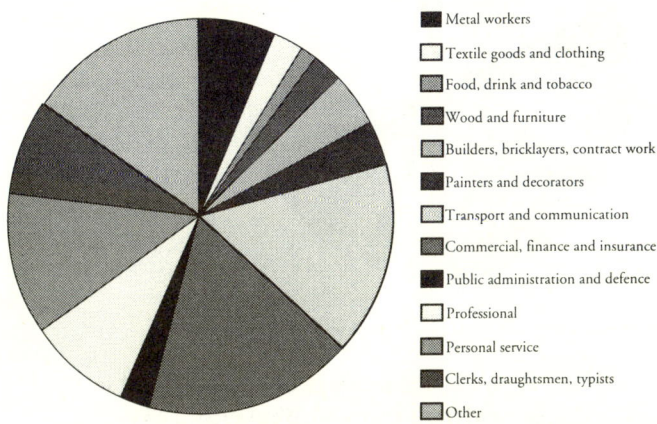

■ Metal workers

☐ Textile goods and clothing

▨ Food, drink and tobacco

▨ Wood and furniture

▨ Builders, bricklayers, contract work

■ Painters and decorators

☐ Transport and communication

■ Commercial, finance and insurance

■ Public administration and defence

☐ Professional

▨ Personal service

■ Clerks, draughtsmen, typists

▨ Other

Source: Census for England and Wales (London: 1931)

The socio-economic base of Stepney was very different from Hampstead and Kensington. During the nineteenth century many newcomers had been attracted to Stepney by the expanding opportunities in the docks and the sweated-workshop trades, such as clothing, footwear and furniture. These industries included a large number of Irish and East European Jewish immigrants as well as English migrants. Stepney's population was largely composed of semi-skilled or casual labourers whose employment was greatly affected by the increasing competition in the dock industries and the seasonal fluctuations in the sweated trades in these years. Although residents in Stepney could find more secure work through local breweries and distilleries, unemployment and underemployment were a continual problem from the late nineteenth century through to the 1930s. In the inter-war years Stepney remained relatively unaffected by the development of new industries such as engineering, the chemical and electrical trades, and by the expansion of the white collar and more middle-class professional occupations. In the 1920s cabinet making, the clothes trade, transport and warehousing, and the distributive trades still dominated Stepney's industrial base.[7] Figure 2.3 highlights that the sweated trades of textile and clothing were the largest employers of men in Stepney in 1931.

**Figure 2.3: Percentage of men occupied in
different trades in Stepney, 1931**

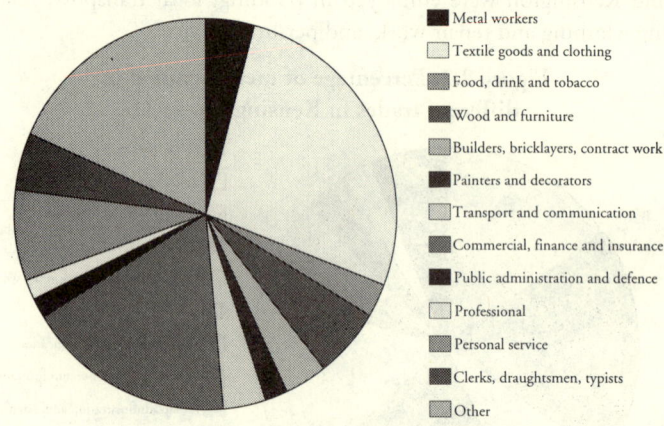

Metal workers

Textile goods and clothing

Food, drink and tobacco

Wood and furniture

Builders, bricklayers, contract work

Painters and decorators

Transport and communication

Commercial, finance and insurance

Public administration and defence

Professional

Personal service

Clerks, draughtsmen, typists

Other

Source: Census for England and Wales (London: 1931)

**Figure 2.4: Percentage of men occupied in
different trades in Woolwich, 1931**

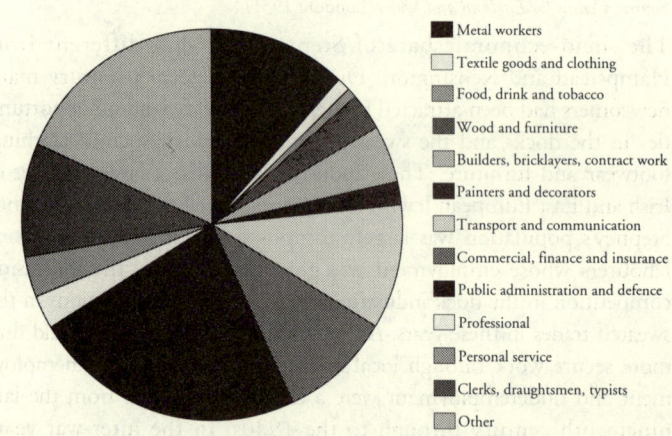

Metal workers

Textile goods and clothing

Food, drink and tobacco

Wood and furniture

Builders, bricklayers, contract work

Painters and decorators

Transport and communication

Commercial, finance and insurance

Public administration and defence

Professional

Personal service

Clerks, draughtsmen, typists

Other

Source: Census for England and Wales (London: 1931)

Like Stepney, Woolwich had a much larger industrial sector than
Hampstead or Kensington. By contrast, however, the industrial base of
Woolwich provided a more secure existence than the one in Stepney.
The chief employer in Woolwich was the Royal Military Arsenal. In
1901 20,000 of the 118,000, or 17 per cent of the inhabitants of

44

Woolwich laboured in the Arsenal, and many more were involved in businesses sustained by workers at the Arsenal.[8] Those employed by the Arsenal tended to be skilled workers who were guaranteed more regular work, greater trade union representation, higher wages and fewer hours than most workers in Stepney.[9] Despite the shortages of munitions' work in the years immediately following the South African War and the First World War, the Arsenal continued to be a major employer in Woolwich through to the 1930s. In 1931 a large percentage of Woolwich's male workforce were employed in the defence industry or public administration (Figure 2.4). By the 1930s industrial work was also available through the dockyards and engineering firms as well as the chemical industries, electric cable works, and building construction schemes in the district. Many were also involved in transport work, commerce or employed as clerks.[10]

Table 2.3: Percentage of working-class families with weekly income either below or within 10s. of the standard poverty line set by *The New Survey of London (NSL)*, 1929, in four London boroughs

Borough	% w-c families below *NSL* standard	w-c families within 10s. per week of *NSL* standard
Hampstead	6.4	16.3
Kensington	12.4	26.2
Stepney	19.3	30.1
Woolwich	7.0	20.6
London (average)	9.8	19.5

Source: H. Llewellyn Smith, *The New Survey of London*, Vols 3 & 4, (London: 1929).

The occupational base and class composition of each area had an important impact on the economic status of their residents. As we can see from Table 2.3 Stepney and Kensington had a much greater proportion of working-class residents who were living either below or within 10s. of the poverty line as assessed by Llewellyn Smith in 1929. This pattern reflected the dominance of unskilled temporary labour among those working and living in these areas, which rendered a much more precarious and insecure existence than the types of work available to the working-class living in Woolwich. Even in Woolwich, however, workingclass families were not immune to poverty. Table 2.3 reveals that while families in Hampstead and Woolwich never suffered the acute deprivation and poverty as those in Stepney and Kensington, many hovered just above the poverty line.

Women's Work

In areas where unemployment and underemployment were common, married women's wages were a major source of income for working-class families. Significantly in 1911 the percentage of employed married women was much higher in Kensington and Stepney than in the other two boroughs, partly reflecting the importance of casual labour among its poorer residents. In Kensington the percentage of such women employed in this year was 19.4 per cent, while in Stepney it was 15.5 per cent.[11] In 1917 approximately 21 per cent of all married and widowed women in Stepney, and 25 per cent of those in Kensington were employed.[12] By contrast, in Woolwich women were remarkably absent from the labour market, reflecting the better incomes of the men employed in the borough as well as the scarcity of work for women. Woolwich had the lowest proportion of married and unmarried women working in London, registering 6.1 per cent in 1911.[13] During the First World War the number of working women rose dramatically in Woolwich, but this trend was short lived.[14] Although the number of married women working was never as low in Hampstead as in Woolwich, it was lower than for Stepney and Kensington.

Much of the work undertaken by working-class married women in all the boroughs was determined by the types of work available. In Hampstead and Kensington most women were employed in some form of domestic service. Figure 2.5 reveals that in 1911 Hampstead and Kensington had the highest proportion of female indoor domestic servants in London, reaching 73.7 and 70.7 per cent respectively.[15] Figures 2.6 and 2.7 indicate that domestic service continued to be the major employer of women in these two boroughs through the inter-war years. Many women were also employed in arduous and poorly paid laundry work in Kensington. In 1917 there were 700 laundries in the borough employing about 7,000 women, of whom about 75 per cent were married.[16] The absence of upper- and middle-class residents in Stepney, meant that domestic services and laundry work were less popular forms of work among women in this borough. In 1911 only 6.4 per cent of employed women worked in domestic service.[17] Avenues of employment open to women in Stepney included the manufacture of cheap and ready-made clothing in large factories such as Schneiders which engaged about 1,000 women. As Figure 2.8 shows this formed a sizeable portion of the women employed in Stepney in 1931. Other work available to women in Stepney included the making of embroidery or artificial flowers, the scraping of lint, the pulling of fur, and the subsidiary tasks of leather and paper manufacture. Jam making, rope making, tent and sack making, rag and paper sorting were also principal employers of women in Stepney.[18] A large proportion of the women working in these industries were single, particularly in the East End tailoring trade in the 1920s,[19] but some of them were also married. In Woolwich few work opportunities were available to women through the local labour economy, except for a very small number of jobs in the personal service sector. In 1911 Woolwich had only 6.4 per cent of its married women engaged in occupations, the smallest proportion in London.[20] This was a pattern that continued into the inter-war years. Figure 2.9 depicts a very large proportion of the women in Woolwich as either retired or not gainfully employed.

Figure 2.5: Map showing the percentage of female indoor domestic servants in London, 1911

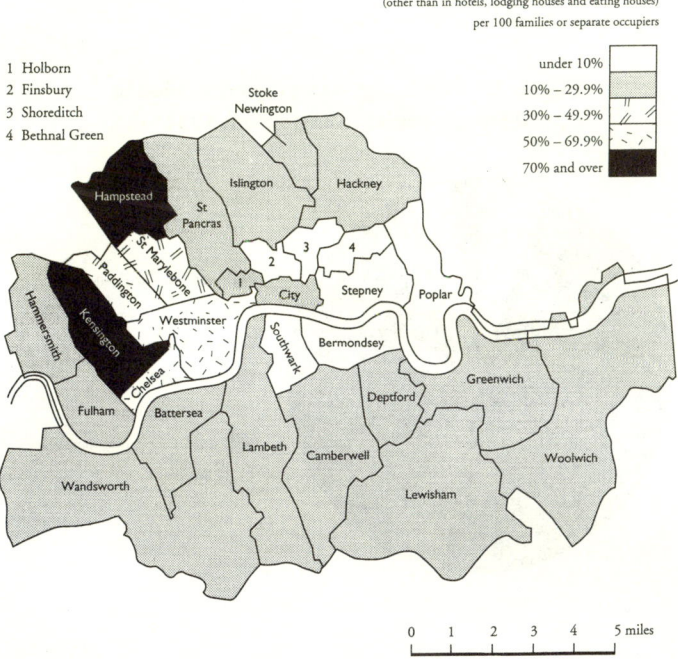

Proportion of female indoor domestic servants
(other than in hotels, lodging houses and eating houses)
per 100 families or separate occupiers

under 10%
10% – 29.9%
30% – 49.9%
50% – 69.9%
70% and over

1 Holborn
2 Finsbury
3 Shoreditch
4 Bethnal Green

0 1 2 3 4 5 miles

Source: LCC, *London Statistics,* Vol. 25 (London: 1914–15).

Figure 2.6: Percentage of women occupied in different trades, Hampstead, 1931

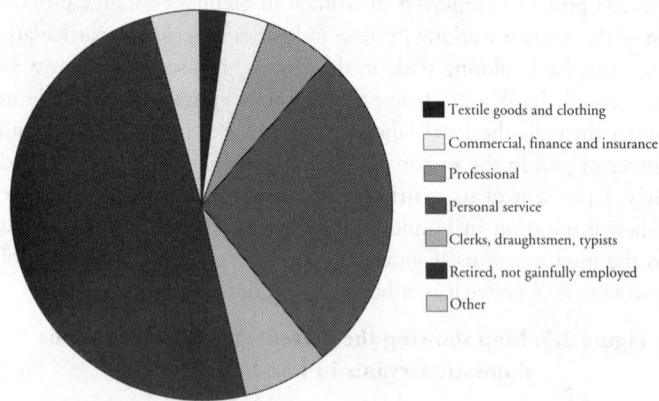

- Textile goods and clothing
- Commercial, finance and insurance
- Professional
- Personal service
- Clerks, draughtsmen, typists
- Retired, not gainfully employed
- Other

Source: Census for England and Wales (London: 1931)

Figure 2.7 Percentage of women occupied in different trades, Kensington, 1931

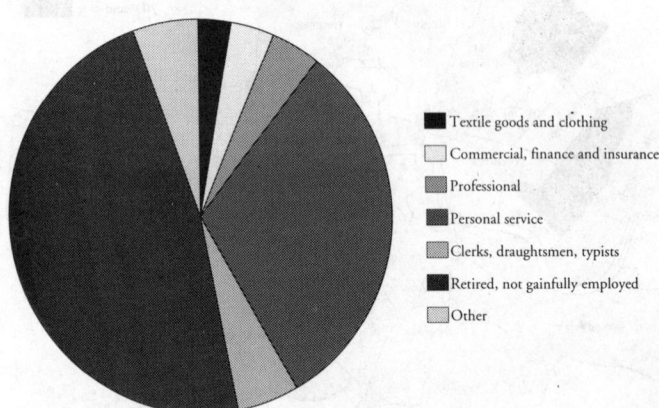

- Textile goods and clothing
- Commercial, finance and insurance
- Professional
- Personal service
- Clerks, draughtsmen, typists
- Retired, not gainfully employed
- Other

Source: Census for England and Wales (London: 1931)

Figure 2.8: Percentage of women occupied in different trades, Stepney, 1931

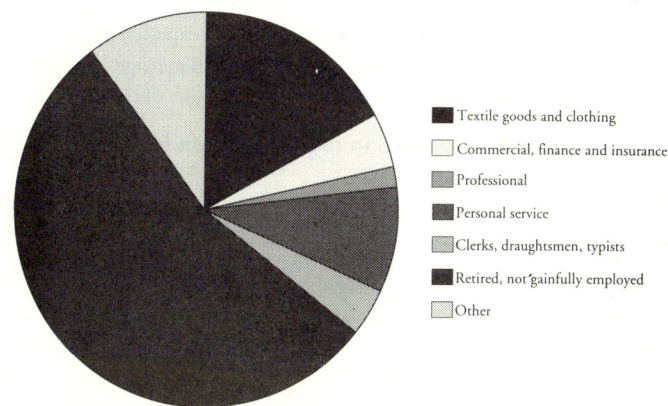

Source: Census for England and Wales (London: 1931)

Figure 2.9 Percentage of women occupied in different trades, Woolwich, 1931

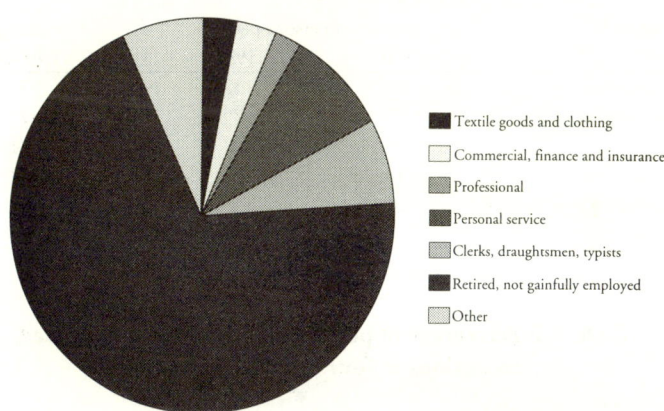

Source: Census for England and Wales (London: 1931)

Residential Conditions

The differences between the boroughs was not only apparent in their patterns of employment and levels of poverty, but also in their levels of population density and conditions of overcrowding. As Table 2.4 shows, Woolwich experienced the largest increase in population of the four boroughs during the years between 1901 and 1931. Yet throughout these years Woolwich had the lowest population density of the boroughs and of London as a whole, reflecting its large acreage of land. This contrasted with Stepney which, although experiencing a decline in population over the years, because of its small acreage continued to be the most densely populated of the four boroughs (Table 2.5).

Table 2.4: Population in four London boroughs

Borough	Population		% change
	1901	1931	1901–31
Hampstead	81,942	88,914	+8
Kensington	176,628	180,681	+2
Stepney	298,600	225,238	−24
Woolwich	117,178	146,881	+25
Administrative County of London	4,536,541	4,397,003	−3

Source: Census of England and Wales (London: 1901, 1931).

Table 2.5: Number of persons per acreage in four London boroughs

Borough	Number of persons per acre		% change
	1901	1931	1901–31
Hampstead	36	39	+8
Kensington	77	79	+2
Stepney	169	127	−24
Woolwich	14	18	+28
Administrative County of London	61	59	−3

Source: Census of England and Wales (London: 1901, 1931).

Table 2.6: Percentage of population living in overcrowded conditions in four London boroughs

Borough	1911	1931	% change 1901–31
Hampstead	7.0	2.4	−66
Kensington	17.1	7.9	−54
Stepney	35	19.7	−44
Woolwich	6.3	3.0	−52

Source: Census of England and Wales (London: 1911, 1931).

The number of persons per acre influenced the level of overcrowding in each area. Not surprisingly Table 2.6 shows that the highest percentage of overcrowding was found in the boroughs with the highest density of population. This trend was not only true for the four boroughs, but for London as a whole. Figures 2.10 and 2.11 indicate that Stepney ranked as among those boroughs with the highest levels of population density and overcrowding in 1911. In all four boroughs the level of overcrowding reduced between the years 1901 and 1931, and was fairly even between them. None the less, a considerable proportion of the population in Kensington and Stepney were housed in common lodge-housing, which had attracted attention from social reformers and politicians because of their appalling conditions since the nineteenth century. Common lodge-houses were notorious for their overcrowding and poverty, and were thus seen as perpetuating the problems of crime and prostitution. While much of this accommodation was demolished by slum clearance schemes carried out in the late nineteenth and early twentieth centuries, a number of such dwellings continued to exist in Stepney and Kensington through to the 1930s.[21]

Figure 2.10: Map showing the density of population in London, 1911

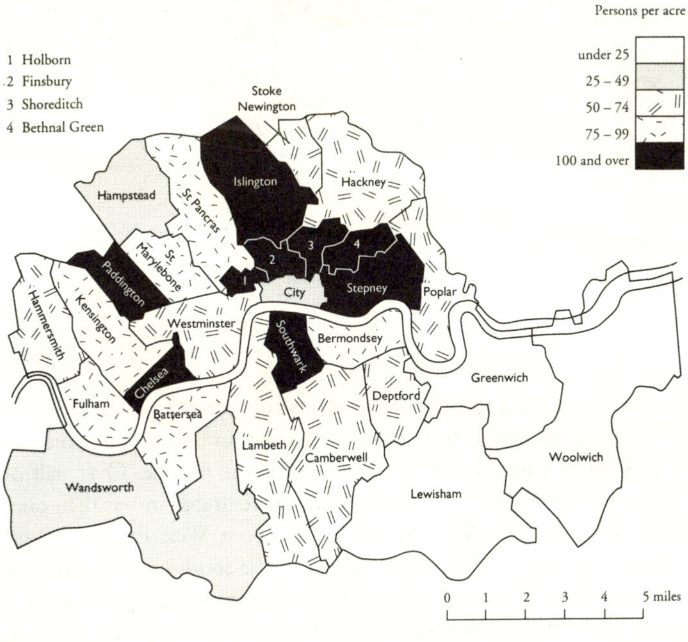

Persons per acre

1 Holborn
.2 Finsbury
3 Shoreditch
4 Bethnal Green

under 25
25 – 49
50 – 74
75 – 99
100 and over

0 1 2 3 4 5 miles

Source: LCC, London Statistics, Vol. 25 (London: 1914–15).

Population density and overcrowding not only differed between the boroughs, but also within the boroughs themselves and were reflected in the residential patterns found among the different classes. In all areas the rich and the poor tended to be segregated from each other, with the poor generally dwelling in locations which had the highest levels of overcrowding. The residential variations within all the boroughs are illustrated in Figures 2.13 to 2.15.

Figure 2.11: Map showing the percentage of population overcrowded in London, 1911

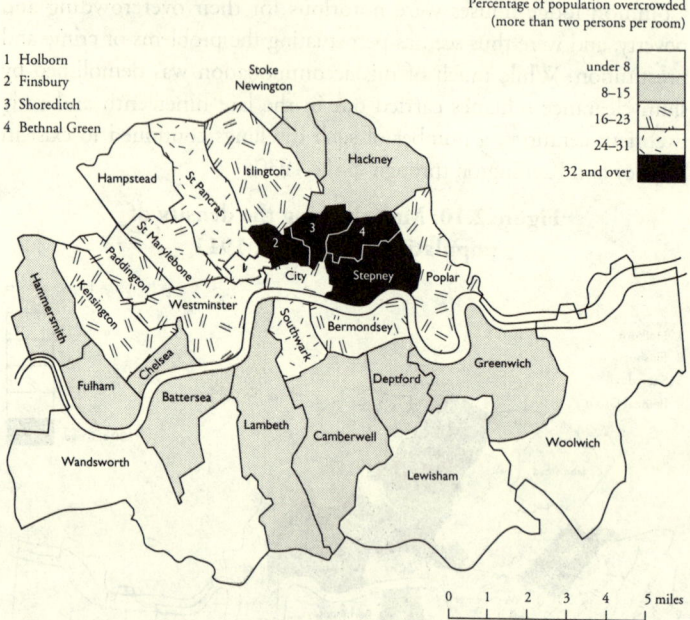

Percentage of population overcrowded
(more than two persons per room)

1 Holborn
2 Finsbury
3 Shoreditch
4 Bethnal Green

under 8
8–15
16–23
24–31
32 and over

0 1 2 3 4 5 miles

Source: LCC, *London Statistics*, Vol. 25 (London: 1914–15).

Within Hampstead the affluent residents congregated primarily in the areas where the houses were most spread out and the population was small such as Town, Belsize Park and Fitzjohn's Avenue. Over half of Hampstead's inhabitants, however, were concentrated in less than one-third of its area; in West Hampstead between West End Lane and Kilburn, and in the Fleet Road district in the south-eastern corner of the borough (Figure 2.12). Most of the accommodation in these areas was in high-density housing. In 1901 while the richer wards of Town, Belsize, Adelaide and Central had 28 persons and 3½ houses on each acre of land, the three western wards of West End, Kilburn and Priory had 53 persons and 8 houses to each acre.[22]

**Figure 2.12: Map of poorest and richest areas
in Hampstead, *c*.1930**

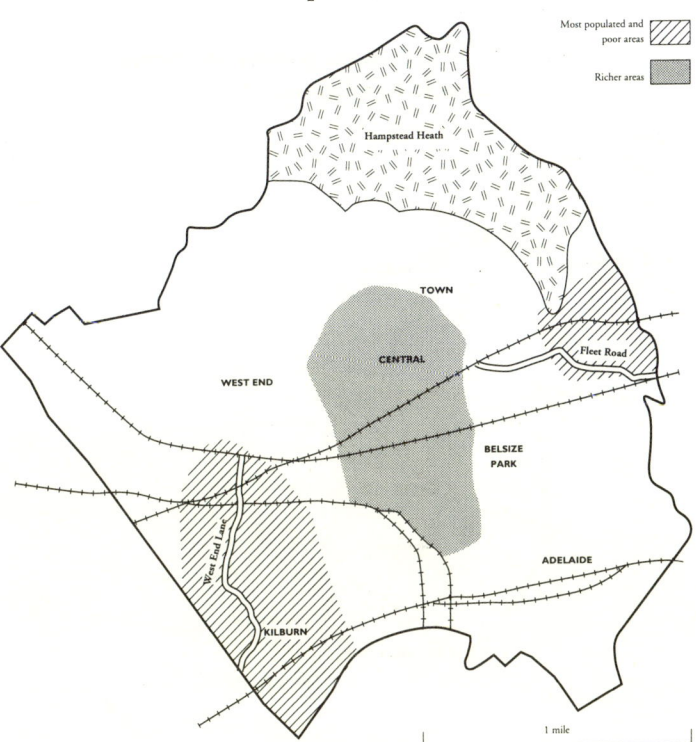

Source: H. Llewellyn Smith, *The New Survey of London,* Vol. 6 (London: 1934), 423–5.

Similar divisions appeared in Kensington (figure 2.13). Most of the
richer residents lived in large houses or great blocks of expensive
flats in the district lying south of Kensington High Street, known as
South Kensington, and to the north of Kensington High Street as
far as Holland Park Road and Notting Hill High Street.[23] To the
north and west of Notting Hill High Street there was a more mixed
middle- and working-class population, the poorest living in Notting
Dale where some of 'the most notorious slums in London' were
located from the mid-nineteenth century through to the 1930s.[24]
Poverty and overcrowding also characterized the extreme north of
Kensington, particularly in the area that lay between the gasworks,
railway lines and a canal. An investigation of 24,296 families in
Kensington revealed that overcrowding was greatest in the wards of
North Kensington, where the number of families overcrowded in

Golborne, was 15 per cent, the highest for the whole borough. This contrasted with 3 per cent for Queen's Gate the least crowded ward, based in South Kensington.[25]

**Figure 2.13: Map of the poorest and richest
areas in Kensington, *c*.1930**

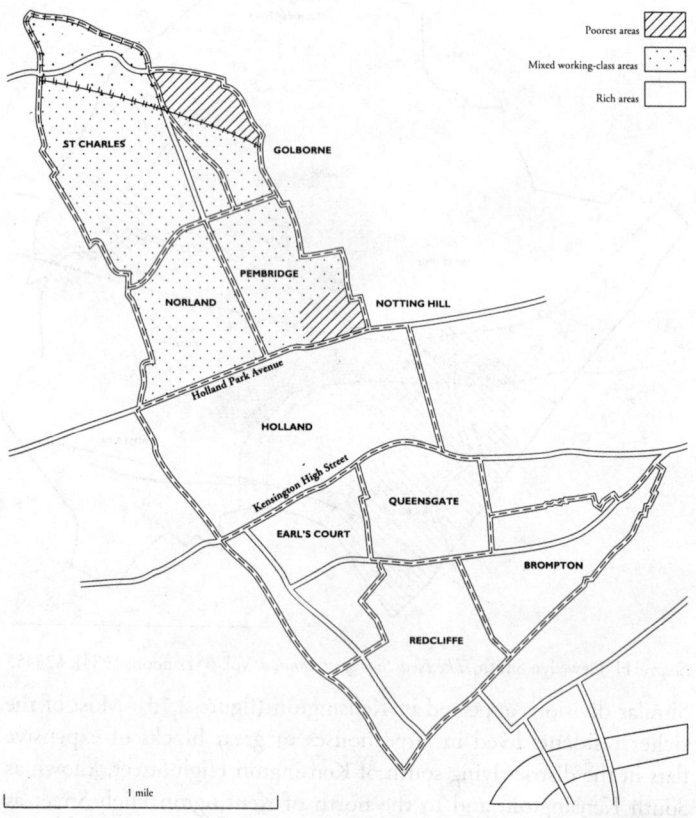

Source: H. Llewellyn Smith, *The New Survey of London,* Vol. 6 (London: 1934), 427–9.

As in Hampstead and Kensington, poverty and overcrowding unevenly distributed in Stepney and Woolwich (Figures 2.14 and 2.15). In Stepney the poorest inhabitants lived south of Commercial Road near the docks and in the eastern part of the borough near the gasworks and the Regent's Canal, while in Woolwich they were housed near the river between the ferry pier and the Royal Arsenal (Rodney Street, Warren Lane, Rope Yard Rails).

Figure 2.14: Map of poorest areas in Stepney, *c*.1930

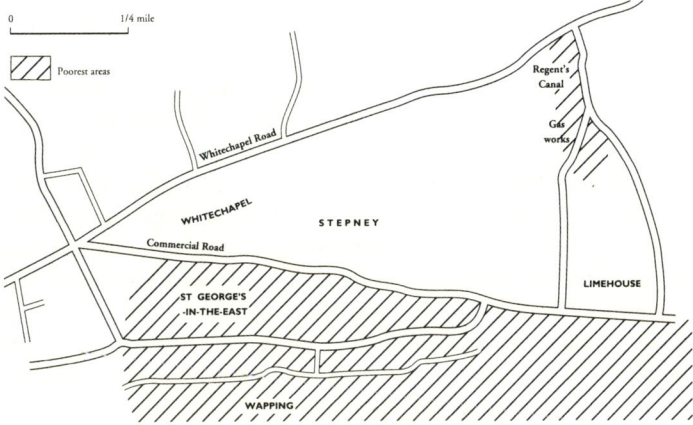

Source: H. Llewellyn Smith, *The New Survey of London,* Vol. 3 London: (1934), 353–5.

Figure 2.15: Map of poorest areas in Woolwich, *c*.1930

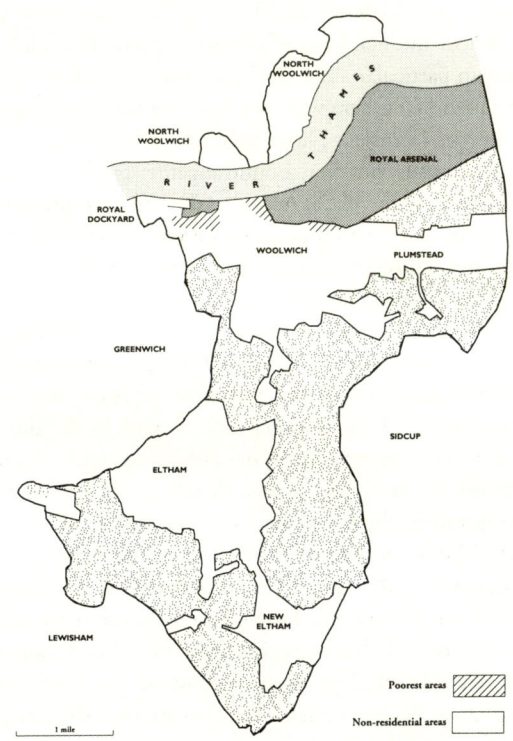

Source: H. Llewellyn Smith, *The New Survey of London,* Vol. 3 (London: 1934), 385–8.

Neighbourhood Relations and Networks

While such differences in the residential patterns highlight the uneven spread of poverty and the variability of housing conditions in each borough, it was also a powerful component in determining social relations and networks within them. On the surface it might be assumed that those who came from the same socio-economic status were more likely to share a sense of common identity and solidarity. Ross has shown that in many working-class neighbourhoods of London poverty could draw residents together through informal networks of mutual assistance and the sharing of limited resources. Yet, it is difficult to determine to what degree neighbours with a common socio-economic background will relate to each other. As Ross has pointed out, while poverty could act as a unifying force, it could also divide people. Sharing tap water and toilets, for instance did not always promote the most harmonious relationship between neighbours.[26] Similarly those who were rich did not always see eye to eye. The social relations within an area, therefore, were subject to highly complex dynamics which operated beyond the issue of class.

Some idea of the manifold of factors that affected solidarity and conflicts within particular areas can be gauged from North Woolwich. Most of the men living here were employed in the Tates' sugar works, rubber and other factories. These residents not only had a common socio-economic status, but were bound together by the particular geographical isolation of the place. Access to the area was difficult because it was shut in by the Thames on one side and traversed by the docks on its north side. Those needing to enter or leave the district either had to wait for a free ferry which ran constantly except for eight hours on Saturday nights and during bad fogs, or go through the docks, but here the dock gates were a major hindrance. On occasions foot passengers and carts had to wait between two and three hours in order to get out. One district midwife, Evelyn Walter, who worked in the area in 1906 indicated that this created impossible conditions when calling for a doctor in times of emergency. It was, therefore, not surprising that in such an environment the atmosphere was one of a small provincial village. This had both positive and negative effects. On the one hand the relative geographic isolation of the place as well as the shared socioecnomic status of the residents fostered a very warm sense of community. Indeed, Evelyn Walter's description of the place is one in which the very closely knit social and welfare networks provided crucial help in times of crisis. None the less, she also showed the environment could be stifling making the spread of 'low malicious gossip' very easy.

As she stated, no man or woman could be seen speaking together without a rumour being started. She herself faced scrutiny and criticism from the local clergy for not partaking in parish work and found them obstructing her ability to establish her midwifery practice.[27]

When looking at the overall relations of each borough rather than from particular districts within them, it would seem that the dominance of particular classes played an important part in neighbourhood relations. This dominance had implications for the political affiliations of each borough as well as their responses to welfare provision. In areas like Hampstead and Kensington, the social relations and political attitudes towards welfare provision were largely influenced by the fact that the poorer residents were confined to domestic service and isolated from other workers. They were also small in number and greatly dependent on their richer neighbours for their employment and welfare. This dependence resulted in particular paternalistic relationships, which were also important in shaping the provision of these two boroughs. In both areas the residential segregation of the poor from the rich reinforced the paternalistic relationship between the two classes. One advantage that the poor in Kensington had over those in Hampstead was that they were much larger in number (Table 2.2), which made it more difficult for the rest of the borough to ignore their plight. Such social relations sharply contrast those of Woolwich and Stepney where the overwhelming majority of working-class residents allowed the working class more formal cultural and political autonomy. In both places the shared experience of poverty was an important political force which drew on the notion of mutual assistance developed at the more localized level of the street and the neighbourhood. Sharing between neighbours and friends was, therefore, taken as a crucial underpinning for justifying larger collective provision by the borough as a whole.[28]

Just as important as the internal class dynamics, was the interaction that residents had with the outside world.[29] The importance of external agents in fostering neighbourhood relations is most apparent in the case of Stepney and Woolwich. Based in the East End, which was renowned as the poorest part of London and attracted a great deal of attention from statesmen and social reformers concerned with the threat of social degeneracy and disorder, Stepney was an area of extensive middle-class philanthropic investment from outside. Settlements of middle-class welfare workers and charitable agencies, therefore, were prolific in Stepney.[30]

Middle-class and voluntary intervention was less strong in Woolwich than in Stepney. Although the presence of the Royal Arsenal and barracks made Woolwich the subject of intense state attention in the interest of national defence, it did not attract the same degree of outside philanthropic interest as Stepney, partly because its poverty was not as striking and also because, as has been described in the case of North Woolwich, it was geographically more isolated from the rest of London. The working class in Woolwich, therefore, because they were less subject to outside interference and largely composed of skilled workers with a more regular income and a stronger trade union base, had stronger cultural and political autonomy from early on than those in Stepney, as manifested by the early strength of trade unionism in Woolwich.

Political Mobilization

The differences in the neighbourhood relations between each borough had important implications for the overall political mobilization and affiliations of each area. Figures 2.16 and 2.17 show that of the four boroughs Woolwich had the greatest percentage of its electoral population turning out for parliamentary and borough council elections, reflecting the high degree of political involvement among its population. Although the percentage of population who voted in elections was not as large in Stepney, the mean average of population voting was slightly higher here than in Hampstead and Kensington. This voting pattern suggests that the political mobilization and interest in the day-to-day running of the borough, was slightly greater in the poorer boroughs than in the richer ones.

It would be too simplistic, however, to attribute such differences in the proportion of population voting in each borough to their variations in class composition. One vital factor which needs to be taken into consideration was the strength of the various political parties and the degree to which they could mobilize the population within each area. Woolwich, which was the most cut off from London and the most cohesive working-class community was the most unusual of the four boroughs and indeed from the rest of London. It not only had a powerful trade union base from the nineteenth century, but also a strong Labour Party from the early twentieth century. In 1903 the Labour Party gained an overwhelming majority on the Woolwich borough council, and in 1904 Woolwich became the first constituency in the country to be represented by an independent Labour Party at all elected levels: MP, local council and Board of Guardians. The strength of the Woolwich Labour Party was rooted in the fact that it allowed individual members to join, a model which the national party adopted in 1918. Until the late 1930s the Woolwich Labour Party was the largest local party in Britain, having 3,380 individual members in

1925, a number unsurpassed anywhere else in these years. This represented 5.3 per cent of the electoral population. By 1939 the membership had risen to 5,199 (Table 2.7).[31] Although in 1906 the Labour Party lost their majority on the Woolwich borough council, they continued to have a strong representation on the council.[32] Throughout the inter-war years, with the exception of 1931, the borough council was Labour (Tables 2.8 and 2.9), and Labour candidates were returned at parliamentary elections.

Figure 2.16: Percentage of the electoral population voting in borough council elections

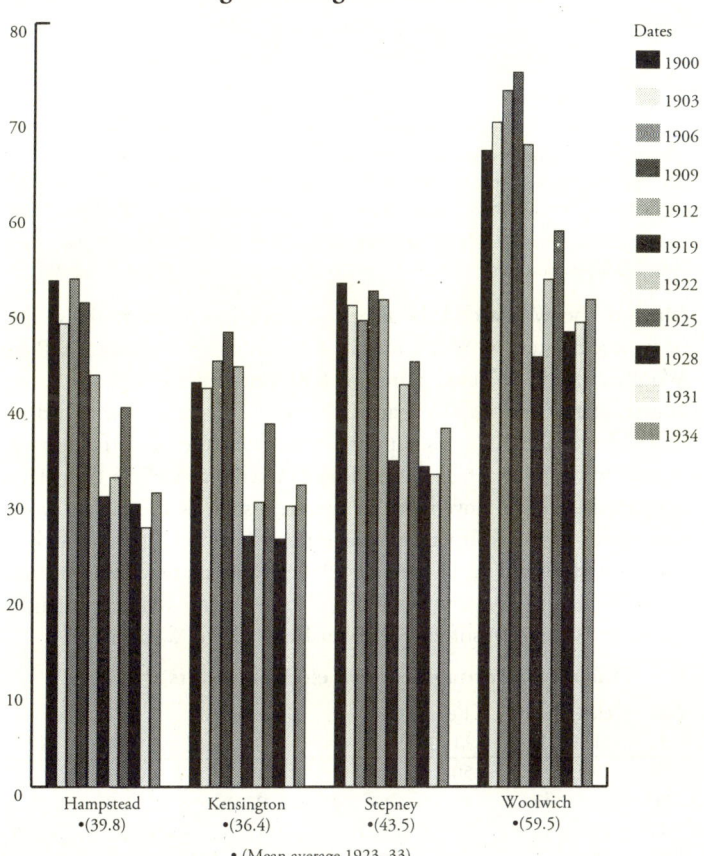

Source: LCC, *Statistical Abstract for London,* (London: 1923–33), Table 30.

Table 2.7: Membership of the local labour parties in four London boroughs

Borough	1925	1929	1934	1939
Hampstead	150	190	120	445
	(0.41%)	(0.47%)	(0.29%)	(1%)
Kensington North	240	540	734	850
	(0.63%)•	(0.91%)•	(1.2%)•	(1.4%)•
Kensington South	160	120	240	240
	(0.5%)•	(0.17%)•	(0.35%)•	(0.34%)•
Kensington Total	400	660	974	2,064
	(0.22%)	(0.52%)	(0.71%)	(1.6%)
Stepney	360	1,780	3,096	6,010
	(0.51%)	(2.28%)	(4%)	(7.81%)
Woolwich	3,380	4,327	4,735	5,199
	(5.34%)	(5.9%)	(6.3%)	(6.9%)

* Based on the number of parliamentary electors 1918 and 1934.
All figures in brackets are the number of members of the Labour Party as a percentage of the number of electors estimated for local government elections, 1925, 1931, 1934.

Sources: J. White, 'Old Worlds for New', unpublished MS, Table 8.3, London Labour Party, A/Rs; LCC, Statistical Abstract for London, 1923–33 (London: 1934), Tables 29 and 26.

Much of the Woolwich Labour party's strength was due to the vitality of its leaders such as Will Crooks (who was the first Labour MP for Woolwich) and William Barefoot (chairman of the Labour Party) whose energy and visions shaped the party's organization and drew votes. The Labour Party's support came from the powerful unions, especially those attached to the Royal Arsenal as well as from local grassroots pressure movements in the area, such as the radical workmen's clubs, the co-operative societies, radical clergymen such as Canon Escreet and C. H. Grinling,[33] and women's organizations such as the Women's Co-operative Guild. These elements were important in building a strong constituency Labour Party within Woolwich.[34]

Table 2.8: Borough council election results, 1900–12

Date	Hampstead			Kensington				Stepney				Woolwich			
	M	P	I	M	P	S	I	M	P	S	I	M	P	S	I
1900	23	13	6	50	10	–	1	37	19	–	4	24	10	–	2
1903	–	–	42	45	15	–	–	21	23	–	16	8	–	25	3
1906	29	13	–	43	5	6	6	42	14	–	4	23	–	12	1
1909	32	6	4	50	8	2	–	35	5	1	19	24	–	10	2
1912	34	6	2	52	2	6	–	31	28	–	1	21	–	15	–

M Moderate P Progressive S Socialist (Labour) I Independent

Source: S. Knott, The Electoral Crucible: The Politics of London 1900–14 (London: 1977), 82–4, 94–6, 109–11, 121–3.

Figure 2.17: Percentage of the electoral population voting in parliamentary general elections

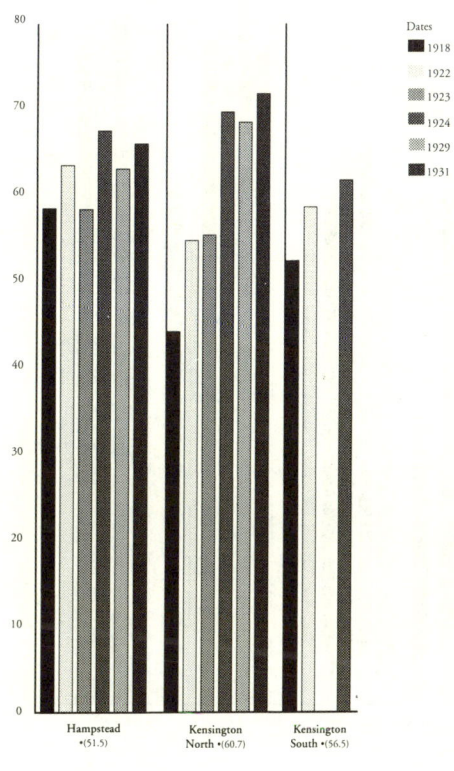

●(Mean Average 1918–1931)

Source: LCC, *Statistical Abstract for London* (London: 1923–33), Table 36.

Figure continued on next page.

Figure 2.17: Percentage of the electoral population voting in parliamentary general elections (continued)

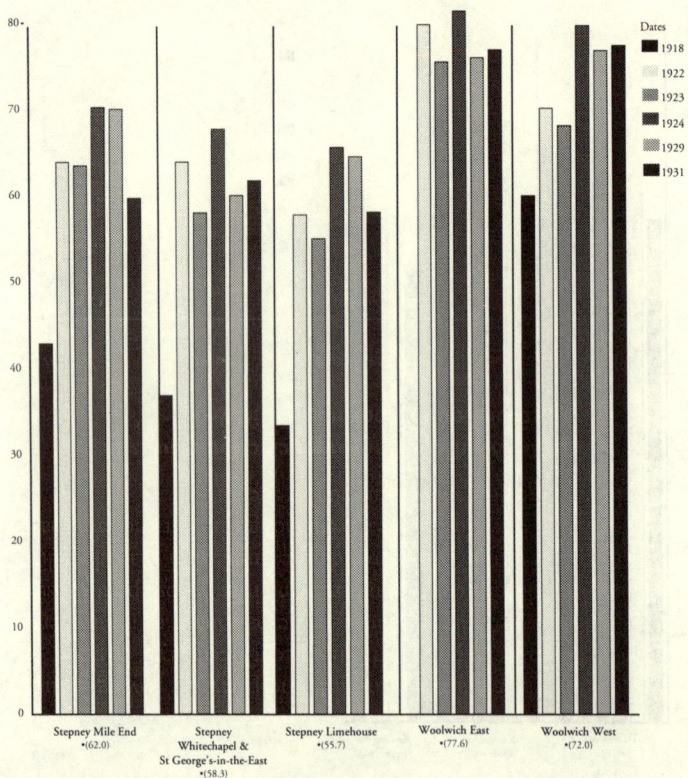

•(Mean Average 1918–1931)

The fortunes of the Labour Party was were much more mixed in the other boroughs. In Stepney the Labour Party was extremely weak in the years before the First World War, despite its overwhelmingly working-class population, but this might be explained by the fact that the majority of them were casual labourers who were more difficult to mobilize politically than those in Woolwich. Before the First World War the majority of MPs in Stepney were conservative, and the Municipal Reform Party (affiliated to the Conservative Party) held the majority of seats on the borough council in these years.[35] Some challenge was posed by the Liberal Party, who won the council elections as the Progressive Party in 1903, and almost half the seats in the 1912 council election. One of the two safest Liberal seats in London before

1914 was in the Stepney ward of Whitechapel. The strength of the Liberals in Stepney in these years and in the 1920s was surprising at a time when overall support for the Liberals was rapidly disappearing, but, in part, can be explained by the loyalty of the Jewish East End to the Liberal Party. Much of the Jewish allegiance to the Liberal Party stemmed from their gratitude towards the party for having granted Jews political emancipation in the nineteenth century.[36] Support for the Liberals was also built up through the patronage of a number of prominent local Jewish community personalities, whose political support of the party in the 1920s 'created the impression that Liberalism was still a viable force in the area even though in fact the local party organizations were little more than hollow shells'.[37]

Table 2.9 Municipal borough election results in four London boroughs, 1919–37

Date	Hampstead		Kensington		Stepney		Woolwich	
	L	O	L	O	L	O	L	O
1919	3	39	6	54	–	–	25	11
1922	5	37	7	53	27	33	23	13
1925	0	42•	6	54	40	20	24	12
1928	0	42	6	54	–	–	33	12
1931	0	42	6	54	39	34	22	33
1934	0	42	14	46	60	–	35	10
1937	6	36	12	48	59	1	35	10

L = Labour Party, O = Other – usually Municipal Reform and Liberal
• Municipal Reform majority
Source: J. White, 'Old Worlds for New', unpublished MS.

Nevertheless, support for the Liberal Party was not unanimous among the Jewish population, and was also extremely weak in non-Jewish areas where the Labour Party was more popular particularly in the years after the First World War. In Stepney as a whole the Labour Party had been growing in strength since the turn of the century, but only set up its own local party in 1918. The following year Labour won the borough council election, and as Table 2.9 shows, with the exception of 1922 continued to capture the polls into the 1930s. The ethnic minorities in the area played a key role in the strength of the Labour Party. The Whitechapel branch of the party had a sizeable number of Irish Catholics as well as Jews. In Mile End the Labour Party was practically all Jewish. Much of the Jewish support for the Labour Party stemmed from the dispersal of wealthier Jews to North-East and North-West London, which left a largely working-class Jewish population in East London in the inter-war years. During the

1920s and 1930s this population, along with the non-Jews, was greatly radicalized by unemployment and terrible poverty, some joining the Labour Party and others the Communist Party.[38] Just as important as the Jews were the Irish, who had a strong voice in the Whitechapel section of the Labour Party. Together the Jews and the Irish played a crucial role in determining policy, especially concerning the provision of birth control as well as the degree to which services should be divided to cater for the ethnic minorities.[39]

In the years between 1934 and 1939 individual Labour Party membership doubled in Stepney, rising from 3,096 to 6,010. By 1939 7.8 per cent of the electorate in Stepney were members of the Labour Party, which was slightly higher than membership in Woolwich.[40] Mile End was the largest and most effectively organized branch of the Stepney Labour Party. This high activity was partly due to the efforts of its full-time election agent, Israel Shafran. In 1930 it had a record membership of 2,000, which accounted for approximately 19 per cent of the electorate in the ward. Figure 2.17 suggests that the strength of the Labour Party in Mile End was able to galvanize a slightly larger proportion of its population into voting in parliamentary elections than in other wards within Stepney. The Mile End branch not only had a Labour club, which was one of the most popular in the East End, but also offered a range of social activities and free legal advice and was responsible for the publication of the *Stepney Labour Times* and the *Stepney Citizen*. Such activities were comparable with the Woolwich Labour Party, which also had the earliest Labour Party newspaper, *The Pioneer*. In both Woolwich and Stepney these newspapers provided a vital voice for local residents, and together with other social activities, were important in drawing support for the Labour Party and for certain issues within each borough, including welfare provision for mothers and babies.

As we shall see in Chapter 4 the strength of the Labour Party in Woolwich and later in Stepney was a key factor determining their high levels of expenditure on municipal provision for maternal and child welfare.[41] By contrast financial funding of such services was more limited in Hampstead and Kensington, which given their larger numbers of wealthy residents, not surprisingly were more politically conservative. In the years before the First World War the Municipal Reform Party held the overwhelming majority of seats on the borough councils of Hampstead and Kensington (Table 2.8). The Municipal Reformers continued to hold the majority of borough council seats and to return conservatives to parliament in Hampstead and Kensington during the 1920s and 1930s (Table 2.9). Parliamentary elections also tended to be won by conservative candidates. The Liberals did mount some opposition to the conservative lobby in both places, but this remained small and limited. In Kensington it was drawn from the residents in the poorer and more socially mixed part of the borough, North Kensington. Much of the Liberal Party's strength in Hampstead came from local progressive intellectual and Fabian circles.

A key supporter of Liberal politics within Hampstead was Thomas Hancock Nunn who came to Hampstead, having originally worked at Toynbee Hall, to serve on the local branch of the Charity Organization Society. From this position he founded the break-away organization, the Hampstead Council for Social Welfare, a voluntary umbrella organization for all the agencies involved in social and welfare relief in 1902. While the Hampstead Council for Social Welfare was a non-political organization, it was none the less a major influence on the politics and direction of services provided in the borough. As chief spokesman for the Hampstead Council for Social Welfare, Nunn ardently campaigned that services within the borough should be funded and initiated by voluntary rather than municipal organizations. His strength in pushing this view not only came from his position on the Hampstead Council for Social Welfare, but through his election as a Liberal candidate to the borough council.[42]

Overall the conservative outlook of Hampstead and Kensington made it difficult for the Labour Party to gain any strong hold in these boroughs. Table 2.7 shows that, with the exception of North Kensington, individual membership of the Labour Party was remarkably small in these areas even in the 1920s and 1930s. In Hampstead the Labour Party was unable to capture any seats in elections for the borough council or the LCC before the First World War, and only a handful in 1919 and 1937. Most of the votes they won were confined to Kilburn, the poorest part of the borough, yet it was an area the Labour Party found hard to mobilize. Few people in Kilburn turned out to vote in the elections. Only 11 per cent of the electorate voted in the parliamentary by-elections in 1932, and the Labour candidate failed to get in by just 58 votes. This contrasted the 1931 parliamentary election for the whole borough when 65.2 per cent of the electorate voted.[43]

The higher number and larger geographical concentration of the poor in North Kensington allowed for greater political mobilization than could be achieved among the poor in Hampstead. The disparity between rich and poor was also much larger in Kensington, fermenting fiercer political debate and contest within the neighbourhood as a

65

whole. Figure 2.17 shows that a higher percentage of population voted in the parliamentary general elections in the North than in the South of the borough. Significantly while many of the borough councillors and LCC representatives in South Kensington gained their seats without any electoral contest, those in North Kensington had to campaign actively to win their seats. In North Kensington much of the contest in the early years was between the Progressives and the Labour Party in the borough council and LCC elections, whereas in South Kensington the Municipal Reformers dominated the political slate unchallenged.[44]

While the Labour Party was weak in South Kensington, it had strong roots in North Kensington from an early stage. As Table 2.7 reveals the numbers joining the Labour Party was much higher in North Kensington than in the South. By 1929 the Labour Party membership in North Kensington was five times greater than in the South. Some of the strongest support for the party was in the Golborne ward, one of the poorest wards in the borough. In the 1903 borough council elections the Labour Party narrowly lost Golborne ward to the Progressives. Three years later Labour won all six borough council seats in the ward and was also successful in 1912, the year when the first Labour parliamentary candidate stood and lost the election in North Kensington.[45] The Labour Party continued to take all the borough council seats in the Golborne ward from 1912 onwards. Labour candidates also secured victories in the elections to the Boards of Guardians in Golborne in these years. The majority of the candidates were skilled artisans, but some were also labourers. A handful of the Labour candidates were also involved in professional occupations, such as medicine.

Part of the success of the Labour Party in the Golborne ward stemmed from the poverty in the area which marked it out from the rest of the borough. Special efforts were also undertaken by the Labour Party within Golborne, such as the establishment of a co-operative trading store, a Socialist Sunday school, and a mother and baby clinic in Telford Road.[46] While Labour candidates were put up for election to the borough council in other wards in North Kensington, they had no real success until the 1934 and 1937 election, showing the general swing to Labour elsewhere in these years.[47] Overall, however, the Labour Party only won seats in North Kensington where there was a greater proportion of working-class voters, and constituted only a small proportion of the total seats on Kensington council.

Women's Social and Political Participation

All four boroughs not only varied in their political composition and organization, but also in the degree to which women participated in their communal and political life. Their presence was important on two fronts, firstly in the more informal world of philanthropy, and secondly in party politics and government administration. Women's participation in these different spheres was a vital determinant of the extent to which their voices were heard, and the ways in which their particular needs and concerns were catered for in each borough.[48]

What role women took in these different worlds was largely shaped by their own social and economic status, as well as the positions allowed to women. In the case of government administration women were forbidden to vote or stand for parliament until 1918. None the less, from the late nineteenth century onwards women could be elected to vestries (later taken over by the borough councils), to school boards (abolished in 1904), Boards of Guardians, and the London County Council. From 1907 women could also stand in borough council elections. Initially this was more strongly supported by the Labour Party than by any of the other political parties.[49]

Part of this opening up of government posts to women resulted from the growing demand for women's political franchise by the suffragette movement in these years. This movement not only challenged the more conventional structures of government to give space to women, but also resulted in raising women's own political consciousness and involvement. For many women, their contact with the suffragette movement constituted their initiation into formal politics. Although very different from the suffragette movement, philanthropic activities were also a vital determinant in boosting women's confidence and pushing them into the public domain and formal politics.[50]

The majority of women who became involved in the suffragette movement or philanthropic work were either upper or middle class, who had more time and money to spare than their working-class sisters. This is not to say that working-class women took less part in political and communal activities, but they faced more constraints. The political participation of married working-class women was particularly limited given the difficulty many of them faced in combining such activity with the tasks of housework and childcare and other forms of employment.[51] While a number of working-class women became involved in politics through the suffragette movement, many had had their political awareness awakened by their participation in the trade union movement or through organizations such as the

Women's Co-operative Guild.

Many of the working-class women's political endeavours stemmed from their experiences as single women. Increased factory work among women in London after the First World War had resulted in a greater mixing between women from slum areas and those who had grown up in the new council housing. While most of the women employed in large factories left once they were married, many of them carried the experience they had learned in the workplace into their married lives. For many of these women, the factory had raised their expectations of what a home should contain, what role their husband should play, and what they were entitled to as citizens in the provision of housing, welfare and maternity care.[52]

The work-place was not only important in raising women's own political consciousness on an individual level, but also determined the extent to which they had a voice within the political domain. One study of the three Northern Towns of Nelson, Preston and Lancaster, has shown that women's political participation within local Labour parties was greatly determined by their numerical and political strength within the work-force. In Lancaster, for instance, where only a very small proportion of women were employed within the work-force and tended to be confined to jobs that were un-unionized and reinforced particular paternalistic relationships, women had a weak role within the Labour party. By contrast women had a strong voice in the Labour party in Nelson, reflecting their strength within the work-force. Here women were not in direct competition with men for employment, and within the work-place women were given a relatively equal role with men and recognized as skilled workers by their male colleagues. This was not the case in Preston, where women's presence in the Labour party was less powerful, reflecting the greater competition between men and women for work, and the rigid sexual division of labour within the work-force and subordinate position of women to their fellow male workers.

Given that the Labour Party controlled the council in all three areas, women's strength within this political party had important implications for the degree to which women's needs and demands were heeded particularly in the context of maternal and child welfare provision. Of all three areas Lancaster had the poorest maternal and child welfare services, reflecting the relative weakness of women in its work-force and the Labour party. Greater commitment was made to maternal and child welfare facilities in Nelson where women had a more active role in the work-place and within the Labour party. Within Preston such services tended to be subordinated to those which were more representative of men's needs, indicating the inferior status of women both within the work-force as well as within the Labour party.[53]

Women's participation in politics and the degree to which they could articulate their needs was dependent, therefore, on a variety of factors. What is most interesting is that it was in Hampstead and Kensington that the suffragette movement seems to have had the strongest support, whose base was drawn from the large numbers of richer women in these areas who had the time and resources to put into suffragette campaigns. In Hampstead the suffragette movement had a high profile from early on with frequent meetings being held by branches of the movement before the First World War.[54] Kensington was also a particularly important stronghold for the suffragettes. Suffragette Meetings were very well attended and sparked great opposition within the borough. Part of the strength of the movement in Kensington was linked to the strong familial and other connections that the Pankhursts had with people in the area.

In Hampstead and Kensington, many of the campaigns run by the suffragette movement also seem to have influenced a wider movement for the election of women to positions of local government. Such campaigns were run by organizations such as the Hampstead Citizen's Union in Hampstead, and the Women's Unionist Association and the Women's Local Government Society in Kensington.[55] These organizations actively sought the appointment of women in posts such as inspectors in workhouses, and the election of women Guardians.[56] The success of their campaigns can be seen from the fact that Hampstead and Kensington were among the first places in the country to have women councillors and women Guardians.[57]

Kensington was unusual in its large number of women who were elected both as Guardians and as councillors from early on and before women had won the vote for parliamentary elections. In 1909 30 women stood as candidates for the 29 borough council elections in the whole of London, ten of whom were in Kensington. Two of the women candidates, both Municipal Reformers who had also won seats on the Board of Guardians in previous years, succeeded.[58] Women were also pushed forward as candidates in the 1910 LCC elections.[59] In 1912 four women were elected to the borough council, two of whom were the previous winners, and two of whom were Labour Party candidates in the Golborne Ward.[60] Many women also stood as Guardians in Kensington, amounting to seven of the 30 contenders in the 1913 elections, six of whom were elected.[61] After the war and the introduction of female suffrage, women continued to

stand in large numbers for the Kensington local government elections, both for the council and the Board of Guardians. In 1919 17
women stood in the borough council elections, and 20 stood in
1922, ten of whom won in each election. Women continued to have
a high profile in the borough council elections through to 1939, and
also in the elections to the Boards of Guardians, 13 standing in the
election in 1922, of whom eight got places.[62]

The suffragette movement was also forceful in Woolwich,
although the type of women involved in political action in the borough differed considerably from Hampstead and Kensington. In
Hampstead and Kensington many of the women who stood for
local government positions tended to be the more prosperous residents who had the resources and free time for such work.[63] In
Woolwich many activists generally came from the working class.
Part of this can be attributed to the scarcity of paid female employment in Woolwich, which gave women more time to devote to such
politics. However, this was not the only cause.[64] Their political activity also stemmed from the presence of the strong radical male work-
force in the Royal Arsenal, as well as the positive encouragement
given to women by the local Labour party. From its foundation, the
Woolwich Labour party saw women as equal members with men
and encouraged them to stand as Labour candidates in borough
council elections as early as 1908.[65] In 1912 two Labour women
were elected to the council.[66] Unlike other local Labour parties, such
as Lewisham, the Woolwich Labour Party was also very supportive
of the suffragette movement indicating the importance it heeded to
women's position in society.[67] By 1919 nearly 1,000 women were
members of the Woolwich Labour Party and by 1926 women's
membership exceeded 1,000 out of a total membership of 5,000.[68]
In 1933 women numbered 1,704 out of a total of 4,013, which
constituted 42 per cent of the membership in the party and 3.7 per
cent of the total female electorate in the borough.[69]

Campaigns for women's suffrage and for the election of women
to local government were much quieter in Stepney than the three
other boroughs. Unlike Kensington and Hampstead, where such
activities were strongly promoted by the presence of a wealthy female
constituency keen to win the vote, or Woolwich which had a Labour
party with a strong sympathy for the suffragette movement, Stepney
had none of these ingredients in the years before the First World
War. In the neighbouring borough of Poplar, where, as in the case of
Woolwich, the Labour party was strong from early on and identified
closely with the women's suffragette movement, women had a higher

political profile in local government.[70] After the First World War women were a more vital component in the political life of Stepney, standing as both Liberal and Labour candidates in the council elections. The Mile End Labour Party had a strong representation of women, with over 600 members in its women's section in 1935.[71]

Whatever the route by which women entered the political domain, the degree to which women could influence the direction of local government provision was greatly dependent on their charisma and personality. This can be seen most clearly in the case of Kensington, where there were a number of formidable women from different political persuasions, all of whom took an active role in local government and speaking out on policies concerning welfare provision. Coming from the Labour Party's ranks were Ethel Bentham and Marion Phillips, who together formed a powerful force within the council chamber. Bentham, who originally trained at the London School of Medicine for Women, had started her political activities in Newcastle where she had been active in the National Union of Women's Suffrage Societies and the Independent Labour Party.[72] Phillips had undertaken a doctorate at the London School of Economics where she had also worked with Beatrice Webb. Bentham first stood as a Labour candidate for the Kensington borough council in 1909 and for the LCC in 1910; finally achieving success in 1912 when she was elected along with Marion Phillips to the borough council. Phillips remained on the council until 1919, after which she left Kensington to be the chief woman officer of the reconstituted national Labour Party. Bentham stayed on the council through to the 1930s.

From 1909 to 1919 Phillips lived in Bentham's house in Holland Park, which formed a central base for Labour Party women activists not only in North Kensington, but also nationally.[73] Alongside their interests in Kensington, these two women were active founders of the Women's Labour League (affiliated to the Labour Party); Bentham taking the semi-permanent chair of the executive committee and Phillips the post of general secretary in 1912. Phillips also edited *The Labour Woman*, the national journal of the Women's Labour League from 1913 through to the late 1920s. In addition, Bentham and Phillips were involved with the Fabian Socialists and the Independent Labour Party. Bentham was also the Fabian representative on the British Section of the Women's International Council of Socialist and Labour Organizations, and was an early elected member of the LCC. Both women were among the first generation of women MPs after the First World War.[74]

Bentham's political standing in the borough stemmed from her role as supervisor of the mother and baby clinic in Telford Road (North Kensington), the first clinic in the country to include medical treatment alongside advice.[75] Originally set up by the Women's Labour League in 1910 as a memorial to the early death of Margaret MacDonald, the clinic was extended to include a baby hospital in 1920. The clinic was not only continually used as a model in national Labour women's campaigns to extend municipal maternal and child welfare provision, but served as a meeting point for many of the key Labour women activists, particularly through its sewing circle which met to raise funds for the clinic.[76] Bentham continued to work for the clinic through to the 1930s, and used it as a constant reference point for her political activities in Kensington, particularly around the issue of infant mortality.[77]

Another figure who had a significant influence on the maternal and child welfare policies pursued in Kensington was Margery Spring Rice, the niece of Dr Elizabeth Garrett Anderson, the first qualified woman doctor to practise in Britain,[78] and Milicent Fawcett, a prominent suffragette. Although Margery Spring Rice failed to be elected to the council on a Progressive slate in 1922, she was extremely active in promoting women's health in the borough and was a co-founder and chairman of the North Kensington Women's Welfare Clinic established in 1924, the third voluntary clinic established in London to provide contraception to married women. The clinic gave contraceptive advice alongside gynaecological help, and was extremely active in pushing the local council to call on the Ministry of Health to agree to municipal provision of such services.[79]

Much of the maternal and child welfare policy pursued by Kensington council was also influenced by women affiliated to the Municipal Reform Party, who were early supporters of women's suffrage. Among these were the first two women elected to the borough council in 1909, Mary Alexander and Amelia Hayne, who respectively represented the wards of Holland and Brompton. Another was Charlotte Keeling, who first won a seat on the borough council in 1912 in the Norland ward and continued to be elected until 1934. All of these women had served as Poor Law Guardians from the turn of the century, and had some previous experience in philanthropic work.[80] As in the case of Bentham and Phillips, all these women saw women's suffrage and the representation of women in local government as a vital force in social reform and welfare provision.[81] Together the presence of Labour women alongside those of the Municipal Reform Party, created an important lobby within the council, making women's issues a high priority on the council's agenda and in other political affairs. Unlike the Labour women, however, who campaigned for more state intervention in welfare and health care, those women who stood on the Municipal Reform platform, were vehemently opposed to state support, seeing it as undermining the independence of the poor they were so keen to educate in the rigours of self help. Such a division of attitude was not only apparent among the different women within Kensington Council, but reflected the overall tension in the council chamber and affected the development of welfare provision.[82]

In Stepney, those women who stood out also came from a variety of political backgrounds. One of the most prominent women in Stepney's political life was the Liberal councillor Miriam Moses. Much of her strength was drawn from her associations with Jewish community work, which she was able to use to capture the council seat for the Spitalfields East Ward between 1921 and 1931. Her presence accounts for the failure of Labour councillors to secure any seats in Spitalfields East Ward until 1931. On the Labour front, two women who were particularly active were Sarah Tobin and Lily Frankel who were elected to the council in 1922 and 1934 respectively. They were leading members of the women's section in Mile End. Lily Frankel served as secretary and chairman of the women's section, and was also a member of various school managing bodies, a co-opted member of the LCC, and chairman of Stepney council's maternity and child welfare committee in the 1930s.[83] Other Jewish women, who did not necessarily have any party affiliations but who were well-known Jewish community figures, also played a key role in the political affairs of the borough, particularly in maternal and child welfare. Among these figures were Alice Model, who set up the Sick Room Helps Society and Jewish Maternity Home; and Caroline Franklin who set up the first Jewish infant welfare clinic.[84] The large profile of Jewish women in the political affairs of Stepney, reflects the dominance of the Jewish immigrant population in the area.

Some of the notable women in the political and social affairs of Woolwich were Alice Gregory, Maud Cashmore and Lelia Parnell. While none of these women were actively involved in any political party, they gained their strength from being the founders of the first maternity hospital in the area, the British Hospital for Mothers and Babies. Their activities stretched beyond the hospital itself to national campaigns for better national training in midwifery as well as increasing state sponsorship of maternity care for poor mothers. Much of their work stemmed from a strong belief both that women could achieve independence through a professional career such as midwifery, and that women should be given the best possible maternity care. Their views and actions were also inspired by a deep sense of Christian morality and the need to help the poor, as well as a strong feminist orientation. Together with the high participation of women in the local Labour party which raised the importance of women's issues within the political affairs of the borough, these three women provided a powerful vision of a good maternity service with well-trained midwives. The founders argued vehemently that the work they carried out was for the good of the whole community. Midwives they stated had an important role in the maternal and child welfare services and were serving their country in a matter of urgent need.[85]

Most of those who were involved in public work within Hampstead were the wives of local councillors or politicians, such as Mrs Hancock Nunn who served on the Distress Committee of the Council. Married to Thomas Hancock Nunn she also was a key organizer in the Hampstead Council for Social Welfare, and visited cases under its auspices. Another example was Mrs Fletcher (wife of the conservative MP Mr J. S. Fletcher) who stood on various committees including Queen Mary's Maternity Home established in Hampstead as a model maternity home by Queen Mary in 1919, and the Infants' Hospital which moved from Hampstead to Westminster in 1907.[86] Margaret Hoare was another notable woman who was particularly active in the public life of the area. She not only participated in the running of the local Red Cross, but for many years was the chair of the house committee of Queen Mary's Maternity Home.[87]

The Medical Profession

The strength and charisma of individual women was only one factor among many influencing the provision of health and welfare in each of the boroughs. One figure who was also important was the medical officer of health, whose main job was to initiate and supervise public health services within each borough. As a number of historians have pointed out, in the early twentieth century many of the medical officers of health tended to come from the more radical section of the medical profession. While their main task was the inculcation of individual responsibility for personal hygiene and cleanliness, which they saw as being achieved by educational measures, many felt that this would remain ineffective against the evils of poverty and poor environmental conditions for which collective state provision was the only answer. In 1905 the Society of Medical Officers of Health, the professional body of medical officers of health, allied itself with the efforts of the Fabian Socialists Sidney and Beatrice Webb to develop a unified health service paid for by the central government, which would replace the existing fragmented health and Poor Law medical services. They hoped that this measure would help to achieve a preventive health scheme in which there would be comprehensive planning for the social, economic and physical environment of health. Part of their ambition was articulated by the Minority Report produced for the Royal Commission on the Poor Law in 1909.[88]

While a unified medical service was never realized on a central level in the early twentieth century, the associations between poverty and ill health and the need for greater collective provision of services was a theme which underlay many of the annual reports written by the medical officers of health in each of the four boroughs. Employed by the borough council, the medical officer of health was primarily an agent of the council and was, therefore, restricted by the levels of expenditure and policies that they established. Yet the individual opinion and judgement of the medical officer of health could play an important role in influencing the direction and level of the services provided. To what extent this happened depended largely on the charisma and personality of individual medical officers, which could be decisive in coaxing the council to undertake more radical policies than they would otherwise have provided.

Among the many medical officers who served in the four boroughs, one of the most memorable and long-serving was James Fenton in Kensington. Born in the Midlands in 1884 Fenton was described on his death as 'one of the most experienced public health administrators in Britain', whose name had become a 'household word in public health'. During his tenure of office in Kensington, Fenton oversaw many pioneering schemes in public health which were used as models elsewhere. As will be explored in greater detail in Chapter 7, one of his major achievements in maternal and child welfare was the establishment of Fathers' Councils, which actively sought the involvement of fathers in the welfare of their family and to take greater responsibility in the initiation and running of public health services in Kensington. In addition to his work as a medical officer, he also presided over the Kensington Medical Society and maintained strong links with the North Kensington Women's Welfare Centre. Within the borough he was extremely popular among both members of the borough council who saw him as a personal friend as well a medical adviser, and was well liked among local doctors. Much of his popularity stemmed from his warm personality, and his 'genius for committee work' and 'ability to counter tension by infectious geniality'. Outside of Kensington, Fenton also had a strong standing, taking a keen role within the Society for Medical Officers of Health of which he became president in 1937. In addition to this he was the chair for the Central Council for Health Education and the Royal Sanitary Institute. On retiring from Kensington he went on to serve as principal medical officer in the Ministry of Health where he used his skill in administration with the National Health Service.[89]

Throughout his career Fenton showed a great passion for public health work, and was adamant to combat the detrimental effects of poverty and bad living conditions on health. From his work within Kensington it is clear that he was keen for people to take health matters into their own hands, and that people should have greater access to collective provision of services provided by the state, including the provision of contraception. The more conservative members of Kensington Council did not necessarily agree with his view, but Fenton had a strong alliance with Margery Spring Rice and other more progressive individuals within Kensington. Fenton, together with these individuals, provided an important lobby in establishing services which, although unable to relieve the terrible poverty and overcrowding in particular parts of the borough and the ill-effects this caused on health, particularly that of infants, were nevertheless ahead of their time in the appreciation and understanding they showed towards their clients.

Fenton's presence in Kensington underlines the important role that medical professionals could make on the direction and quality of services within a borough. This leverage was not confined to medical officers of health or to Kensington. In East London, the obstetrician and general practitioner, Dr William H. Francis Oxley, had a crucial influence on the quality of maternity care offered in the area. After qualifying at St Bartholomew's Hospital in 1897, Dr Oxley set up a general practice in Poplar, which was to be his base for the majority of his life. Alongside his general practice he was obstetric surgeon for the local nursing home, St John the Divine, and obstetric surgeon and lecturer in midwifery at the East End Maternity Home in Stepney where he was initially the only obstetrician, and took complete charge of the hospital's emergency work without the aid of an assistant.

Oxley's stress on the need for minimal obstetric interference dominated the care of the East End Maternity Home, resulting in the remarkably low rates of maternal mortality that brought both him and the hospital high recognition the world over.[90] His policy of 'wait and see' was unusual for many obstetricians and doctors in these years, but as we shall see in the following chapters, this was a

key to his success. Indeed, part of the remarkably low rate of maternal mortality found in Stepney may partly be accounted for by the
good provision of care Oxley offered through his services to the East
End Maternity Home. The influence of his work was not confined
to Stepney. In 1929 he was among the founding members of the
British (later Royal) College of Obstetricians and Gynaecologists,
and in 1931 was the first general practitioner to be permitted membership of the College. His eagerness to raise the standards of obstetric care was seen in his efforts on the Interdepartmental Committee
investigating maternal mortality in the years 1928–32, becoming
known as one of the more militant members of the committee.[91]

Both in his general practice and in his work at the East End
Maternity Home Oxley showed enormous commitment and devo-
tion to his patients and was quick to draw the links between poverty
and ill health. This dedication was clearly stated in his position on
abortion, which he felt could not be prevented when women faced
the continual problem of poverty, household difficulties and the
struggle to maintain the family income. For him it was important to
tackle these issues rather than to castigate women for performing
abortions such as those which involved taking strong aperients or
using soap and water douches to bring on a period. In contrast to
many other medical experts in the late 1930s Oxley also did not
believe that abortion was increasing in these years. He argued that
the noted rise was the result of increasing hospitalization of cases and
more exact certification. Like Fenton, Oxley also felt that one of the
ways to curb abortions was to promote birth control. Such views,
however, were not shared by many at the time.[92]

Conclusion

As we have seen in this chapter, while all four boroughs were situated in
Britain's wealthiest city, they were highly diverse in their socio-economic
conditions and class composition. Of the boroughs, Hampstead had the
most wealth and largest proportion of middle-class residents, and
Stepney had the least prosperity and greatest number of working-class
residents. Falling in between was Kensington which had a high number
of rich inhabitants and also a large constituency of very poor people
confined to the unskilled labouring sector. Closer to Stepney was
Woolwich, which had a very large proportion of working-class dwellers,
but these had a more regular and higher income than those of Stepney
who were less skilled and unionized. Each borough also varied in their
levels of population density and overcrowding, with Stepney recording
the largest number of people per acre and the greatest percentage

of population living in overcrowded conditions. Not far behind was Kensington. By contrast Hampstead and Woolwich had very low densities of population and were relatively unaffected by overcrowding. As we will see in the next chapter this had crucial implications for the health standards found among infants and mothers in each borough.

Just as important as socio-economic conditions in determining the levels of maternal and child health, was the quality of health and welfare care available to them. Following chapters will show that this was highly variable between the boroughs, and largely governed by the political outlook and mobilization of each area described here. As we shall see, while the dominance of the Labour Party in Stepney and particularly Woolwich increased the propensity to municipal spending on maternal and child welfare facilities, the conservative outlook of Hampstead and Kensington tended to curb such expenditure. Yet, as will become clear, the form of services provided was not totally dependent on the general political outlook of each area, but could also be influenced by the efforts of particular individuals, and the overall participation of women within the philanthropic and political arena of each area. Kensington, for instance, which was largely conservative in outlook, provided surprisingly innovative and inspiring forms of care for mothers, which might be explained by the very strong presence of women in the political and philanthropic life of the borough. What form this took and how it compared with other boroughs is the subject of the remaining chapters.

Notes

1. H. Llewellyn Smith, *The New Survey of London: Eastern Area,* 6 (London: 1932), 354. See also G. Stedman Jones, *Outcast London* (London: 2nd edn 1984) and J. A. Gillespie, 'Economic Change in the East End of London during the 1920s', unpub. Ph.D., Cambridge, 1984, for more information on the development of the industries in Stepney and the problems of poverty.

2. C. Booth, *Life and Labour in London* (London: 1902), 1st ser. II, 424–5; F. M. L. Thompson, *Hampstead: Building a Borough, 1650–1964* (London: 1974), 51.

3. Thompson, *op. cit.* (note 2), 27.

4. J. Davis, 'Jennings' Buildings and the Royal Borough: The Construction of the Underclass in Mid-Victorian England', in D. Feldman and G. Stedman Jones (eds), *Metropolis London: Histories and Representations since 1800* (London: 1989), 15.

5. H. Llewellyn Smith, *The New Survey of London: Western Area,* 6 (London: 1934) 424, 428.

6. Thompson, *op. cit.* (note 2), 53.

7. Gillespie, *op. cit.* (note 1), 83–4, 88.

8. D. Weinbren, '"The Peace Arsenal" Scheme: The Campaign for Non-Munitions Work at the Royal Ordnance Factory, Woolwich after the First World War', unpub. Ph.D., Thames Polytechnic, 1990, 22.

9. For more information on the Arsenal and the work it provided in Woolwich see *ibid.*, 29, 33; and D. Thom, 'Women Munition Workers at Woolwich Arsenal in the 1914–18 War', unpub. M.A., Warwick, 1975.

10. 'Woolwich Metropolitan Borough Survey', report by Dr Allan Parsons, December 1934, 3–4 (PRO file: MH66/404).

11. LCC, *London Statistics*, 25 (London: 1914–15), map showing married women engaged in occupations, 1911.

12. E. W. Hope and J. Campbell, *Report on the Physical Welfare of Mother and Children: England and Wales*, 1 (London: 1917), 300, 378.

13. *Census of Great Britain* (1911); LCC, *London Statistics*.

14. Thom, *op. cit.* (note 9), 26–7; Weinbren, *op. cit.* (note 8), 141.

15. LCC, *London Statistics*.

16. Hope & Campbell, *op. cit.* (note 12), 300. Many of the women employed as domestic servants were Welsh migrants, reflecting the lack of popularity of domestic service among London-born women (J. White, 'Old Worlds for New', unpublished MS, 109–10). One woman, who was sent from the Rhondda Valley to work as a domestic servant in North London at the young age of fourteen recalled the loneliness and long hours she had to work. See interview with Mrs A. B. by L. Marks, London, 7 June 1992, transcript.

17. LCC, *London Statistics*.

18. Hope & Campbell, *op. cit.* (note 12), 378; White, *op. cit.* (note 16), 103.

19. Gillespie, *op. cit.* (note 1), 214.

20. By contrast the percentage of married women employed was 15.5 in Stepney, 19 in Kensington, and 10.5 in Hampstead. LCC, *London Statistics*.

21. For more information on the attention such housing attracted in the two boroughs see J. White, *Rothschild Buildings: Life in an East End Tenement Block, 1887–1920* (London: 1980), Ch. 1; and Davis, *op. cit.* (note 4), 11–39.

22. Thompson, *op. cit.* (note 2), 46; Llewellyn Smith, *op. cit.* (note 5), 423.

23. *Ibid.*, 427.

24. For more information on the development of slum housing in Kensington and the attitudes of local residents and the press towards it in the nineteenth century see Davis, *op. cit.* (note 4).

25. Kensington MOH, *A/R* (1935), 44. The equivalent percentage of population living in overcrowded situations in Stepney was 19.7%, and in Woolwich it was 2.75%.

26. E. Ross, 'Survival Networks: Women's Neighbourhood Sharing in

London before World War I', *Hist. Workshop J.* (1983), 4–27. See also J. White, *The Worst Street in North London: Campbell Bunk, Islington Between the Wars* (London: 1986), Ch. 3.

27. British Hospital for Mothers and Babies, Register of the Midwifery School, Nurse Evelyn Walter, 1–2 (GLRO file: H14/BMB/c1/1).

28. G. Rose has shown the success of Poplar Labour Party was not only rooted in the communal solidarity people felt for each other because of the social and economic deprivation they faced, but also because of the cultural and religious traditions they shared. This ranged from the music hall and feeling of neighbourliness to ideologies of Christian socialism, all of which were shaped by the particularities of Poplar. ('Imagining Poplar in the 1920s: Contested Concepts of Community', *J. Hist. Geog.* 16/4 (1990), 425–37).

29. For an interesting discussion on the ways in which the internal social dynamics of a neighbourhood are affected by the social composition of an area see M. Savage, *The Dynamics of Working-Class Politics: The Labour Movement in Preston, 1880–1940* (Cambridge: 1987). Savage has shown that in Preston the collective action of the working class was weaker before the 1890s when there was greater interference from Preston's élite. During this period any popular action tended to be undermined by the erection of churches in working-class neigh-bourhoods by the élite of the town. This measure not only deter-mined the cultural and social life of the working-class areas, but even altered their physical layout. Between 1890 and 1914, however, the social dynamics changed as the more middle-class residents increas-ingly moved out of the working-class neighbourhoods, and institu-tions originally established by the élite were taken over by local resi-dents and finally replaced with their own organizations in the inter-war years (101–15).

30. Stedman Jones, *op. cit.* (note 1), 12, 14, 241, 244–5, 283–4.

31. R. Eatwell, *The Woolwich Labour Party, 1903–1951* (London: 1982), 4; See Table 8.3 in White, *op. cit.* (note 16).

32. S. Knott, *The Electoral Crucible: The Politics of London 1900–1914* (London: 1977), 123.

33. For more information on the involvement of these clergymen with the Labour Party see P. Thompson, *Socialists, Liberals and Labour* (London: 1967), 23.

34. Eatwell, *op. cit.* (note 31), 4.

35. The large number of Jewish immigrants in Stepney, made anti-alienism an important issue during the borough's political campaigns, but this does not explain the conservative success in the area. Liberals, like the conservatives, were champions of the anti-alien cause. Some of the conservative candidates who supported the restric-tion of immigrations were also Jews themselves, such as Harry S. Samuel, elected MP for Limehouse in 1900. (Thompson, *op. cit.* (note 33), 30). The allegiance of some Jews to the issue of anti-

· alienism stemmed partly from 'political opportunism and loyalty and partly out of fear: the presence of Jewish pauper refugees, and the agitation to which it had given rise, threatened (so it was said) to endanger the safety of the entire Anglo-Jewish community, especially since the poor Jews tended to be much less hostile to Socialism than their bourgeois co-religionists'. G. Alderman, *London Jewry and London Politics 1889–1986* (London: 1989), 39–40.

36. James Kiley, a former mayor of Stepney and MP for Whitechapel between 1916 and 1922, for instance, was able to gather votes for the Liberals on the basis of the respect he had won for championing Jewish interests in parliament. E. R. Smith, 'Jews and Politics in the East End of London, 1918–1939,' in D. Cesarani (ed.), *The Making of Modern Anglo-Jewry* (Oxford: 1990), 146.

37. These personalities included Miriam Moses, Ida Samuel, Harry Kosky, Jack Somper and Jack Rosenthal. See Smith, *op. cit.* (note 36), 146.

38. *Ibid.,* 150–3. Jewish Labourism, predated this period and had roots in the socialist circles and trade unions Jewish immigrants brought with them from Eastern Europe and the clubs they established in the 1880s and 1890s. For more information on this see Alderman, *op. cit.* (note 35), 73–8 and W. J. Fishman, *East End Jewish Radicals* (London: 1975).

39. L. Marks, 'Irish and Jewish Women's Experience of Childbirth and Infant Care in East London 1870–1939: The Responses of Host Society and Immigrant Communities to Medical Welfare Needs', unpub. D.Phil, Oxford, 1990, Chs 1 and 8; and *eadem, Model Mothers: Jewish Mothers and Maternity Provision in East London, 1870–1939* (Oxford: 1994), Ch. 6.

40. Local Labour Party *A/Rs* cited in White, *op. cit.* (note 16), Table 8.3.

41. Nationally Labour-controlled councils were a significant factor in raising overall municipal spending. See M. Powell, 'Hospital Provision Before the NHS: Territorial Justice or Inverse Care Law', *J. Soc. Pol.,* 21, Part 2 (April 1992), 145–64, 160.

42. M. J. Moore, 'Social Work and Social Welfare: The Organizations of Philanthropic Resources in Britain, 1900–1914', *J. Br. Stud.,* 16 (1977), 85–104, 99. The HCSW will be discussed in more detail in following chapters.

43. *Hampstead and Highgate Advertiser,* 8 November 1919, 5; *Hampstead Citizen,* October 1932, 4, see also March 1935, 4. White, *op. cit.* (note 16), Table 8.2.

44. *Kensington News and West London Times,* 6 November 1903; 5 November 1909; 3 January 1910, 6; 8 November 1912, 3.

45. Knott, *op. cit.* (note 32), 81–3, 96; *Kensington News and West London Times, 3* January 1910, 6.

46. P. Hollis, *Ladies Elect: Women in English Local Government 1865–1914* (Oxford: 1987), 413; *The Labour Woman,* July 1920, 106.

47. *Kensington News and West London Times,* 7 November 1919, 3; 17

November 1922, 2; 23 October 1925, 5; *North Kensington Citizen,*
November 1934. In 1934 the Labour Party took over control of the
LCC from the Municipal Reformers. In 1937 there were 75 Labour
councillors on the LCC as opposed to 49 Municipal Reform councillors. (A. Saint (ed.), *Politics and the People of London : the LCC
1889–1965,* (London: 1989)).

48. Many historians have shown that women's involvement in both the
informal networks of philanthropy and government were an important
force in building state welfare provision. This was not only true within
Britain, but also elsewhere. For the most recent discussions on this subject and for a comparative perspective see the collection of essays in S.
Koven and S. Michel (eds), *Mothers of a New World: Maternalist Politics
and Origins of Welfare States* (London: 1993); and G. Bock and P.
Thane (eds), *Maternity and Gender Policies: Women and the Rise of the
European Welfare States, 1880s–1950s* (London: 1991).

49. *Kensington News and West London Times,* 14 June 1912, 6. Women's
participation in local government was also promoted by the Fabian
Women's Group, which tackled the education of 100,000 women
within London County Council boundaries to enable them to have the
necessary qualifications for becoming electors. The campaign successfully enabled women to be elected to Poor Law Boards and occasionally to local councils. See S. Alexander, 'The Fabian Women's Group,
1908–52', in S. Alexander, *On Becoming a Woman and Other Essays in
19th and 20th Century Feminist History* (London: 1994), 153.

50. For more information on this see A. Summers, 'A Home from Home
– Women's Philanthropic Work in the Nineteenth Century', in S.
Burman (ed.), *Fit Work for Women* (London: 1979); and J.
Walkowitz, 'Jack the Ripper and the Myth of Male Violence', *Fem.
Stud.,* 8/3 (1982), 543–75.

51. For a particularly interesting account of one working-class woman's
struggles to balance family life with suffrage political activities see H.
Mitchell, *The Hard Way Up* (London: 1968, 1984).

52. White, *op. cit.* (note 16), 127–8. See also S. Alexander, 'Becoming a
Woman in London in the 1920s and '30s', in Alexander, *op. cit.* (note
49), 205.

53. J. Mark-Lawson, M. Savage and A. Warde, 'Gender and Local
Politics: Struggles over Welfare Policies' 1918–39', in Lancaster
Regionalism Group, *Localities, Class and Gender* (London: 1985).

54. *Hampstead Advertiser,* 21 February 1907, 10; 14 March 1907, 3; 31
October 1912; *Kensington News and West London Times,* 11 March
1910, 3.

55. Louisa Twining, a key social activist in workhouse reform who was a
resident in Kensington took an active part in the Women's Local
Government Society. *Kensington News and West London Times,* 24
March 1905, 2.

56. Together with other moves to get women appointed as inspectors or

relieving officers in the workhouse, or as a medical doctor for the council, this stand raised considerable objections from the more male conservative circles within Kensington, such as the Middle Classes Defence Organization or male councillors, who argued that either women were incapable of the ruthlessness required in such positions or that they threatened men's jobs. In 1913 after a meeting with suffragettes and anti-suffragettes, 44 councillors voted against sending a petition to parliament calling on the government to give women the vote. Only 14 were in favour of the petition. *Kensington News and West London Times,* 24 March 1905, 2; 15 November 1907, 6; 3 May 1907, 5; 10 May 1907, 3; 29 October 1909, 3; 17 January 1913, 3.

57. *Ibid.,* 22 October 1909, 5; Hollis, *op. cit.* (note 46), 207, 412.

58. *Ibid.,* 22 October 1909, 5; 29 October 1909; 5 November 1909; 3 February 1911, 6.

59. *Ibid.,* 11 February 1910, 6.

60. *Ibid.,* 8 November 1912, 3.

61. *Ibid.,* 14 March 1913, 5.

62. *Ibid.,* 7 November 1919, 3; 7 April 1922, 5; 3 November 1922, 3. In some wards women won their seats with no ballot contest as there were no other contenders.

63. In Oxford much of the voluntary maternal and child welfare services in the area were shaped by the contribution made by the wives of the Oxford dons, who had a great deal of free time to devote to such causes. Such voluntary provision inhibited the growth of municipal provision. E. P. Peretz, 'Regional Variations in Maternal and Child Welfare between the Wars: Merthyr Tydfil, Oxfordshire and Tottenham', in D. Forster and P. Swann (eds), *Essays in Regional Local History* (Hull: 1992).

64. In the Northern town of Lancaster, for instance, which had a low rate of female employment, women's political action was very weak. Mark-Lawson, Savage & Warde, *op. cit.* (note 53).

65. W. Barefoot, *Twenty-Five Years' History of the Woolwich Labour Party 1903–1938* (Woolwich Labour Party: c.1928), 23–4. In 1910 the Women's Labour League supported Margaret Bondfield as a candidate for the LCC elections in Woolwich. (Hollis, *op. cit.* (note 46), 414).

66. *The Labour Woman,* May 1913, 10; Hollis, *op. cit.* (note 46), 412.

67. For more information on women's role in the Woolwich Labour Party and the support given by the Labour Party to the suffragette's cause see I. Dove, 'Women's Suffrage and the Woolwich Labour Party 1908', *South London Record: Southwark and Lambeth History Workshop,* 1 (1985), 24–32; *idem, Yours is the Cause: Suffragettes in Lewisham and Woolwich* (London: 1988). The extent of the support for the suffragette cause is revealed in the Woolwich Labour Party's Minutes, see particularly 30 January 1912.

68. Woolwich Labour Party, *A/Rs* (1919), and (1926); *The Labour Woman*, 1 February 1926, 29.

69. Eatwell, *op. cit.* (note 31), 20. 1933 was the first year the party gave a gender breakdown of the figures.

70. Poplar was particularly well-known for figures such as Susan Lawrence, originally a councillor in Poplar and later the first woman MP (in East Ham in 1922); Minnie Lansbury who was one of the Poplar Labour councillors imprisoned during the Poplar rates dispute in 1921; and for the political and social activities of Sylvia Pankhurst, Daisy and Jessie Lansbury and Doris Lester. Women's association with political affairs in East London had roots stretching back to 1888 when Annie Besant was elected to the London School Board in Tower Hamlets and can also be linked to the social reforming activities of figures such as Octavia Hill, Henrietta Barnett and Beatrice Webb. E. Vallance, 'Women in Politics', *East London Record*, 5 (1982), 2–12; and G. Rose, 'The Struggle for Political Democracy: Emancipation, Gender, and Geography', *Society and Space: Environment and Planning*, 8 (1990), 8, 395–408; Hollis, *op. cit.* (note 46), 343, 353.

71. Smith, *op. cit.* (note 36), 153.

72. Bentham left the National Union of Women's Suffrage Societies in 1911 when it insisted she put women before her Labour Party loyalties. (C. Collins, 'Women and Labour Politics in Britain, 1893–1932', unpub. Ph.D., LSE 1991, 153, 173.) None the less this did not dampen her calls for women's right to vote. In an address to a Women Workers Conference, Bentham made it clear she wanted a determined battle to win women's right to vote, but that this should be done by the peaceful means of the ballot box, and not by any 'injudicious or futile action'. (*Kensington News and West London Times*, 31 January 1913, 6.) Bentham was also active in the Fabian Women's Group, helping Maud Pember Reeves in her investigation of mothers and their family budgets in Lambeth to compile the book *Round About a Pound a Week* (London: 1913). See Alexander, *op. cit.* (note 49), 152.

73. Among those who gathered at the house were Mary Longman, Susan Lawrence and Aino Malmberg.

74. Collins, *op. cit.* (note 72), 161, 173; P. Thane, 'Women in the British Labour Party and the Construction of State Welfare, 1906–45', in Koven & Michel, *op. cit.* (note 48), Hollis, *op. cit.* (note 46), 9, 412; *The Labour Woman*, 1 November 1922, 171; 1 May 1927, 67; J. M. Bellamy & J. Saville (eds), *Dictionary of Labour Biography* (London: 1979) 173–9.

75. *The Labour Woman*, December 1913, 139; March 1915, 1; October 1915, 327–8; July 1920, 106.

76. Letter from Isabel Peterkin to Lucy, 15 October 1976, in papers relating to Mary Middleton and Margaret MacDonald Baby Clinic and

Hospital (National Museum of Labour History archives, Box BAB 429). The work of the clinic is explored in more detail in Chs 4 and 8.

77. *Kensington News and West London Times,* 21 February 1913, 5; 27 November 1914, 3; 4 June 1920, 5; Hollis, *op. cit.* (note 46), 413.

78. In 1865 Elizabeth Garrett Anderson had connections with Kensington, attending some of the first meetings of the Kensington Society, a group of about fifty women who met to discuss issues relating to women. J. Manton, *Elizabeth Garrett Anderson* (London: 1965, 1987), 160, 170.

79. M. Spring Rice, *Working-class Wives* (London: 1939, repr. 1981), x; 'Kensington Public Health Survey' (PRO file 52/177). The history of this clinic and its role within Kensington is explored in more detail in Chs 4, 7 and 8.

80. Charlotte Keeling, for instance, had served as manager of the Kensington and Chelsea District Schools, was a member of the Old Age Pensions Sub-committee, and had been a school manager for different schools in London since the early 1890s. She was also the district secretary of the Children's Care Committee, and worked for the Country Children's Fund. *Kensington News and West London Times,* 29 October 1909, 5. Mary Alexander was the daughter of a city merchant (Hollis, *op. cit.* (note 46), 210).

81. *Kensington News and West London Times,* 3 February 1911, 6.

82. *Ibid.,* 4 July 1902, 5; 5 November 1907; 29 October 1909, 5; 17 January 1913, 3.

83. Smith, *op. cit.* (note 36), 153.

84. L. Marks, '"Dear Old Mother Levys": The Jewish Maternity Home and Sick Room Helps Society, 1895–1939', *Soc. Hist. Med.,* 3/1 (1990), 61–88; *Caroline Franklin 1863–1935 – An Appreciation,* written by friends (printed for private circulation, 1936), (British Library: 1086 cc.15).

85. British Hospital for Mothers and Babies, *A/R* (1905), 6.

86. *Hampstead Advertiser,* 28 March 1907, 3; 18 April 1907, 3; 26 November 1907, 7; 23 July 1908, 3.

87. *London Hospital Illustrated* (1950), 4; E. H. Benjafield, 'Queen Mary's Maternity Home, Hampstead' (LH file: QM/A/7/15). Originally created from the funds raised by Queen Mary's Needlework Guild during the First World War, the Home was intended to serve the wives and children of servicemen and be a model for other maternity homes.

88. J. Eyler, 'The Sick Poor and the State: Arthur Newsholme on Poverty, Disease and Responsibility', in D. Porter and R. Porter (eds), *Doctors, Politics and Society: Historical Essays* (Amsterdam: 1993); F. Honigsbaum, *The Struggle for the Ministry of Health* (Social Administration Research Trust: 1970); J. Lewis, *What Price Community Medicine? the Philosophy, Practice and Politics of Public Health Since 1919* (Brighton: 1986), Ch. 1; D. Porter, '"Enemies of

the Race": Biologism, Environmentalism, and Public Health in
Edwardian England', *Vict. Stud.,* 34/2 (1991), 160–77.
89. *Br. Med. J.,* 17 March 1962, 804–5; *The Lancet,* 17 March 1962,
599.
90. *Br. Med. J.,* 14 February 1959, 443–4; 14 March 1959, 728; *The Lancet,* 7 February 1959, 319.
91. *Br. Med.* J., 14 February 1959, 443–4; 14 March 1959, 728; *The Lancet,* 7 February 1959, 319.
92. Letter from Dr Oxley to Secretary of the Interdepartmental
Committee on Abortion, 10 October 1937, 5 (PRO file: HO
326/29).

3

Infant and Maternal Health in Four London Boroughs

As highlighted in the introduction, much of the social and political discourse of the early twentieth century centred on the physical well-being of the nation. The health of the infant lay at the heart of this debate. Seen as the future generation, their health was seen to require special attention. In 1915 Ashby, a medical expert on infant mortality, emphasized the careful treatment that infants needed,

> Just as hot-house plants are exceedingly sensitive to their surroundings and only thrive when placed in the most favourable surroundings as regards light, warmth and soil, and quickly show by drooping the slightest departure from favourable conditions, so do infants respond favourably or unfavourably to feeding, housing, and general environment, according as these are good or bad.[1]

This obsession for the health of the infant was manifest not only in the writings of medical professionals but also in the legislation of these years. In 1902, for instance, a Midwives Act was passed which regulated midwives for the first time. Alongside this legislation various educational schemes were also developed, including the establishment of health visiting and schools for mothers, later known as infant welfare centres. For many medical practitioners and policy makers these measures accorded with their belief that the solution to infant mortality lay in the education of mothers. Various maternal and infant welfare schemes were also created by voluntary and municipal agencies.[2] The First World War, like the South African War, again prompted anxieties about the reproduction of the nation and led to the Maternity and Child Welfare Act of 1918, which enabled local authorities to establish grant-aided child welfare clinics.

The Maternal and Child Welfare Act also provided money for antenatal care, reflecting the increasing shift in emphasis towards the health of the mother.[3] While maternal mortality had been a source of concern in a number of reports from 1875, unlike infant mortality, it was not accorded the same national priority until the 1920s and 1930s when persistent and even rising rates of maternal mortality fuelled public outcry over the standards of midwifery care for mothers.[4] Throughout the early twentieth century, whether it be the health of the infant or that of the mother, the burning issue was whether an amelioration of social and economic deprivation was the answer to poor health, or whether the solution lay in more extensive medical and educational measures. These questions were closely tied to wider political and social considerations.

Here I focus on the determinants of infant and maternal mortality. In assessing these determinants, it is important that proper weight should be given to social and economic conditions as well as to medical and preventative schemes. This is difficult given that the determinants of maternal and infant health are multifarious and often overlap and cannot be isolated. In addition, each borough experienced very different social and economic conditions. The boroughs not only varied greatly from each other in their degree of poverty and wealth, but also in their housing density and demographic profiles. These differences, together with the diverse social relations, political complexion and maternal and infant welfare services are examined in other chapters, all had an important impact on the differing levels of infant and maternal mortality found in each borough. Here I provide a general account of the ways in which the social, economic and demographic conditions in each area affected their rates of infant and maternal mortality. In doing this, however, it is difficult to weight the importance of different risk factors because I do not intend to evaluate the risk of mortality on an individual level. Reflecting the distinct determinants of health for the two groups, the first section of this chapter considers the different factors affecting infant health and the last section considers those affecting maternal health.

Infant Health

An infant's chance of survival is dependent on a wide range of factors and on its age. Those deaths which occur within the first 28 days of life (the neonatal period) are most commonly associated with the conditions experienced during foetal development and birth. Some neonatal deaths are attributable to the quality of maternity care during delivery, although historically this is hard to prove. In recent years intensive neonatal care has been documented as having some impact on neonatal health. Clearer associations can be seen historically between prematurity and congenital defects and neonatal mortality. The earlier an infant death occurs in the neonatal period, the more likely it is associated with one of these factors which are often described as 'endogeneous' causes of infant mortality. By contrast those deaths which occur in the 11 months after birth (the post-neonatal period) are more closely linked to the quality of the environment in which they are cared for, and the access their families have to health services and effective treatment for life-threatening experiences. While the determinants of neonatal and post-neonatal mortality can overlap, the overall difference in the cause of death makes it important to distinguish between these two categories. Historically it is difficult to separate post-neonatal from neonatal mortality because the Registrar General only began to distinguish between these categories from 1906, and in the case of the four boroughs in this study only from 1911.[5] Accurate assessment of the causes of infant mortality are also hindered by the changes that occurred in medical diagnosis during these years. The relatively small number of deaths recorded for each borough also makes the accurate assessment for every year difficult, thus necessitating the need for taking an average over five rolling years. In addition to these problems, the boroughs experienced a shift in population which cannot be controlled for in undertaking an assessment of mortality patterns.[6]

From the evidence available, it would seem, however, that much of the decline in infant mortality in England and Wales and in London in the early twentieth century resulted from a reduction in post-neonatal mortality, primarily from diarrhoeal causes.[7] Neonatal deaths, which accounted for a much smaller proportion of the overall rates of infant mortality, declined more slowly. As post-neonatal mortality fell, however, neonatal mortality began to constitute a greater proportion of infant deaths, becoming the major component of infant death by the 1950s, with the majority of these deaths taking place close to the time of birth.[8]

Before examining how these trends in post- and neonatal mortality related to those found in the four boroughs in the years 1902–36, it is important to view the overall pattern of infant mortality in each borough. The rate of infant mortality was much higher in Stepney and Kensington than the two other boroughs and that for London as a whole (Figure 3.1). What is most striking is the overall decline in infant mortality from 1911 to the early 1920s in all of the boroughs, and the sharp divergence and increase in the rates shown for Kensington from the late 1920s. Woolwich, and to some extent Stepney, showed a slight incline in infant mortality in the late 1920s, but this was less striking than that for Kensington. Given the correlation between social and economic deprivation and infant mortality, it might be argued that the rise in infant mortality was due to some extent to the economic recession in the late 1920s and 1930s which caused grave unemployment particularly among unskilled labourers of whom there were many in Kensington and Stepney and to some extent in Woolwich.

Figure 3.1: Infant mortality rates in four London boroughs and the whole of London, and England and Wales, 1911–39

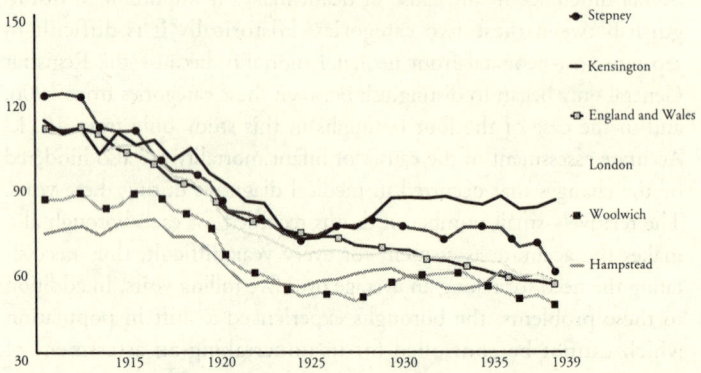

Infant deaths per 1,000 live births over an average of 5 rolling years.

Source: Registrar General, *Annual Returns of Births, Deaths and Marriages for England and Wales* (London: 1911–39).

None the less, while the economic recession might explain part of the upsurge in infant mortality in the late 1920s, it does little to clarify the overall differences in infant mortality between the boroughs for the whole period. Similarly some researchers would argue that unemployment is not a true indicator of deprivation and that levels of family income are a more accurate gauge for understanding the correlation between economic circumstances and rates of infant mortality.[9] Such debates over the importance of unemployment and family income are still a live issue today. Unfortunately there is not sufficient material to understand the degree to which the economic recession of the early twentieth century affected the family income in each of the boroughs and how they differed from each other. Llewellyn Smith's survey of London in 1929, however, indicated that the percentage of working-class families who were living either below, or within 10s. of his poverty line, was greatest in Stepney and Kensington where infant mortality was highest. Much of the deprivation in these areas was coupled with poorer housing and a higher degree of overcrowding which, when combined, as we shall see in greater detail below, were not favourable to good infant health. Yet which of these factors was more important than another is difficult to determine. As health experts continue to debate today it is hard to discern the precise components of poverty that cause ill health. Does damp housing play a greater or lesser role in causing sickness, for instance, than living in squalid and overcrowded conditions, or is it the demoralization caused by poverty that results in a greater susceptibility to poor health? Many medical experts at the turn of the century would have argued that poor infant health was most attributable to the immediate environment in which the infant lived.

While part of the differences in infant mortality rates can be explained by their varying levels of socio-economic conditions, what is less explicable is the fact that the rate of reduction, i.e. the extent to which infant mortality dropped over the years, was greater in Stepney and Woolwich than in Kensington and Hampstead. Infant mortality frequently falls most sharply in areas already experiencing very high numbers of infant deaths. Once it has reached a lower level the rate of reduction is usually more gradual. Nevertheless, this phenomenon cannot explain the greater reduction of infant mortality recorded in Stepney and Woolwich than in the two other boroughs. The underlying rate of infant mortality in Stepney almost matched that of Kensington, and yet Stepney experienced a greater decline (Table 3.1). Similarly, Woolwich which experienced a rate of reduction for infant mortality almost equal to that of Stepney, had a lower underlying mortality level. By contrast, Hampstead, which showed comparable underlying rates of infant mortality to those of Woolwich, did not witness as great a reduction.

It would therefore seem that Stepney and Woolwich, despite being among the poorer boroughs of London, experienced more improvement in their rates of infant mortality than did Hampstead and Kensington. This pattern of reduction is found in both neonatal and post-neonatal mortality (which together go to make up infant mortality). Tables 3.2 and 3.3 both indicate that in all the boroughs the reductions in infant mortality as outlined in table 3.1 was attributable to the fall in post-neonatal deaths. Both Stepney and Woolwich showed a greater reduction in post-neonatal mortality than the two other boroughs (Table 3.2). In the case of neonatal mortality the differences between the boroughs were less perceptible, both in the case of the underlying trend and in the rate of reduction (Table 3.3). Yet even here it would seem that Stepney and Woolwich showed slightly greater reductions than the other two boroughs. Why these two boroughs witnessed a greater reduction in both post-neonatal and neonatal mortality, despite starting at very different levels, raises important questions not only about the complex nature of infant health and its relationship to medical provision, but also to socio-economic conditions. These issues can only be explored by examining the different components to each category of mortality. As we shall see, the reasons behind the fall in infant mortality in Stepney and Woolwich differed in relation to post-neonatal and neonatal mortality.

Table 3.1: Underlying trends and rates of reduction in infant mortality in four London boroughs, London, England and Wales, 1911–39

Area	Underlying rate of IMR•	Rate of reduction
Hampstead	61.6	1.4%
Kensington	88.71	1.3%
Stepney	86.6	2.7%
Woolwich	63.7	2.3%
London	76.82	2.7%
England & Wales	73.7	1.8%

• All figures are calculated using standard linear regression, with 1925 as the midpoint for the underlying rate.

Source: Registrar General, *Statistics for England and Wales, A/Rs* (London: 1911–39).

Table 3.2: Underlying trends and rates of reduction in post-neonatal mortality in four London boroughs, London, England and Wales, 1911–39

Area	Underlying rate of PNNMR	Rate of reduction
Hampstead	33.48	1.28%
Kensington	60.48	1.36%
Stepney	61.03	3.03%
Woolwich	37.43	3.01%
London	50.22	3.36%
England & Wales	45.41	4.05%

All figures are calculated using standard linear regression, with 1925 as the midpoint for the underlying rate.

Source: Registrar General, *Statistics for England and Wales, A/Rs* (London: 1911–39).

Table 3.3: Underlying trends and rates of reduction in neonatal mortality in four London boroughs, London, England and Wales, 1911–39

Area	Underlying rate of NNMR	Rate of reduction
Hampstead	29.08	0.55%
Kensington	29.64	1.31%
Stepney	27.96	1.97%
Woolwich	27.40	1.53%
London	28.06	1.69%
England & Wales	33.80	1.15%

All figures are calculated using standard linear regression, with 1925 as the midpoint for the underlying rate.

Source: Registrar General, *Statistics for England and Wales, A/Rs* (London: 1911–39).

Post-neonatal Mortality Patterns

As stated above the health of an infant in the post-neonatal period is chiefly determined by the conditions under which it is reared. Recent studies of infants' health in the late nineteenth and early twentieth century have shown that while poverty greatly decreased an infant's chance of survival, this was outweighed by environmental conditions such as overcrowding and high population densities, poor water supplies, and inadequate sewerage and refuse disposal. From her research into infant mortality in 97 great towns between the years 1895 to 1910, Watterson has shown that 'raising private incomes without changing environmental conditions would do little to improve infant mortality levels. On the other hand, environmental improvement without change in incomes, would have some effect, especially in better-off communities.'[10] Watterson's conclusions are to some extent reflected in the patterns of mortality found in Hampstead, Kensington, Stepney and Woolwich. Figure 3.2 illustrates the different rates of post-neonatal mortality in each of the boroughs for the years 1911 to 1936. From this we can see that Hampstead had the lowest rate of post-neonatal mortality in these years, closely followed by those of Woolwich. Indeed, both these boroughs had much lower rates of mortality than those found for England and Wales and the whole of London. Table 3.4 indicates that the post-neonatal mortality rates registered in Hampstead and Woolwich for the years 1911–39, were some of the lowest recorded for the 29 boroughs in London. By comparison Kensington and Stepney ranked as having some of the highest rates of post-neonatal mortality in London.

93

Table 3.4: Post-neonatal mortality rates of four London boroughs compared with the highest and lowest rates in other boroughs in London, 1911–39

	1911–20			1921–30	
Borough	PNNMR	PNNMR	Borough	PNNMR	PNNMR
		rank within London			rank within London
Bermondsey	90.77	1	Shoreditch	61.32	1
Stepney	79.08	7	Kensington	54.04	2
Kensington	70.82	9	Stepney	52.85	4
Woolwich	51.26	25	Hampstead	30.21	26
Hampstead	41.42	29	Woolwich	29.42	28
			Lewisham	26.45	29

	1931–39	
Borough	PNNMR	PNNMR
		rank within London
Kensington	57.55	1
Stepney	47.21	4
Woolwich	30.65	25
Hampstead	27.49	27
Stoke Newington	25.92	29

Sources: Registrar General's, *Statistics for England and Wales* (1911–39); *Census for England and Wales* (London: 1911, 1921, 1931).

Figure 3.2: Post-neonatal mortality rates in four London boroughs, London as a whole, and England and Wales, 1911–39

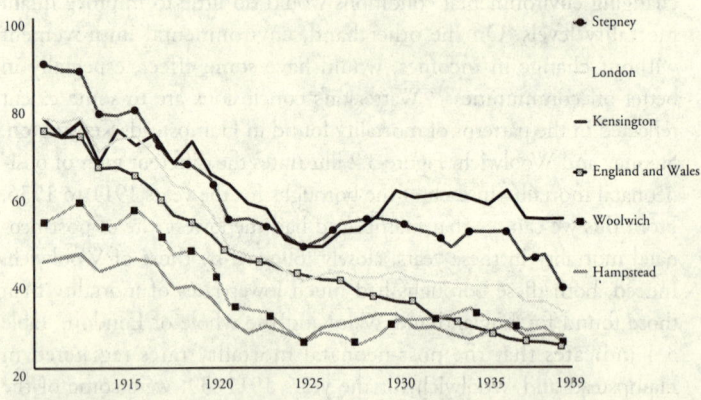

Post-neonatal deaths per 1,000 live births over an average of 5 years.
England and Wales figures do not include London.

Source: Registrar General, *Annual Returns of Births, Deaths, and Marriages for England and Wales* (London: 1911–39).

Social and Economic Conditions and Post-neonatal Mortality

One explanation for the low rate of post-neonatal mortality in Hampstead was the relative prosperity of the borough, but this was not the case for Woolwich. As we have seen in Chapter 1, while Hampstead had the lowest percentage of population living in poverty in London, Woolwich had a much greater number of poor residents. What these boroughs shared in common was a low density of population and relatively low rates of overcrowding. Thus, while infants in Woolwich were born to many families living in poverty, this disadvantage was countered by the relatively good environmental conditions in which they were reared. This, however, was not the case in Kensington and Stepney where many infants not only suffered the disadvantage of being born to parents experiencing great poverty, but of being raised in a very densely populated and overcrowded area. Table 3.5 shows that Kensington and Stepney suffered some of the highest rates of overcrowding and density of population of the 29 metropolitan boroughs in 1911 and some of the worst rates of post-neonatal mortality in London. In this respect they were not dissimilar from Bermondsey which had the highest rate of post-neonatal mortality in the capital. By contrast the table shows that the rate of post-neonatal mortality in Woolwich and Hampstead ranked much lower, reflecting their better housing conditions and sparser population. It would seem, therefore, that the rates of post-neonatal mortality found in each borough reflected the complex relationship between poverty, population density and overcrowding.

Table 3.5: Post-neonatal mortality rates of four London boroughs compared with other areas of London and with density and overcrowding, 1911

Borough	Overcrowding		Density of Population		PNNMR, 1911–20	
	% of population	as rank within London	Density	as rank within London	rate	as rank within London
Bermondsey	23.4	7	83.9	11	90.77	1
Stepney	35.0	2	159.0	4	79.08	7
Kensington	17.1	11	75.2	15	70.82	9
Woolwich	6.3	27	14.7	29	51.26	25
Hampstead	7.1	26	37.7	24	41.42	29

Sources: Registrar General, *Statistics for England and Wales, A/Rs* (London: 1911–20); LCC, *London Statistics*, 25 (London: 1914–15).

Table 3.6: Infant mortality by size of tenement in Finsbury, 1905–6

Size of tenement	Census population 1901	Infant mortality per 1,000 births			
		All causes		Diarrhoea and other zymotic diseases	
		1905	1906	1905	1906
1 room	14,516	219	211	53	67
2 rooms	31,482	157	178	42	56
3 rooms	21,280	141	188	34	43
4 rooms & upwards	33,185	99	121	19	26
Borough	101,463	148	157	37	45

Source: G. Newman, *The Health of the State* (London: 1907) 113.

The association between poverty, housing conditions, and population density is not only apparent in the overall trends of post-neonatal mortality for each borough but also when examined on a more localized level. Without a detailed and painstaking search through census material and death certificates it is difficult to explore this issue on a familial or street basis. In 1907, however, George Newman, medical officer of health for the London borough of Finsbury, showed that in his borough infant mortality was much greater for those living in one room tenements than for those able to rent four or more rooms. As Table 3.6 shows this was not only true for infant deaths from all causes, but also for those from diarrhoea and other zymotic (infectious) diseases. Even in Hampstead, where infant mortality was remarkably low, the number of infant deaths was substantially greater in the more overcrowded and densely populated areas of the borough. In 1906, for instance, the medical officer of health for Hampstead commented that while the overall rate of mortality for the borough was only 77 per 1,000 births, the rate for the ward of Kilburn was 113. Within particular sub-wards of the Kilburn ward, infant mortality climbed to an even higher rate of between 140 and 222. Similar differences were reported in later years. Much of this was attributed to the overcrowding and densely packed population in these areas. In 1921 the average number of persons per house in Hampstead was 3.8, whereas in Kilburn, where some of the highest rates of infant mortality were found, it was 8.4.[11]

The strongest links between poverty, housing conditions and infant mortality rates can be seen in evidence from Kensington. When broken down by sub-wards we can see that those areas in Kensington which experienced the highest percentage of overcrowding also had some of the worst records in infant mortality. As Table 3.7 shows, the likelihood of an infant dying before its first birthday in the 1930s was almost two times greater in the wards of Golborne and Norland than in Brompton or Holland where the percentage of overcrowding was less. The mortality differential was even more striking when considered in relation to the cause of death. In 1932 an enquiry was undertaken of each of the 232 infant deaths in the borough. This investigation revealed that while the overall rate of infant mortality in North Kensington was approximately double that of South Kensington (the richer part of the borough), the disparity was even greater for cause of death. It showed that 'the number of infant deaths from common infectious diseases in North Kensington was ten times as many as that in South Kensington. Infant deaths from pneumonia and bronchitis were five times, from enteritis (diarrhoea) thirteen times, and from wasting diseases nine times more frequent in North than in South Kensington.' Table 3.7 compares the rates of the total number of infectious deaths (without wasting diseases) for each of the sub-wards, showing the worst rates for these diseases were found in the wards of Golborne and Norland.

The investigation also revealed a close association between poverty and infant mortality, showing that in 52 per cent of the households where the infant died, the income was below the unemployment benefit level for the size of family involved, and in 21.5 per cent the family income was less than 50 per cent above the unemployment level. In 16 per cent of the households the family income was double the rate of unemployment benefit, but even here wages were below £3 a week.[12]

Family income was not the only element found to be an important cause of infant death. According to the investigation the most vulnerable infants were those who were born to those families who were the most mobile. North Kensington had a very large migrant population who had come to the area in search of the cheap accommodation Kensington offered in the way of tenement housing. Of the total deaths 45 per cent were found among such families, and of that 32 per cent were among those who left their address in the 'period varying from five to eighteen months after the death'. Many of these families were the poorest of the poor, and possessed no furniture. Out of their meagre resources they were expected to pay high rents for inadequate accommodation, leaving little money over to purchase other needs.[13]

When we break down the rates of post-neonatal mortality by cause of death we can begin to see why overcrowding and poverty were such important determinants of infant health. Changes in medical diagnosis and knowledge about disease prevents an accurate assessment of the causes of infant mortality in the four boroughs, but from the evidence available from the Registrar General from 1911 onwards it would seem that diarrhoea, bronchitis, pneumonia, whooping cough and measles took a heavy toll on infants' lives in these years. Of these diarrhoea was the most common cause of infant death, accounting for approximately a quarter of all deaths in England and Wales and London in the late nineteenth and early twentieth centuries (Figure 3.3).

Table 3.7: Percentage of families found to be living in overcrowded conditions and infant mortality rates in different parts of Kensington

Ward	% families overcrowded 1935	IMR 1931–5	No. births 1932	Deaths from infectious diseases• 1932	
				No.	IMR
North Kensington:					
Golborne	15	99	569	42	74
Norland	14	110	330	25	76
St Charles	10	88	576	39	68
Pembridge	8	80	158	10	63
South Kensington:					
Brompton	5	22	92	1	11
Holland	4	87	157	7	44
Earl's Court	4	35	179	1	6
Redcliffe	4	68	157	3	19
Queen's Gate	3	48	84	1	12

• infectious diseases includes measles, whooping cough, diphtheria, bronchitis, pneumonia and enteritis (diarrhoea).

Sources: Kensington MOH, *A/Rs* (1931–5); Meeting of Sub-Committee of Kensington Council, 17 October 1933, Minutes, 8.

Diarrhoea is a gastro-intestinal disease, the causes for which are complex. The determinants of diarrhoea are related not only to the general health of the infant, its resistance to disease, dental development and degree of breast-feeding, but also to the external factors such as climate, excrement removal and general sanitary conditions. The importance of climatic and environmental conditions is most clearly seen in the years after 1885, when, despite sanitary improvements and a general rise in living standards, diarrhoeal deaths rose dramatically. In the late 1890s the number of infants dying from this disease was twice as high as it had been in 1885. Much of this rise can be attributed to the very hot dry summers of the years which encouraged the breeding of flies and contamination of food.[14]

Figure 3.3: Infant deaths from all causes and diarrhoea in London and England and Wales, 1902–38

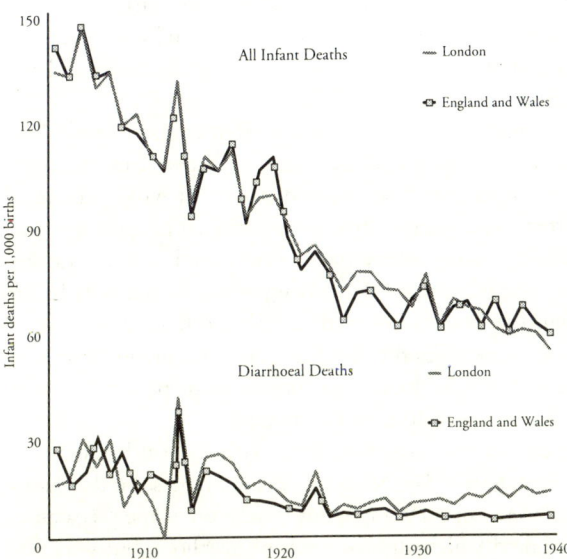

Source: Registrar General, *Annual Returns of Births, Deaths and Marriages for England and Wales* (London: 1911–39).

The spread of the disease under these climatic conditions was made worse in an insanitary environment and where food storage was limited.[15] The difficulties this caused were highlighted by the medical officer for Woolwich in 1906. He pointed out that cow's milk was frequently

> stored in unclean jugs, exposed to flies and dust, mixed in the wrong proportions and administered through a foul tube bottle. Apart from such an extreme instance of mismanagement of cow's milk, there is no doubt whatever that women of the poorer classes have great difficulty, not only of purchasing milk of sufficient purity for their infants, but also in storing it properly at home, although they may be exceedingly careful in mixing it in proper proportions and administering it through tubeless bottles.[16]

In these circumstances it is not surprising that much of the supplementary food given to infants was infected. Unlike adults and older children, infants have a digestive system which is too underdeveloped to cope with food infected by bacterial organisms (especially some strains of Escherichia coli) which can result in fatal diarrhoeal attacks.[17] Those infants living in an insanitary environment who are breast-fed

99

have an advantage because this provides them with their mother's antibodies for fighting infections[18] and they are less likely to consume milk infected by bacteria. Contemporaries in the early twentieth century constantly noted that infants who were hand and bottle-fed were more susceptible to epidemic diarrhoea, especially in dry and hot summer weather.[19]

Not all supplementary feeding was dangerous. Newsholme showed that such feeding could be safe if prepared in the right conditions. He highlighted the contradiction that while infants of wealthier parents were more liable to be given supplementary food than their working-class counterparts, they were less likely to die. From this he concluded that infants from richer homes were better protected from the hazards involved in artificial feeding because of their parents' income. Wealthy families were not only more able to afford a better quality of food, but could also prepare it in much safer conditions than in working-class homes.[20]

Housing conditions and their links with ill health remains a controversial issue to this day. None the less, it would seem that housing conditions were not only important in relation to the preparation and storage of food which affected levels of diarrhoea, but were also crucial determinants in the major causes of other infant deaths, particularly bronchitis and pneumonia, and to some extent also measles and whooping cough. Figure 3.4 shows that these diseases accounted for as large a proportion of infant deaths in England and Wales and London as did diarrhoea.

The causes of these diseases are multifarious, but cold, damp climatic conditions have a strong impact on promoting their incidence, particularly in the case of bronchitis. Atmospheric pollution, allergies to mould and a host of other factors also play an important role.[21] The strength of these elements can be seen in England and Wales and London today by the higher rates of infant mortality in winter months and the greater incidence of respiratory disease among working class infants. The difficulties poorer people have in covering heating costs, of the bad state of their housing, were no less real for the working-class in the early twentieth century than they are today. In addition many working parents had, and still have, considerable difficulty in affording adequately warm clothing.[22] Measles and whooping cough, although not directly linked to a cold environment, were often fatal among those infants already weakened by respiratory complaints such as bronchitis and pneumonia. Overcrowding and the fact that most working-class families were confined to one-roomed accommodation, also meant that such infectious diseases spread very easily for there was no way of isolating the victim.[23]

Figure 3.4: Infant deaths from bronchitis, pneumonia, whooping cough and measles per 1,000 births in London and England and Wales, 1912–38

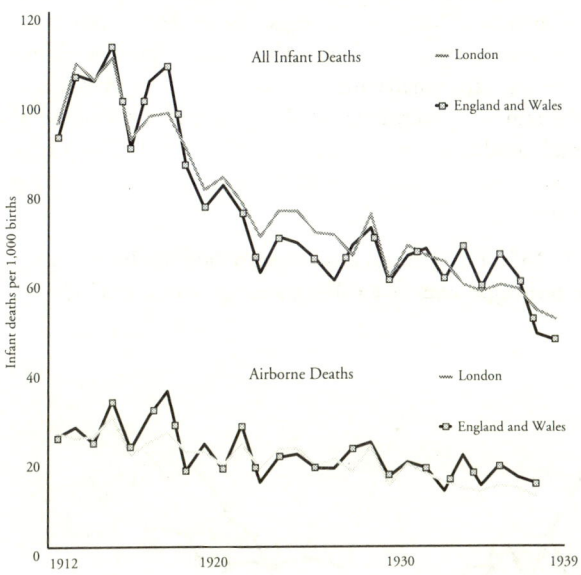

Source: Registrar General, *Annual Returns of Births, Deaths and Marriages for England and Wales* (London: 1911–39).

Hardy has also shown that the threat of measles and whooping cough was more severe where a child was suffering from rickets. At the turn of the century rickets was widely prevalent among working-class children all over the country, and was particularly common in the large towns, and industrial and mining areas, as well as in the southern rural areas. Chiefly afflicting the poor, rickets tended to be rare or non-existent among the middle classes. Of the four boroughs in the late nineteenth century, Hampstead and Woolwich had a much lower incidence of rickets than the other two boroughs, reflecting the fact that they were less urbanized and had greater amounts of open space.[24]

Rickets is a disease which is caused by a deficiency in vitamin D, which can be avoided by adequate exposure to sunlight. In the late nineteenth century air pollution from dense palls of smoke from industry and domestic heating reduced the amount of sunlight. In addition many of the dwellings people lived in were poorly designed to let sunlight in. Hardy claims that this, together with 'popular concepts of respectability; and the constraints which kept young children indoors – young mothers lacking in vitality, tenement accommodation, poverty and ignorance', all contributed to a very high incidence of the disease.[25] Part of the problem could have been rectified by the consumption of a diet rich in vitamin D, consisting of fish oils, fish extracts, animal fats, eggs, cheese, butter and milk. Such foods, however, were not in the staple diet of most working-class homes in the late nineteenth and early twentieth centuries.[26] Deprived of vitamin D, both because of a poor diet and because of environmental conditions, working-class children not surprisingly frequently had rickets, making them that much more susceptible to respiratory infections.

Figure 3.5: Infant diarrhoeal deaths per 1,000 births in four London boroughs over five rolling average years, 1913–36

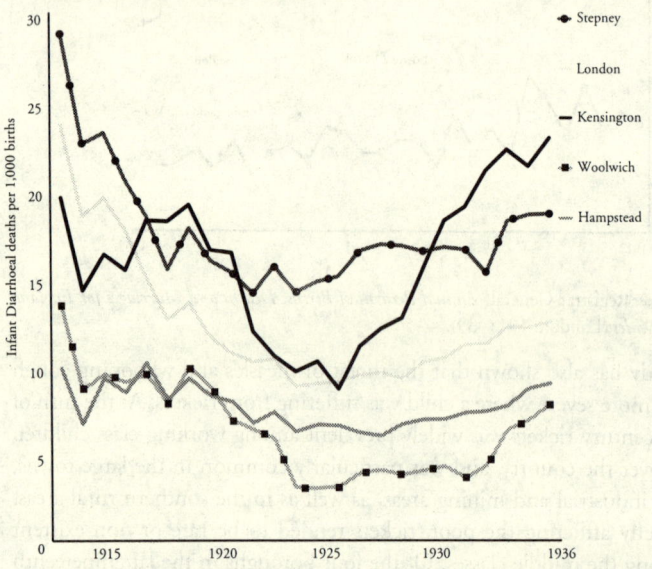

Source: Registrar General, *Annual Returns of Births, Deaths and Marriages for England and Wales* (London: 1911–39).

Poverty, bad sanitation, overcrowding and inadequate housing, and diet therefore all played a vital role in varying degrees in determining the major causes of post-neonatal infant mortality. How was this reflected in the four boroughs? If we examine the rates of diarrhoeal infant death and those of respiratory diseases for the four boroughs we can see that the higher rates of post-neonatal mortality found in

Kensington and Stepney were also reflected in the high number of infant deaths from these diseases. As Figure 3.5 shows the incidence of diarrhoea was much greater in these boroughs than in Hampstead or Woolwich and well above that of London as a whole. The rise in the post-neonatal mortality in Kensington in the late 1920s and the early 1930s illustrated in Figure 3.2, is also reflected in a higher incidence of diarrhoeal deaths for these years in Figure 3.5. Such a correlation is not so perceptible in the case of the respiratory diseases, but as Figure 3.6 indicates these diseases were still found to be much higher in Stepney and Kensington than the other two boroughs and for London as a whole. In the case of diarrhoea and the respiratory diseases it would seem, therefore, that the higher density of population, poorer sanitary and housing conditions as well as poverty in Stepney and Kensington was a crucial determinant in the health of their infants.

Figure 3.6: Infant deaths from bronchitis, pneumonia, whooping cough and measles per 1,000 births in four London boroughs over five rolling years, 1913–36

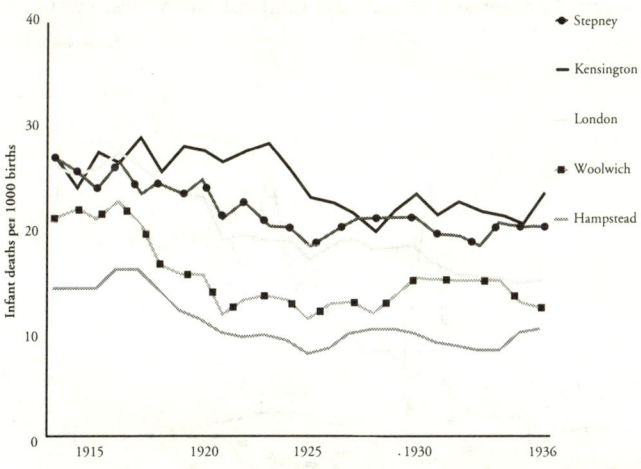

Source: Registrar General, *Annual Returns of Births, Deaths and Marriages for England and Wales* (London: 1911–39).

Illegitimacy and Post-neonatal Mortality

Social and economic conditions also seem to have outweighed other factors commonly associated with high infant mortality such as illegitimacy. Factors associated with illegitimacy had an influential impact on infant mortality. This included the shame attached to illegitimacy which forced many unwed mothers to hide their condition, which prevented them from getting medical and social assistance during and after the birth. Until the mid-1930s illegitimate infants faced a much greater risk of dying, particularly in the post-neonatal period.[27] Throughout the 1920s and 1930s the number of illegitimate infants dying in the four boroughs was much higher than that of legitimate infants. Even in an area like Woolwich, which had low rates of both infant mortality and illegitimacy, the number of illegitimate infants dying before their first birthday was triple that of legitimate infants in these years.[28] Only in the 1930s did the gap begin to narrow. The very small number of births and infant deaths among the illegitimate group might be exaggerating the rate of infant mortality among the illegitimate infants in the boroughs, but figures from England and Wales and London as a whole indicate that illegitimate infants had a much greater risk of dying than legitimate ones. Many of these deaths were caused by the scarcity of social and medical resources for unmarried mothers and their infants.

Figure 3.7: Percentage of illegitimate births in four London boroughs, London as a whole, and England and Wales, 1901–19

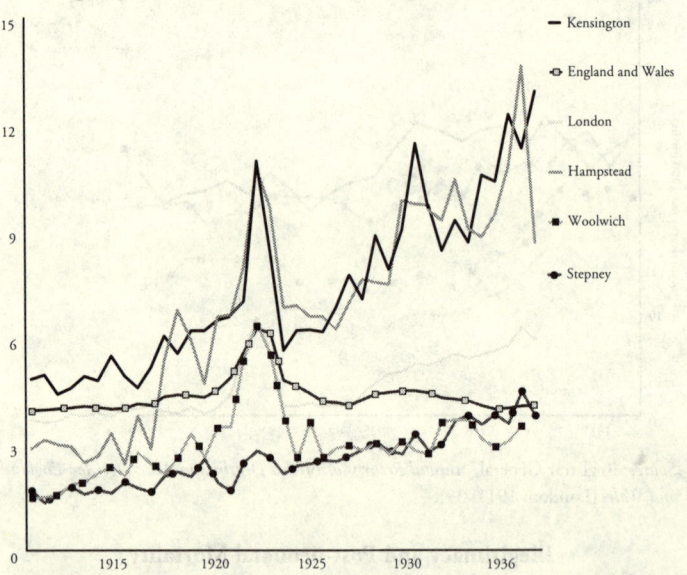

England and Wales figures do not include London.

Source: Registrar General, *Annual Returns of Births, Deaths and Marriages for England and Wales* (London: 1911–39).

Figure 3.8: Births per 1,000 females aged 15–44 in four London boroughs, 1901–39

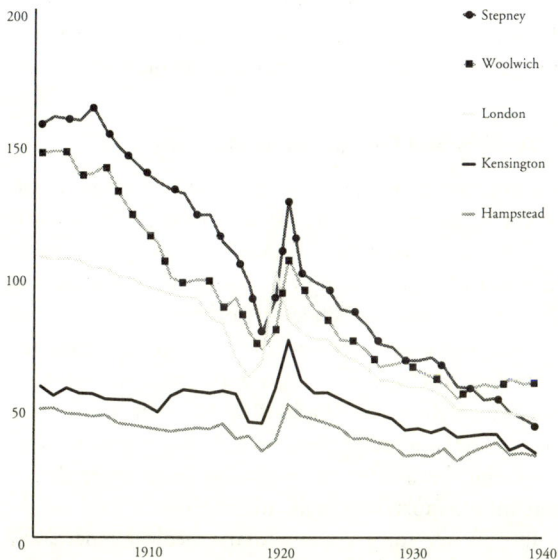

Source: Registrar General, *Annual Returns of Births, Deaths and Marriages for England and Wales* (London: 1911–39).

It might be expected, therefore, that areas which had a higher rate of illegitimacy faced higher rates of infant mortality. Evidence from the four boroughs, however, indicates that the overall rate of infant mortality was not greatly affected by the rate of illegitimacy. Figure 3.7 shows the different levels of illegitimacy as a percentage of total births for the four boroughs. Stepney, which had a high rate of infant mortality, had a very low rate of illegitimacy, never rising to more than 3 per cent of the total births. In Woolwich, illegitimacy was also rare, except in the war years, when it briefly rose to similar levels for London as a whole. The relative absence of illegitimacy in Stepney and Woolwich might be linked to the scarcity of domestic servants in these areas as highlighted in Chapter 2.[29] Hampstead and Kensington, which had a large proportion of female domestic servants in their populations, had much higher rates of illegitimacy. Other studies of illegitimacy in London have shown that the precarious position of female domestic servants gave them a greater propensity to falling pregnant outside marriage than other female workers. The difficulties of caring for a child and keeping employment as a domestic servant made the risk of infant death that much greater. Many of these unmarried mothers were forced to hand their infants over to foster-mothers who often bottle-fed and neglected the infants.[30] While for an individual infant illegitimacy could mean a greater risk of death, illegitimacy cannot be taken as a major contributor to the overall trends of post-neonatal mortality in the four boroughs.

Fertility and Post-neonatal Mortality

Sharply contrasting the trends in illegitimacy illustrated in Figure 3.7, is that of the birth rates for each of the boroughs depicted in Figure 3.8. Stepney and Woolwich, which had lower illegitimacy rates than Hampstead and Kensington, had greater numbers of births than these two boroughs. While no correlation can be made between the trends in illegitimacy and the number of births, fertility, like illegitimacy, also has to be taken into consideration when examining infant mortality. The relationship between fertility and infant mortality is the subject of great historical controversy. One difficulty in isolating the impact of fertility on infant mortality, is that the fall in infant mortality itself might have influenced the decline in fertility. While some contemporary medical experts and historians have argued that there was no real correlation between fertility and infant deaths,[31] more recent research has indicated a connection. Woods *et al.* have shown that while fertility declined greatly in the years 1876 to 1899 infant mortality did not fall over-all. None the less, they have shown that when 'the diarrhoeal component of infant mortality is ignored because it was critically influenced by short-run meteorological variations, then the under-lying long-run trend of infant mortality began to move downward from 1891, if not earlier'. They argue that this means that there could be a positive link between the decline in fertility and rates of infant mortality and suggest that

> the decline of fertility could have exerted a powerful influence on the subsequent decline of infant mortality not only by relieving the mother of caring for large numbers of offspring, but also because longer birth intervals would tend to improve the chances of an older child receiving adequate care while the mother was nursing a newly born baby (i.e. the high-parity and short birth-interval effects).[32]

In comparing Figure 3.2 with 3.8, however, it would seem that by the early twentieth century there was no clear association between the rates of post-neonatal mortality in each of the boroughs and their birth rates. Stepney which had a very high rate of fertility, experienced high post-neonatal mortality, and Hampstead which had a low birth rate and had a low rate of post-neonatal mortality both point to some connection. However, Woolwich had a high birth rate and yet a low rate of post-neonatal mortality and similarly Kensington which had very high numbers of post-neonatal deaths had low fertility. It would seem, therefore, that other factors were more important in determining the post-neonatal mortality patterns of each borough other than their levels of fertility.

Breast-feeding and Infant Mortality

One added complication in unravelling the connection between infant mortality and birth rates is their relationship to breast-feeding. High levels of breast-feeding are commonly associated with low rates of fertility. Fertility is thus difficult to separate from breastfeeding habits. The problems involved in distinguishing between fertility and breast-feeding therefore make it hard to isolate which of the two factors were more influential in determining levels of infant mortality. Yet it is clear that breast-feeding did have an impact on infant mortality. As we have seen, infants of poverty-stricken working-class families living in conditions of bad housing and poor sanitation stood a much fairer chance of survival if they were breast-fed.[33] This correlation, however, is not clear cut. Fildes has shown that infant mortality was particularly high in working-class areas of London where breast-feeding was widespread, contrasting the low rates of infant mortality in the wealthier districts where breast-feeding was slightly less common. Within the context of the four boroughs there does not seem to have been any great difference in the percentage of infants who were breast-fed. As Fildes' research reveals, the percentage of infants who were wholly or partially breast-fed in the first month of life in Stepney and Kensington, ranged between 91 and 97 per cent in the years 1905 to 1919, while in Hampstead and Woolwich the percentage ranged between 86 and 96 per cent. Trends in the percentage of infants who were breast-fed therefore do not explain the different rates of post-neonatal mortality recorded in each of these boroughs.[34]

Much depended on the length of time the infants were breast-fed. As Fildes has pointed out, those infants who are breast-fed for long spans of time are more able to withstand disease than those who are fed for only a short period, or those who receive no breast milk at all.[35] Unfortunately the duration of lactation was not routinely recorded for all the boroughs in Fildes' survey, which makes it difficult to measure the number of months the mothers nursed their infants. Evidence for eight of the boroughs examined by Fildes, however, displayed a relatively consistent pattern.

> By 3 months of age between 78% and 84% of children were still
> receiving some breast milk, with between 65% and 72% receiving
> no additional food. At 6 months over 70%, and at 9 months over
> 50%, were still wholly or partially breastfed. Early supplementation
> and premature weaning seems to have occurred most in the poor
> boroughs of Finsbury, Stepney and St Pancras.

In Stepney in 1911–12 the overall number of infants being wholly or
partially breast-fed tended to decline in the same way as the other
seven boroughs, but the number of infants who were exclusively
breast-fed dropped much more dramatically in Stepney than elsewhere among infants aged over three months, and fell to a very low
percentage in the ninth and tenth month of life. In the first month of
life 90 per cent of all infants in Stepney were exclusively breast-fed,
but this fell to 75, 44 and 4 per cent in the third, sixth and ninth
months respectively. By comparison, in Paddington in 1907–11, the
percentage of infants exclusively breast-fed, although initially smaller
among neonates, fell less dramatically from 88 in the first month to
60 per cent in the seventh month. A similar pattern was also shown in
Fulham in 1906 and 1925.[36] Sadly no evidence remains on the levels
of exclusive breast-feeding in Hampstead and Woolwich. Nor does
such material on exclusive breast-feeding exist for Kensington, but in
this borough the percentage of infants aged 1 and 3 months who were
wholly or partially breast-fed in the years 1909 and 1910 was slightly
smaller than in Stepney.[37]

Evidence suggests that while breast-feeding was widespread among
infants aged 1 month, premature weaning occurred from a young age in
many of the boroughs. Part of the reason for the widespread use of
premature supplementary feeding in Stepney and in Kensington was
the large numbers of women who were working in these areas which
limited the time that they had for breast-feeding. Indeed, women's work
was cited by many medical experts as one of the major causes of infant
mortality in these years.[38] Such assertions were subject to much debate,
and many other contemporaries pointed out that women's work,
because it raised the family income, rather than being detrimental to
infant health actually enhanced their chances of survival.[39]

Much depended on the type of work that women undertook. In
1911 and in 1917 Kensington showed a much higher number of its
married women working in occupations outside the home (such as
laundry work) than in the other boroughs. This abundance of
married women working was also reflected in its greater number of

voluntary day nurseries from early on. Such work was difficult to combine with intensive breast-feeding. Stepney also had a number of women who worked in factories in Limehouse who would have experienced difficulties in breast-feeding. None the less, a large proportion of the women who worked in Stepney undertook home piece-work or, as in the case of those in Hampstead, some form of domestic labour, which was easier to combine with childcare. By contrast the number of mothers working outside the home in Woolwich was very small. Here mothers' work accounted for only 5.5 per cent of the factors contributing to premature weaning in the years 1905 to 1909.[40] In Kensington, and to some extent in Stepney, the higher proportion of women working outside the home, probably accounted for a greater degree of premature weaning of infants and could be one explanation for their higher rates of post-neonatal mortality than in Woolwich and Hampstead.

Nevertheless, it would be wrong to link the high rates of post-neonatal deaths in Kensington and Stepney solely to premature weaning as a result of women's work. Evidence from Woolwich for instance showed that the lack or insufficiency of breast milk accounted for 74 per cent of the reasons given for premature weaning and the illness or debilitation of the mother accounted for over 20 per cent.[41] Such difficulties in breast-feeding raise questions which go beyond the time and extent women devoted to breast-feeding, and relate more generally to the mother's health as a whole which can affect not only the health of the foetus, but also the quantity and composition of breast-milk. Although still unproven, some research has suggested that while undernourished women can continue to breast-feed, their milk has 'a lower calorific value containing smaller quantities of protein and particularly fat'.[42] Similarly such women also tend to produce less quantity of milk.

Infants of undernourished women who are fed solely on their mother's milk are, therefore, more likely to be underfed. Fildes claims that many of the infants in early twentieth century London were disadvantaged in this way, showing that while breast-feeding was undertaken on a wide scale, the benefits of such a practice were weakened by the mother's inability to continue the feeding for a long period of time. In most families mothers tended to go without food in favour of their husbands or their children, and the poorer the family the worse the diet for the mother. No extra provision was made for lactating mothers. Thus most of these women survived on a staple diet of 'white bread and a scrape of margarine, butter or jam, and weak tea with a dash of milk' with very little fresh milk, vegetables or meat.[43] In

1905 a health visitor in Kensington commented that much of the malnutrition of infants in her area was related to the inadequate nutrition of nursing mothers.

> Thus it happens that when the mothers get up and about, the little milk they had disappears, or becomes almost valueless as food for their offspring. Unable to provide cow's milk, or another good substitute, the infant is fed with bread as a supplementary article of diet, and sometimes as the sole article, malnutrition, disease often, and sometimes death, being the result.

She reported seeing at least 50 mothers in this state.[44]

Breathlessness and exhaustion were common complaints among mothers. Similarly anaemia, pulmonary tuberculosis and breast disease frequently prompted doctors to advise against breast-feeding. Many mothers also suffered breast abscesses for which, in the absence of antibiotics, there was no effective treatment; and these could cause long-term debilitation or in some cases cause scarring which could impair a mother's ability to nurse subsequent children.[45] In such circumstances supplementary feeding could help those infants not receiving adequate nourishment from their mothers. Even so, as already highlighted, conditions under which such food would have been prepared, and the inferior nutritional quality of foods used to supplement or replace breast-milk in the early twentieth century probably countered the benefits of such feeding, resulting in higher rates of infant mortality from diarrhoea.[46]

Although many poor women in London in the early twentieth century suffered poor health which could have undermined the quality and quantity of milk they produced, it is unclear what impact this had on the overall trends in post-neonatal mortality in the four boroughs. A number of health visitors in London noted that many of the poor infants failed to double their weight within a year of being born, which they expected for most infants in such a period from birth.[47] These observations, however, do not reveal whether there was any link between women's health and the quality and quantity of breast-feeding and what impact this had on the survival of the infant. Some research suggests the greatest advantage of breast-feeding as opposed to artificial feeding is seen when the infant is 3–6 months old.[48] No evidence remains for the degree to which this was practised in Hampstead and Woolwich, but between 88 and 76 per cent of infants in this age group in Kensington, and between 72 and 68 per cent of those in Stepney, were wholly or partially breast-fed in the years 1909 and 1913. None the less, it is hard to link these feeding

practises to the overall health of the infants in this age category in the
boroughs. Recent research has also shown that only in conditions of
acute starvation, such as in Holland during the hunger-winter of
1944–5, would the health and breast-feeding capacities of the
mother have affected the life of the infant, but even here the
connections are complex and were usually more apparent in the
health of the next generation.[49]

Neonatal Mortality Patterns

From Fildes' work it would seem that breast-feeding was most
intensively carried out within the first month of an infant's life.
While breast-feeding might have been useful in protecting neonates
from gastro-intestinal or respiratory infections, these diseases were
not the major causes of death for infants in this age group. Most
neonatal deaths are attributable to prematurity, congenital defects,
or birth injuries. Given the very different causes of death for these
infants than those who were older we would therefore not expect the
patterns of neonatal mortality in each of the boroughs to reflect the
rates of post-neonatal mortality.

**Figure 3.9: Neonatal mortality rates in four London boroughs,
London, and England and Wales, 1911–39**

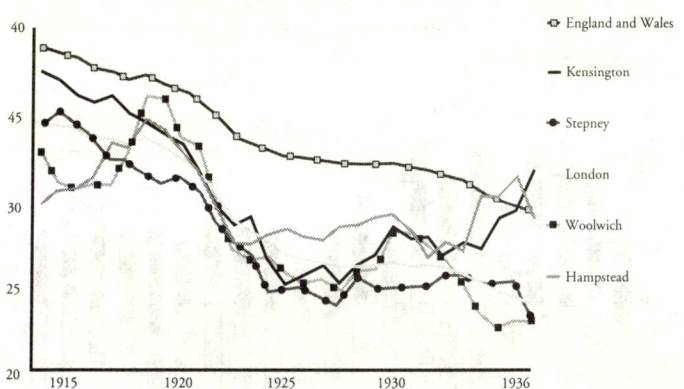

Neonatal deaths per 1,000 live births over an average of five years.
England and Wales figures do not include London.

Source: Registrar General, *Annual Returns of Births, Deaths and Marriages for England
and Wales* (London: 1911–39).

Figure 3.9 and Table 3.3 show that the trends in neonatal mortality in
the four boroughs diverged considerably from those of post-neonatal
deaths. Firstly, rates of neonatal mortality recorded for England and
Wales were greater than for London. This rate contrasted with

post-neonatal mortality where the rates were higher for London. Secondly, in the case of the four boroughs the gap in the underlying trends of neonatal mortality shown in Table 3.3 was much less marked than that of post-neonatal mortality.

What is most striking in Figure 3.9 is the higher levels of neonatal mortality in Hampstead than in Stepney, especially when we remember that in the case of post-neonatal mortality there was the reverse pattern. Stepney also showed a greater overall reduction than Hampstead in its neonatal rate. Indeed, Table 3.8 indicates that the neonatal mortality rate in Stepney not only compared favourably with Hampstead, but that it ranked among some of the lowest in the 29 boroughs of London. While neonatal mortality was also initially relatively low in Hampstead, by 1931–9 it was ranked as among some of the highest rates in London. Part of this might be offset by the great disparity in the confidence levels of neonatal mortality found in Hampstead.

Figure 3.10 Neonatal and post-neonatal infant mortality per 1,000 births in Hampstead, 1912–32

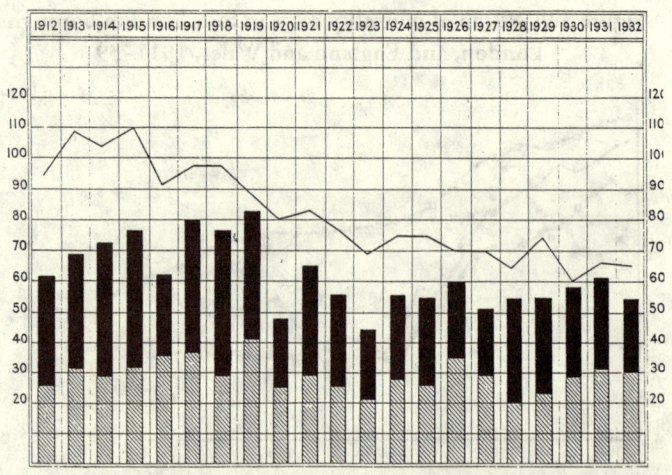

The Infant Death Rate per 1000 births for the Borough is represented by the chimneys, the lined portion of which shews the death rate amongst newly-born babies (*i.e.* under 1 month old).
The Infant Death Rate for England and Wales is represented by the line.

Source: Hampstead MOH, *A/R* (1932).

Whatever the reason, the high rate of neonatal mortality in Hampstead caused much concern for medical professionals in the area. In 1919 the medical officer of health for Hampstead calculated that 43 per cent of the infants in his borough died in the first month of their lives, and 27 per cent of them within seven days of being born.[50] This percentage was similar to those recorded in Woolwich between 1912–19, where the percentages were respectively 42 per cent and 28 per cent.[51] In Kensington in 1932 the percentage of infants dying within the first month of life was lower than in Hampstead at 30 per cent, but the percentage of infants dying within the first seven days was almost the same at 22.[52] No equivalent evidence exists for Stepney.

Table 3.8: Neonatal mortality rates of four boroughs compared with the highest and lowest rates in other boroughs in London, 1911–39

	1921–20			1921–30	
Borough	NNMR	NNMR rank within London	Borough	NNMR	NNMR rank within London
Shoreditch	54.90	1	City	42.39	1
Kensington	34.87	7	Hampstead	26.95	12
Woolwich	32.82	21	Kensington	26.05	19
Stepney	32.38	22	Woolwich	24.49	26
Hampstead	31.95	23	Stepney	24.35	27
Chelsea	29.23	29	Chelsea	22.88	29

	1931–39	
Borough	NNMR	NNMR rank within London
City	47.19	1
Hampstead	28.25	4
Kensington	27.49	6
Woolwich	24.30	15
Stepney	23.96	17
Camberwell	20.20	29

Sources: Registrar General, *Statistics for England and Wales, A/Rs* (London: 1911–39); *Census for England and Wales* (London: 1911, 1921, 1931).

Figure 3.10 shows how even though infant mortality dropped in Hampstead over the years 1912 to 1932, there was no significant drop in the proportion of deaths taking place in the neonatal period. By contrast, post-neonatal mortality, which constituted a larger proportion of the deaths in the earlier years, increasingly began to decline from 1923. Such a pattern is not only true for Hampstead but can also be found elsewhere.[53]

Determinants of Neonatal Mortality

Why neonatal mortality did not fall as rapidly as post-neonatal mortality has been the subject of much historical discussion. One difficulty in understanding this phenomenon is lack of historical evidence we have on the major causes of neonatal mortality particularly in relation to congenital malformations and prematurity. Some experts have linked the occurrence of prematurity to socio-economic deprivation, but this is by no means conclusive.[54] A closer link exists between socio-economic status and stillbirths, but these are unrelated to the incidence of prematurity.[55]

While it is difficult to find a historical cause for the incidence of prematurity and congenital defects, it is easier to find an explanation for birth injuries, the third most common cause of neonatal death. Loudon has shown that where there were numerous doctor deliveries and a tendency by doctors towards a high rate of interference, the result could be high rates of neonatal mortality due to birth injury. Evidence from the US supports this theory.[56] From this you might expect London to have had a higher rate of neonatal mortality than England and Wales, because it had a much higher proportion of births delivered by doctors compared to the rest of the country.[57] Yet Figure 3.9 and Table 3.3 show that this was clearly not the case.

One explanation is that many of the deliveries in London were undertaken by medical students working under the supervision of voluntary teaching hospitals. As we shall see in Chapter 6 many of these hospitals provided a very high quality of maternity care with minimal interference and a good standard of antenatal provision. However, as Chapter 6 will highlight, the standard and quality of maternity care was highly variable within London, which could partially explain the differences in the neonatal mortality found for the four boroughs. Hampstead, which had a higher rate of neonatal mortality had a greater number of births delivered by general practitioners who were under less supervision and therefore had more potential for increased interference and birth injury. Stepney, by contrast, which had a remarkably high number of voluntary teaching hospitals which offered stricter supervision of deliveries, had a lower rate of neonatal mortality indicating a slightly better standard of care than that found in Hampstead.

Maternal Health

Good quality care during childbirth was not only an important determinant of neonatal health, but was also vital to the survival of the mother herself and was a crucial factor determining maternal mortality. Maternal deaths differ from many other kinds of mortality, because they are not necessarily the result of a pathological process, but more usually the result of a normal physiological process going wrong, the occurrence of which should be more readily prevented than disease. It was this viewpoint which formed much of the discussion during the inter-war period concerning the persistence of high maternal mortality.[58] Many specialists in the 1930s believed that at least 40 per cent of maternal deaths were preventable through good obstetric care.[59] Yet by the 1930s, when the training and licensing of doctors and midwives had improved, and antiseptic practice had been adopted in most deliveries, the maternal mortality rate remained as high as it had been in the mid-nineteenth century. Deaths in childbed were the second most common cause of death among women of childbearing age after tuberculosis.[60] Although there were variations over the years, between 1855–1934 the maternal death rate in England and Wales averaged around 4.6 per 1,000 live births, totalling some 3,000 to 4,000 maternal deaths a year.[61] By the early 1920s the obstinacy of maternal mortality caused much concern not only among the medical professionals but also among politicians, the general public, and the daily press.

Regional studies carried out by medical practitioners and health officials at the time investigated the impact poverty and social deprivation had on maternal mortality rates, but the importance of these factors was sometimes denied for political reasons.[62] Malnutrition and anaemia certainly weakened many women and made them unable to sustain haemorrhaging they might otherwise have coped with.[63] Some contemporaries also believed that obstructed labours were caused by deformed pelvises resulting from rickets, which as we have seen above was widespread in the population in these years. In general, however, pelvic malformation and poor health accounted very little for the maternal mortality figures during this period.

Determinants of Maternal Mortality

If we consider what the major causes of maternal mortality were in these years, it will become clear that clinical factors probably had a greater impact on the statistics than social and economic ones. Once abortion is excluded, which, although a major cause of maternal mortality, was highly variable in the years 1902 to 1936, most maternal deaths in this period were caused by puerperal fever, toxaemia and haemorrhages.[64] While rates of maternal mortality varied over the years, the proportion of deaths by cause remained the same, with puerperal fever accounting for between 33 and 50 per cent of all maternal deaths, toxaemia 20 per cent, and haemorrhages, between 15 and 20 per cent.[65]

Puerperal Fever

Of the three major causes of death, puerperal fever (also known as puerperal sepsis) was the greatest killer, causing the death of approximately 12,500 women in England and Wales in the years 1920 to 1929.[66] Medical classification of the disease changed over the years, but puerperal fever was defined as an infection of the uterus during or after delivery, usually caused by streptococcus pyrogenes. Once the uterine cavity was infected the infection could spread to other areas of the body, such as the pelvis causing pelvic cellulitis, pelvic thrombophlebitis, or sometimes a pelvic abscess, or could enter the peritoneal cavity leading to peritonitis. The infection could also enter into the bloodstream resulting in puerperal septicaemia. Fatal cases of puerperal fever were usually due to septicaemia or peritonitis or both together.

One of the major problems in curbing such infections was the difficulty of preventing the spread of streptococcal bacteria (the main cause of puerperal fever) as many birth attendants could be asymptomatic carriers of streptococcus in their noses and throats. Middle-class mothers had no more protection against septic infection from doctors who attended them than working-class mothers had from midwives. While the aetiology of puerperal sepsis was little understood until the 1920s, certain precautions could be taken to curb the spread of the disease. Antisepsis, first introduced in the 1880s, and minimal medical interference during delivery were the best measures that birth attendants could take to guard against puerperal fever before the introduction of sulphonamides in the late 1930s.[67] Failure to adhere to such precautionary procedures could have fatal consequences.

Obstetric Haemorrhages

Like puerperal fever, the incidence of obstetric haemorrhages was largely linked to the standard of attention provided by the birth attendant. The cause of obstetric haemorrhages can be divided into the two main categories of ante-partum haemorrhage and post-partum haemorrhages. Of these post-partum haemorrhages was the one most affected by the quality of maternity care. In most deliveries haemorrhages are prevented by the firm contraction of the uterus once the baby is born. This contraction not only causes the separation of the placenta from the wall of the uterus and its expulsion, but also brings the walls of the uterus into apposition, which is vital in preventing haemorrhage from the massive blood-vessels which supply blood to the placenta. Most cases of post-partum haemorrhage occur where the

116

uterus is unable to contract fully and strongly 'either because the placenta has separated from the uterine wall but has not been expelled from the uterus; or because the uterine contraction is feeble' as in the case of women whose muscles have been weakened from frequent childbearing.[68]

While some cases of haemorrhage are caused by a torn cervix, over 90 per cent are caused by bleeding from the placental site. Where post-partum haemorrhage is caused by a retained placenta, the placenta should be removed as soon as possible, When this should occur, however, is difficult to judge because the expulsion of the placenta is tied up with the physiological process of the third stage of labour which can be slow. Thus it is important to wait. Similarly the manual removal of the placenta is not an easy procedure to perform and was particularly dangerous before the introduction of blood transfusion and antibiotics in the 1940s and 1950s.[69]

The cause of ante-partum haemorrhage was less preventable than post-partum haemorrhage, but its treatment was just as dependent on the dexterity and skill of the birth attendant. Ante-partum haemorrhage can be divided into those classified as 'accidental haemorrhage' (or placental abruption) and those called placenta praevia. The cause of accidental haemorrhage, which is a condition in which part of the placenta becomes detached during pregnancy, is unknown. In such circumstances the best treatment is a simple rupture of the membranes and sedation. Placenta praevia is when the placenta lies so low in the uterus that its lower edge either lies adjacent to the internal os or lies across and covers the os. This condition is easily missed in pregnancy and was only recognized in the past once labour had commenced and haemorrhaging had begun. It is particularly difficult to treat because it can only be stopped once the baby and placenta has been delivered, and often the placenta is blocking such a delivery. One solution was to perform a caesarean section, but this was largely unsafe until the 1930s.[70]

Taken together it would seem that the incidence and outcome of ante- and post-partum haemorrhage was to some extent dependent on the quality of care a mother received during pregnancy and her delivery. The degree to which this had an impact varied. As Loudon has argued,

> Ante-partum haemorrhage could not be prevented and its treatment required a high degree of skill which, before the Second World War, was usually available only in a few hospitals staffed by specialist obstetricians. Post-partum haemorrhage, however, could usually be prevented by ordinary skill and judgement (which often consisted of

waiting patiently) which should have been attainable in home deliveries by midwives and general practitioners.[71]

Toxaemia and Eclampsia

Of the three main causes of maternal mortality, toxaemia was the least susceptible to the standard of maternity care. This disease occurs in the last three months of pregnancy. The first symptoms of the disease are usually high blood pressure, followed by albuminuria and oedema. At a more dangerous stage the symptoms can be malaise, blurred vision, severe headache and convulsions which are known as eclamptic fits or eclampsia. In the past toxaemia and eclampsia were put in the same category, but each are separate from each other. Deaths resulting from toxaemia are caused by damage to the kidneys or to cerebral haemorrhages, while those from eclampsia are the result of eclamptic fits. Those most at risk from toxaemia are first-time mothers, those with multiple pregnancies, and those who are older. Eclampsia is more evenly spread throughout the population of childbearing age. In both cases treatment is largely ineffective once a woman is in labour. The best precautions for toxaemia and eclampsia is the termination of pregnancy, but this was often dangerous and required a well coordinated and high quality of antenatal supervision, which as we shall see in Chapter 6 was not necessarily provided in the early twentieth century.[72]

Maternal Mortality Patterns in the Four Boroughs

When considered as a whole, it would therefore seem that clinical factors were the primary cause of maternal mortality in the years 1902–36. The remaining part of this section considers to what extent such clinical causes affected the rates of maternal mortality in the four boroughs. A word of caution is needed before examining the trends in each borough. Maternal deaths are uncommon in the context of total births, which necessitates a large number of births before any accurate estimate can be made for maternal mortality.[73] In the context of the four boroughs, this is difficult to obtain because the total number of births in each area, particularly in Hampstead, was very small, which could distort the figures for rates of maternal mortality. The small numbers involved also hinder any accurate assessment of the exact causes of maternal mortality in each borough. For this reason I have focused on the overall patterns of maternal mortality rather than particular causes. An additional problem in reading the differences between the boroughs was the wide annual fluctuations in their rates of maternal mortality. For greater clarity in comparing the patterns of maternal mortality in each borough I have measured, therefore, all maternal deaths over an average of nine rolling years.

Figure 3.11: Maternal deaths per 1,000 births over nine folling average years in four London boroughs, London, England and Wales, 1905–36

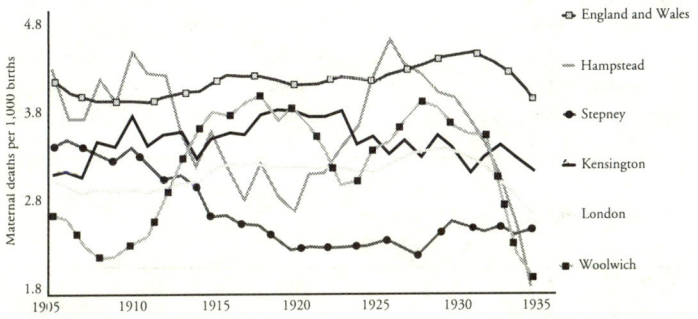

Source: Registrar General, *Annual Returns of Births, Deaths and Marriages for England and Wales* (London: 1911–39).

From Figure 3.11 we can see that there were very wide differences in the rates recorded in each of the boroughs. In some respects the differing rates of maternal mortality registered for the four boroughs reflected the rates of neonatal mortality. While the causes of neonatal mortality differ widely from those of maternal mortality,[74] the echo of the trends in Figure 3.9 with Figure 3.11 suggest a tentative link. Although probably stronger in the case of maternal mortality, the quality of maternity care was one factor which influenced the outcome of both neonatal and maternal health. It is this factor which could explain the similarities found in Figures 3.9 and 3.11. The comparative trends of neonatal and maternal mortality can be most clearly seen in the case of England and Wales and in London. Just as the neonatal mortality rate was lower in London than in England and Wales so was the rate of maternal mortality. Parallels can also be seen in the rates of neonatal and maternal mortality in Stepney. The high fluctuation in maternal and neonatal mortality for the other boroughs makes this comparison difficult to determine.

Table 3.9: Maternal mortality rates of four boroughs in relation to the highest and lowest rates in London as a whole, 1911–39

| | 1911–20 | | | 1921–30 | |
Borough	MMR	MMR rank within London	Borough	MMR	MMR rank within London
City	4.44	1	Westminster	5.13	1
Woolwich	3.64	5	Hampstead	4.26	5
Kensington	3.47	9	Kensington	3.40	11
Hampstead	3.31	13	Woolwich	3.39	12
Stepney	2.60	26	Stepney	2.41	29
Holborn	2.37	27•			

| | 1931–9 | |
Borough	MMR	MMR rank within London
City	5.44	1
Kensington	3.13	8
Stepney	2.58	19
Woolwich	2.07	26
Hampstead	2.01	28
Finsbury	1.32	29

• 29 is the lowest rank for all years except for 1911–20 when missing figures for Stoke Newington make 27 the lowest rank.

Sources: Registrar General, *Statistics for England and Wales, A/Rs* (1911–39); *Census for England and Wales* (London: 1911; 1921; 1931).

Table 3.10: Underlying trends and rates of reduction in rates of maternal mortality in four London boroughs, London, England and Wales, 1901–39

Area	Underlying rate of MMR•	Rate of reduction
Hampstead	3.4	0%
Kensington	3.2	0%
Stepney	2.8	1.16%
Woolwich	2.99	0%
London	2.95	0%
England & Wales	4.0	0%

• All figures are calculated using the standard linear regression, with 1920 as the midpoint for the underlying rate.

Source: Registrar General, *Statistics for England and Wales, A/Rs,* (London: 1901–39).

More important than the association between neonatal and maternal mortality is what was happening to maternal mortality itself. As we can see in Figure 3.11 Stepney had a lower rate of maternal mortality than any of the other boroughs and than London as a whole (see also Table 3.9). Not only was maternal mortality lower in this borough, but it was also dropping more consistently and substantially than in the other boroughs. This is more clearly seen from Table 3.10 than in Figure 3.11 which is difficult to read because of the wide variations caused by the annual fluctuations. Using standard linear regression to estimate the underlying rate of maternal mortality in any year assuming a linear decline in maternal mortality per year, it would seem that of the four boroughs the underlying rates in 1920 (the mid year) are lowest in Stepney and highest in Hampstead. In addition the underlying annual reduction was significant for Stepney (and could not be explained by chance variation), but not for any other borough or for the rest of the country or London as a whole. The maternal mortality rates for all four boroughs and London as a whole are significantly lower than the rates for England and Wales.

The low rate and consistent reduction of maternal mortality in Stepney is striking given the socio-economic deprivation of the area, and when contrasted with the higher underlying rates of maternal mortality found in the more prosperous boroughs of Hampstead and Kensington. Given the overwhelming importance of clinical factors in determining the high level of maternal mortality it could be argued that the lower rate of maternal mortality in Stepney stemmed from the fact that the borough hosted a better quality of maternity services than elsewhere. What this consisted of and what impact this had on maternal health is the subject of Chapter 6.

Parity and Age in Determining Maternal Mortality

The difference in the rates of maternal mortality recorded in Stepney from elsewhere might not only be a reflection of its good standard of maternity care, but could also be linked to the demographic profile of the childbearing population in the area. Those women who are at greatest risk of dying at childbirth tend to be those who are giving birth for the first time (primipara) or have had more than three previous pregnancies (multipara), or who are older than average.[75] An absence of suitable statistical material makes it difficult to know the extent to which this affected the trends of maternal mortality in the four boroughs.

One way of tackling this problem is to correlate the fertility patterns of each borough with the maternal mortality rates. Overall in these years working-class neighbourhoods were known to have a much higher birth rate than those which were more middle class.[76] In Chapter 2 we saw that Stepney and Woolwich had a much larger proportion of working-class residents than the two other boroughs, which seems also to have been reflected in their higher fertility rates (Figure 3.8). Women in Stepney and Woolwich were, therefore, more likely to be producing more children than in the two other boroughs, making the number of first-time (primiparae) mothers small. By contrast Hampstead and Kensington probably had a very large number of primiparous women. Within the category of first-time mothers, Hampstead and Kensington, therefore, seem to have had a larger group who were at risk than Stepney or Woolwich. The London County medical officer of health pointed to this fact when considering why maternal mortality was much higher in the West End boroughs than those in the East End. The difference he argued lay in the fact that the districts in the West End had a higher proportion of primiparae than those in the East End.[77]

Nevertheless, while the risk of maternal mortality diminishes with the second and third birth, it then rises steadily for each subsequent delivery. This risk is particularly important in Stepney and Woolwich where the high fertility rates suggests a large proportion of women had more than three previous pregnancies. In addition to this a large number of women would have had large families, making the possibility of spacing their children difficult, and often undermined their recovery and general health when faced with another birth. Thus the advantage Stepney and Woolwich had of not having many primiparae women would have been countered by their higher number of multiparae women.

Just as important as parity was also the age of the mothers in each of the areas. Older mothers are usually at greater risk of dying in childbirth. Unfortunately no statistics remain for the age at which most women in these boroughs were giving birth. What is known is that the age at marriage was usually lower in working-class neighbourhoods, suggesting that first-time mothers in these areas probably gave birth at a younger age than those in the more middle-class areas such as Hampstead and Kensington.[78] Yet the big family size in Stepney and Woolwich suggests that women in these areas probably continued to bear children well into their later years. From this it could therefore be said that the age of the mother in each of the boroughs varied between those who were primiparae and who had had three previous pregnancies, thus balancing each other out in their impact on the overall rates of maternal mortality.

Illegitimacy and Maternal Mortality

Another factor which has to be taken into consideration in relation to the rates of maternal mortality in each of the boroughs is that of illegitimacy, which was not only often associated with higher rates of infant mortality but was also linked to greater numbers of maternal deaths. As we have seen from above, Kensington and Hampstead had much higher rates of illegitimacy than Stepney or Woolwich, thus increasing the number of women at risk in childbirth. The overall impact of illegitimacy on maternal mortality, however, cannot be disentangled from the other factors outlined above. Indeed, illegitimacy, just as much as parity and age of mother, while important in influencing the outcome of an individual mother's experience of childbirth, could still have been countered by skilled obstetric care. Overall, it would seem, that in all cases maternity provision, rather than the demographic characteristics of the population, were more important in determining the levels of maternal mortality within each borough.

Abortion and Maternal Mortality

One factor not considered above, but which might have played a role was also the incidence of abortion in each borough. Abortion was one of the major contributors to maternal death in these years. One of the reasons for the low rate of maternal mortality in Stepney in these years could be the large proportion of Irish immigrants living in the borough, whose Catholic ties might have reduced the number of abortions in the area. Evidence on this issue, however, is hard to find. Nuns working in East London remembered that Irish immigrants were less likely to seek abortion, but it was not unknown.[79] Similarly, to what extent the reluctance to use abortion was widespread among other residents in Stepney is difficult to determine. In addition, no records are available for showing whether there was any difference in the abortion rates between the boroughs. It is, therefore, difficult to see to what extent abortion influenced the patterns of maternal mortality in each area.

Conclusion

Overall it would seem that in all the boroughs the rates of infant and maternal mortality dropped in the years 1902 to 1936. The speed with which this happened, and the degree to which it occurred, however, varied showing the complexity of the determinants of maternal and infant health and the great variability in social and economic conditions as well as medical and welfare provision available in each borough. As we have seen the decline in infant mortality took place much earlier than maternal mortality, reflecting the distinct determinants of each type of mortality.

Within the context of infant mortality, whether it be post-neonatal or neonatal mortality, it would seem that overall the standards of infant health in all four boroughs improved most in Stepney. This improvement is particularly interesting given that Stepney had one of the highest rates of post-neonatal mortality, caused primarily by its very poor socio-economic circumstances. Yet this borough managed to achieve the greatest reductions of post-neonatal mortality, standing in marked contrast to Kensington which had equally high rates of infant mortality and poor living conditions. Stepney's rate of reduction also contrasted with Hampstead, where there was greater economic and social prosperity and a low rate of post-neonatal mortality.

While the reduction in post-neonatal mortality in Stepney might be related to an improvement in living and economic conditions in the borough, it might also be linked to the strong commitment to infant welfare services in the borough. Woolwich, which also experienced a comparable rate of reduction in post-neonatal mortality, had equally good infant welfare provision from an early stage. The nature of the infant welfare services in Stepney and Woolwich and how they differed from the two other boroughs is the subject of following chapters. Clearly, however, it would seem these services had an important role to play in countering the detrimental effects that poor socio-economic conditions so often caused to infant health.

Good provision of services was also an important determinant of neonatal and maternal health. The type of care this involved, however, was very different from that needed to secure the health of a post-neonatal infant. As we have seen the life of a mother and her neonatal baby was heavily dependent on the quality of medical attention provided during pregnancy and childbirth. That this was more important than socio-economic considerations is most clearly illustrated in the case of Stepney where maternal and neonatal mortality was low despite the acute deprivation of the area. Indeed, Stepney stood out in contrast to the other boroughs, particularly in the case of maternal mortality, and was the only area to experience any significant reduction over the years.

While the differences in neonatal mortality between the boroughs are smaller than in the case of maternal mortality, it would seem that Stepney was also the borough to experience the greatest reduction in neonatal mortality. This pattern contrasted with that of the more prosperous borough of Hampstead where maternal and neonatal mortality was greater and did not decline as significantly as in

Stepney. What this suggests is that the quality of medical provision for mothers and their new-born infants in Stepney was probably the best for the standards of the time and better than anywhere else. Following chapters will explore why this was so and what implications it had for maternal and neonatal health.

Notes

1. H. J. Ashby, *Infant Mortality* (Cambridge: 1915), 10.
2. School medical inspections were another way to ensure that from childhood to adulthood the nation's population would remain healthy and provide both a good work-force and army.
3. For more information on the development of maternity and child welfare services see A. Davin, 'Imperialism and Motherhood', *Hist. Workshop J.,* 5 (1978), 9–66; C. Dyhouse, 'Working-Class Mothers and Infant Mortality in England, 1895–1914', *J. Soc. Hist.,* 12, (1979), 248–67; J. Lewis, *The Politics of Motherhood* (London: 1980); *eadem,* 'The Working-Class Wife and Mother and State Intervention,' in J. Lewis (ed.), *Labour and Love: Women's Experience of Home and Family 1850–1940* (Oxford: 1986).
4. I. Loudon, 'Deaths in Childbed from the 18th Century to 1935', *Med. Hist.,* 30 (1986), 1–41, 2; Lewis, *op. cit.* (note 3), 35–6.
5. Not included in this study are stillbirths which only began to appear as a separate category from 1926. These deaths were those occurring from the 28th week of pregnancy to the time of birth. For more information on trends in stillbirths see I. Loudon, *Death in Childbirth: An International Study of Maternal Care and Maternal Mortality 1800–1950* (Oxford: 1992), 19–21.
6. Prior to 1911 there were also changes in the boundaries of the boroughs, most especially in the case of Stepney. This might again distort the figures, but from 1911 the boundaries remained consistent to 1939.
7. I. Loudon, 'On Maternal and Infant Mortality, 1900–1960', *Soc. Hist. Med.,* 4/1 (1991), 29–74. See also R. I. Woods, P. A. Watterson and J. H. Woodward, 'The Causes of Rapid Infant Mortality Decline in England and Wales, 1861–1921', Parts I and II, *Popul. Stud.,* 42 (1988), 343–66 and 43 (1989), 113–32, see particularly Part II, 114–15; N. Williams, 'Infant and Child Mortality in Urban Areas of Nineteenth Century England and Wales: A Record Linkage Study', unpub. Ph.D., Liverpool, 1989, 23–5; M. Tew, *A Safer Childbirth: A Critical History of Maternity Care* (London: 1990), 5–6.
8. For a detailed analysis of this trend see Loudon, *op. cit.* (note 7), 37–40.
9. C. Webster, 'Health, Welfare and Unemployment During the Depression', *P & P,* 109 (1985), 204–29; C. Webster 'Healthy or Hungry Thirties?, *Hist. Workshop J.,* 13 (1982), 110–29; J. M.

Winter, 'Unemployment, Nutrition and Infant Mortality in Britain, 1920–1950', in J. M. Winter (ed.), *The Working Class and Modern British History* (Cambridge: 1983); M. H. Brenner, 'Fetal, Infant and Maternal Mortality During Periods of Economic Instability', *International Journal of Health Services,* 3 (1973), 145–59. See also Loudon *op. cit.* (note 7), 48–50; and Loudon *op. cit.* (note 5), 42–6.

10. P. A. Watterson, 'Role of the Environment in the Decline of Infant Mortality: An Analysis of the 1911 Census of England and Wales', *J. Biosoc. Sci.,* 18 (1986), 457–70. See also Woods *et al., op. cit.* (note 7), Part II, 114–15; N. Williams, 'Death in its Season: Class, Environment and the Mortality of Infants in Nineteenth-century Sheffield', *Soc. Hist. Med.,* 5/1 (1992), 71–94.

11. Hampstead MOH, *A/Rs* (1906) 33; (1925) 9.

12. Meeting of Sub-Committee of Kensington Council, 17 October 1933, Minutes, 8.

13. *Ibid.*

14. E. W. Hope, 'Autumnal Diarrhoea in Cities', *Publ. Hlth,* July 1899, 660–5; Woods *et al., op. cit.* (note 7), Part I, 361–2, and Part II, 120; D. Dwork, *War is Good for Babies and Other Young Children: A History of the Infant and Child Welfare Movement* (London: 1987), 49–50; Williams, *op. cit.* (note 7), 30 and ch. 5.

15. A. S. Wohl, *Endangered Lives: Public Health in Victorian Britain* (London: 1983), 22–5.

16. Woolwich MOH, *A/R* (1906), 90–1. See also Hampstead MOH, A/R (1905), 23 and (1906), 48.

17. S. Szreter, 'The Importance of Social Intervention in Britain's Mortality Decline', *Soc. Hist. Med.,* 1/1 (1988), 1–38, 31.

18. J. M. Leventhal *et al.,* 'Does Breastfeeding Protect against Infections in Infants less than 3 months of age?', *Paediatrics,* 78 (5 November 1986), 896–903.

19. At the turn of the century numerous medical experts showed that infant mortality rose dramatically in the years of hot, dry summers. Kensington MOH, *A/R* (1922), 10. In 1921 the Woolwich MOH reported that the incidence of summer diarrhoea was 1.25% among breast-fed infants; 3.32% among infants who were partially bottle-fed and 8.91% among those who were totally hand-fed. Woolwich MOH, *A/R,* (1921). See also V. Fildes, 'Breastfeeding in London, 1905–1919', *J. Biosoc. Sci.,* 24 (1992), 53–74.

20. See Newsholme, cited in Woods *et al., op. cit.* (note 7), Part II, 116–17. Supplementary feeding was fairly widespread in the Jewish community, and yet this did not have an adverse impact on the health of their infants despite the fact that they were living in comparable poverty and overcrowded conditions to their neighbours. Part of the reason for the low Jewish infant mortality was the Jewish rituals concerning cleanliness and diet which ensured that any supplementary food was prepared in the best hygienic conditions

possible. For more information on this see L. Marks, *Model Mothers: Jewish Mothers and Maternity Provision in East London 1870–1939* (Oxford: 1994), Ch. 2.

21. A. Hardy, 'Rickets and the Rest: Child-care, Diet and the Infectious Children's Diseases, 1850–1914', *Soc. Hist. Med.* 5/3 (1992), 389–412, 394.

22. Wohl, *op. cit.* (note 15), 19–20.

23. A. Hardy, *The Epidemic Streets: Infectious Diseases and The Rise of Preventive Medicine, 1856–1900* (Oxford: 1993), Ch. 10. See also P. Aaby, 'Social and Behavioural Factors Affecting the Transmissions and Severity of Measles Infection', in J. Caldwell, *et. al.,* (eds), *What We Know about Health Transition: The Cultural, Social and Behavioural Determinants of Health* (Canberra: 1990), 826–42; and *idem,* 'Patterns of Exposure and Severity of Measles Infection. Copenhagen 1915–1925', *Ann. Epidemiol.,* 2 (1990), 257–62.

24. Hardy, *op. cit.* (note 21), 398, 403.

25. Hardy, *op. cit.* (note 23), Ch. 9. See also Hardy, *op. cit.* (note 21). Air pollution not only blocked out the necessary sunlight, but was also probably an important determinant of the higher levels of respiratory diseases. Recent research has shown a strong correlation between air pollution and respiratory diseases among young infants and children. See N. Graham, 'The Epidemics of Acute Respiratory Infections in Children and Adults: A Global Perspective', in *Epidemiol. Rev.,* 12 (1990), 149–78, 157.

26. The importance of these foods in reducing the incidence of rickets can be seen in the case of Jewish children living in East London at the turn of the century. Despite the lack of sunlight in many of their dwellings, Jewish children rarely experienced rickets, which can be attributed to their diet which was very rich in vitamin D. See Marks, *op. cit.* (note 20), Ch. 2, and Hardy, *op. cit.* (note 21), 404–6.

27. 'Report of the Infant Committee', *Trans. Obstet. Soc. of London,* 13 (1870), 132–49, 142–3; L. Rose, *The Massacre of the Innocents: Infanticide in Britain 1800–1939* (London: 1986), 23.

28. Woolwich MOH, *A/R* (1906–38) and *Registrar General's Annual Statistics for England and Wales* (London: 1918–20).

29. One of the reasons for the low rate of illegitimacy in Stepney was also the presence of Irish and East European Jewish immigrants who many commentators saw as having a higher level of chastity and morality than the local population. L. Marks,'"The Luckless Waifs and Strays of Humanity": Irish and Jewish Immigrant Unwed Mothers in London 1870–1939', *Twentieth Cent. Br. Hist.,* 3/2 (1992), 113–37.

30. J. R. Gillis, 'And the Risks of Illegitimacy in London, 1801–1900', *Fem. Stud.,* 5/1, (1979), 142–73, Table 1, 145, 147, 149, 151; A. R. Higginbotham, 'The Unmarried Mother and her Child in Victorian London 1834–1914', unpub. Ph.D., Indiana, 1985, 54, 159, 179–80.

31. J. M. Winter, 'Aspects of the Impact of the First World War on Infant Mortality in Britain', *J. Eur. Econ. Hist.,* 11 (1982), 713–38, 723.
32. Woods *et al., op. cit.* (note 7), Part II, 121–6.
33. *Ibid.*
34. This study was based on the nutritional information for 222,989 infants, which represented 39.2% of all registered births in the 23 boroughs during the years for which figures were available between 1905 and 1919. In the first month of life over 92% of these children received some breast milk with almost 86% of these having been breast-fed exclusively. Only 7.6% were artificially fed from birth. Fildes, *op. cit.* (note 19), Table 1, 53–74.
35. *Ibid.*
36. *Ibid.,* Table 4.
37. Kensington MOH, *A/R* (1913), 12. The evidence does not make clear whether this was exclusive or partial breast-feeding.
38. Kensington MOH, *A/R* (1910), 11; Stepney MOH, *A/R* (1913), 65 and 68.
39. Davin, *op. cit.* (note 3), Dyhouse, *op. cit.* (note 3), Wohl, *op. cit.* (note 15), 23–4.
40. Fildes, *op. cit.* (note 19), Table 6; Woolwich MOH, *A/Rs* (1909).
41. Woolwich MOH, *A/R* (1909).
42. Fildes, *op. cit.* (note 19), 67. For more information concerning the controversy over maternal and infant mortality see J. D. Wray, 'Maternal Nutrition, Breastfeeding and Infant Survival', and A. Lechtig *et al.,* 'Effect of Maternal Nutrition on Infant Mortality', both in W. H. Moseley (ed.), *Nutrition and Human Reproduction* (New York & London: 1977); R. Morley *et al.,* 'Mother's Choice to Provide Breast Milk and Developmental Outcome', *Archives of Disease in Childhood,* 63 (1988), 1382–5; J. Illingworth *et al.,* 'Diminution in Energy, Expenditure During Lactation', *Br. Med. J.,* 292 (15 February 1986), 437–41. See also Great Britain, Committee on Medical Aspects of Food Policy, *Present Day Practice in Infant Feeding: Third Report* (London: 1988), 8–10 for nutritional value of human milk.
43. Fildes, *op. cit.* (note 19), See also a detailed study of the budgets of working-class families in Lambeth 1909–13 in M. Pember Reeves, *Round About a Pound a Week* (London: 1913, repr. 1979).
44. Kensington MOH, *A/R* (1905), 59. See also Woolwich MOH, A/R (1906), 89.
45. Fildes, *op. cit.* (note 19), M. Llewellyn Davies, *Maternity: Letters from Working Women* (London: 1915, repr. 1978).
46. Machine-skimmed condensed milk was a popular supplement in working-class areas. Often this was fed through long-tube feeding bottles which were impossible to clean. Fildes *op. cit.* (note 19), 67, 68.
47. Fildes, *op. cit.* (note 19), 67. For more detail on the staple diet of working-class mothers see Pember Reeves, *op. cit.* (note 43), ch. 7.

48. A. S. Cunningham, 'Breastfeeding and Morbidity in Industrialized Countries: An Update', in D. B. Jelliffe and E. F. P. Jelliffe, *Advances in International Maternal and Child Health* (Oxford: 1981), 128–68.

49. L. H. Lumley, 'Obstetric Performance of Women after in Utero Exposure to the Dutch Famine', unpub. Ph.D., Columbia, 1988; L. H. Lumley, and F. W. A. Van Poppel, 'Health and Demographic Effects of the Dutch Famine of 1944–45', unpub. paper presented to Society for Social History of Medicine Annual Conference on Famine and Disease, 5–7 July 1991, Cambridge.

50. Hampstead MOH, *A/R* (1919), 75.

51. Woolwich Council, MCW Committee Minutes, 4 January 1922, 26.

52. Kensington Council Meeting of Sub-Committee Minutes, 17 October 1933, 7.

53. Loudon, *op. cit.* (note 7), 39.

54. Wohl, *op. cit.* (note 15), 15–16. Research based on a study of mothers and daughters who experienced the Dutch famine during the Second World War, has shown that only in acute situations of starvation is there any real link between prematurity and social and economic conditions, and that this association is most marked among the first-born infants born to those mothers who had been exposed to the famine during the first and second trimester of their own intrauterine life. Lumley, *op. cit.* (note 49).

55. Figures from the Registrar General however indicate no real difference in rates of stillbirth in the four boroughs for the years 1928 to 1939, and no rise in the years of economic recession. *Registrar General's Annual Statistics for England and Wales* (London: 1928–39), Table 18.

56. Loudon, *op. cit.* (note 7), Table 4, 41.

57. For more information on the number of doctor deliveries see Ch. 5.

58. In 1924 Sir George Newman wrote: 'Not less than 700,000 mothers in England and Wales give birth to children each year. Of this number approximately 3,000 per annum have died during the last 10 years in the fulfilment of this maternal function. That is a serious and largely avoidable loss of life at the time of its highest capacity and its most fruitful effort....The death rate among women in childbirth has shown but little proportional lessening in the past 20 years.' Preface to a report by Dr Janet Campbell (Senior Medical Officer to MCW Department) to the MH 1924, cited in *Onward,* 3 April 1924, 57, (newspaper issued by City of London Maternity Hospital).

59. I. Loudon, 'Maternal Mortality: 1880–1950. Some Regional and International Comparisons', *Soc. Hist. Med.,* 1/2 (1988), 183–228, 184–5. In 1930 a MH Committee investigating 2,000 maternal deaths concluded that 48% of the causes of maternal mortality were preventable (cited in *Onward,* October 1930).

60. S. Ryan Johansson, 'Sex and Death in Victorian England', in M. Vicinus, (ed.), *A Widening Sphere* (Indiana: 1977), 163–81, 169–70;

Loudon, *op. cit.* (note 59), 184.

61. Maternal mortality appears to have declined in England and Wales from 1650 to 1850 before levelling out from about 1850 to 1934. R. Schofield, 'Did Mothers Really Die? Three Centuries of Maternal Mortality, in "The World We Have Lost"', in R. Smith, L. Bonfield and K. Wrightson (eds.), *The World We Have Gained* (Oxford: 1987), 254. 'Even when the rate of maternal mortality was unusually high, at least 96–7% of all deliveries ended successfully. In the context of total deliveries, therefore maternal deaths were uncommon events.' Childbirth however was a common event in society, which made people more aware of the danger of maternal mortality. Loudon, *op. cit.* (note 59), 184.

62. Many in the Ministry of Health, such as Newman, denied that social and economic factors had any bearing on maternal mortality and morbidity so as to avoid the necessity of making wider state welfare provision. Webster, *op. cit.* (note 9), 122–3.

63. Loudon, *op. cit.* (note 59), 198. Webster suggests that the high rate of anaemia and toxaemia among mothers in depressed areas shows that the vast expansion in maternal and child welfare clinics had little impact on the poor standards of health and nutrition in such areas. More radical solutions were needed in state welfare but ministers were reluctant to undertake them (*op. cit.* note 9, 122–3).

64. All information described on the causes of maternal mortality is drawn from a much fuller account in Loudon, *op. cit.* (note 5), Chs 3, 4 and 5.

65. *Ibid.,* 43.

66. *Ibid.,* 43, 50.

67. For a more detailed account of puerperal fever, and its origins and treatment see *ibid.* Ch. 4.

68. *Ibid,* 99.

69. *Ibid.*

70. *Ibid.,* 100–2.

71. *Ibid.,* 102.

72. *Ibid.,* Ch. 5.

73. For the difficulty in measuring maternal mortality *ibid.,* Chs 1 and 2, and Appendix 4.

74. For a good discussion of the difficulties of connecting neonatal and other forms of infant mortality with maternal mortality trends see Loudon, *op. cit.* (note 7).

75. The same risk can be applied to neonatal mortality. *Ibid.,* 56.

76. The differentiation in fertility trends is also perceptible in terms of occupation. Those at the top of the occupational social scale such as the professions had much smaller families than those at the bottom. See Registrar General, *Decennial Supplement for England and Wales* (London: 1931–9), Appendix.

77. LCC, *Maternity Services of London: Report by the County MOH to the*

Hospitals and Medical Services Committee, (London: 1934), 17
(GLRO library [LP] 26.8 LCC).

78. For the differential in ages at marriage and fertility patterns between
the different classes see Registrar General, *Decennial Supplement for
England and Wales* (London: 1931–9), Appendix.

79. Sister P. and Sister T., interviewed by L. Marks, London, 14
December 1987, notes. The Irish immigrant presence in Stepney was
important in determining the provision of contraception in the area.
See ch. 4. For more information on attitudes to abortion see Ch.1.

4

Politics and Provision

'Whatever we squander and whatever we save – we must save the
baby life of the British race.'[1] Appearing as part of a campaign for the
first Baby Week in Hampstead in 1917, these words were not unique
to Hampstead nor were they merely a phenomenon of the First
World War. As Chapter 1 has already shown, many statesmen, social
reformers and medical experts anxious about Britain's economic,
military and physical strength had made similar calls since the end of
the nineteenth century. The extent to which these ideas were trans-
lated into reality can partly be seen by the unprecedented rise in the
number of maternal and child welfare facilities in these years. Such
provision, however, disguises the complex dynamic between politics
and health care provision during this period. It also hides the constant tension in these years over who should take responsibility for
the provision of services, the state or the individual, and the debates
over which services would be the most effective. Such questions not
only arose in heated parliamentary sessions, but also among those
working on a more localized grassroots level.

What stand was taken was highly variable and greatly dependent
on the gender, class and political persuasion of those involved.
Building on Chapters 2 and 3, this chapter explores the ways in
which the different socio-economic conditions and political com-
plexions of each borough, and their particular infant and maternal
health profiles, shaped the debates over maternal and child welfare
and considers what implications this had for policy and its implementation. As Chapter 2 has already highlighted, each borough,
while integrally part of London, had their own distinct socio-
economic and political characteristics and could be considered communities in themselves united by their formal geographical and

132

political boundaries. Even within each borough there were multiple layers of communities, each with their own needs and demands. This did not always make for the most harmonious of relations.

Where the conflict of interest was most perceptible was in the context of the political parties. While the Labour Party, primarily concerned with the poorer residents, was more likely to prioritize the funds and welfare provision of the borough in their direction, the Municipal Reform (Conservative) Party, and to some extent the Liberal Party, more closely identified with the ratepayer, seeing their interests as taking precedence in deciding the level and mode of welfare services to be provided.[2] Different political parties, therefore, appealed to very distinct groups of voters, which entailed contrasting notions of who should be protected and provided for.[3]

To what extent each political group was listened to and represented in policy formulation depended on their overall political strength within the borough. As Chapter 2 has already shown, the high proportion of upper- and middle-class residents in Hampstead and Kensington meant that the overall political outlook and mobilization of services was dominated by conservative groups whose power within the council chamber allowed greater voice for the interests of the ratepayer than those of the poor. By contrast the political outlook of the two other boroughs, especially Woolwich, was more radical and in tune with the needs of the poor, reflecting their larger working-class constituency.

While the different political groups played an important role in determining the level of services in each area, their interests, however, were only one among many in each borough. As I argued in Chapter 2, the social and political mobilization of women, and the presence of certain charismatic medical professionals and other individuals, each of whom had their own political agendas and constituencies, were also crucial in the formulation and implementation of maternal and child welfare provision. This chapter focuses on the extent to which the perceptions of and arguments used by different individuals and groups were shaped by the particular constituency they represented. It also examines the degree to which their views shaped the maternal and child welfare policies formulated within each borough.

The vast number of individuals and groups who were involved in maternal and child welfare and the number of issues which were raised under its umbrella, makes this a difficult subject to cover in detail. This chapter, therefore, only examines a minority of the services provided in these years and the debates that took place over

133

their implementation. These include the provision of milk depots, the Kensington Baby Clinic, milk and food for poor mothers and infants, and contraception. Such areas were chosen not only because of the importance they were accorded in debates on maternal and child welfare, but also because they were services which fuelled particularly fraught conflicts that highlight the complexities involved in the development of welfare provision. Much of my exploration of these issues will be from the perspective of the rhetoric used in galvanizing such services. In the final part of the chapter, however, I consider what implications this had in the practical sense, focusing on the overall structure and funding of services in each borough.

Milk Depots, 1902–10

One of the most burning questions in the early twentieth century was the persistence of infant mortality. Yet despite the gravity of concern the problem generated, no consensus existed on how it might be resolved. Some of the fiercest contests over this issue can be seen in Kensington which had the highest rate of infant mortality in London.[4] Many within the borough were appalled by the problem. In 1902 Orme Dudfield, medical officer of health for Kensington, summed up the feelings when he reminded his readers that 'Quite apart from general considerations as to the future of the Empire and the like, this in a West London borough more particularly, ought not to be tolerated by the borough itself.'[5]

Yet while many shared Dudfield's horror at the high rates of infant mortality, seeing it as ruining Kensington's prosperous reputation in the rest of the capital, battles raged over how it was to be eliminated.[6] One of Dudfield's suggestions was to set up a municipal milk depot and municipal crèches. Yet such a proposition did not meet universal approval. Many within the borough regarded such municipal provision, as one newspaper editor put it, as the first step towards 'municipal trading in a peculiarly insidious form' and an evasion of responsibility on the part of the individual.[7] While such arguments were justified on the ideological grounds of the need to minimize state intervention and encourage individualism, what lay behind them was also an economic motive. By emphasizing the responsibility of the individual, defenders of these views avoided making any commitment to financing services for the poor. Indeed, the poor were expected to provide for themselves and any help given to them was deemed a charitable cause rather than a right.

In common with Stepney and Hampstead, Kensington never established a milk depot. Part of this might be attributed to the strong conservative forces within these borough councils before the First World War and their resistance to municipally funded services. This conservativism is particularly striking in the case of Hampstead where the presence of George McCleary (Hampstead's medical officer of health from 1906) would on the surface be seen to have been an important force in establishing such a depot. Prior to coming to Hampstead McCleary had established the first milk depot in London in Battersea in 1902 for which he had received national recognition. On coming to Hampstead he continued to be an active campaigner for such provision, yet his attempts to have a similar depot in Hampstead fell on deaf ears.[8] Part of McCleary's success in establishing such a depot in Battersea and not in Hampstead lay in the strength of the Labour movement within Battersea which was sorely lacking in Hampstead. One of McCleary's strongest supporters in Battersea had been the Socialist worker and Labour leader, John Burns, whose presence firstly on the London County Council (from 1889) and then in parliament from 1892 was important in galvanizing the establishment and acceptance of the milk depot and other maternal and child welfare services.[9]

Within Woolwich the Labour movement also played a crucial role in the provision of a milk depot. In 1906 a milk depot was established in the wake of the Labour Party's victory in the borough council's election that year. Following the example of those that had been established elsewhere in the country, the depot in Woolwich provided milk for necessitous nursing mothers and those infants whose mothers were unable to breast-feed. Those setting up the clinic were explicit that the depot 'was not to supplant natural feeding' and every effort was 'made to encourage breast-feeding and prevent the depot milk being used for children who can be naturally fed'.[10]

The chief aim of the depot was to provide pure modified milk free from germs at the same price as ordinary milk, thus enabling the very poor to purchase good clean milk at an affordable price. This goal was seen as crucial given that about half of the parents of the infants in the borough who were hand-fed did not have the financial means to purchase modified milk and were forced to use condensed milk, often resulting in infantile diarrhoea.[11]

While most infants in the borough were breast-fed, in 1908 it was estimated that about 19 per cent of the infant population in Woolwich were being hand-fed.[12] The depot was, therefore, not serving a small minority. Within months of opening, the depot was reporting a rapid increase in numbers and that the depot was obviously fulfilling a public need.[13] By 1908 328 infants were being provided with milk, approximately 12 per cent of the infant population of the borough.[14] A great majority of those supplied were those who otherwise would not have been able to pay the costs to sufficiently feed their children.[15] Woolwich was unusual in that it supplied milk to the family's doorstep.[16] In common with other depots it also had an extensive health visitors' scheme and established infant consultations for infants to be weighed and checked by a medical officer. Thus the depot was not only seen as a supplier of milk but also encouraging the education of mothers on infant rearing and feeding.[17]

While the establishment of the milk depot in Woolwich partly arose as a result of pressure from the Labour Party within the council chamber and can be seen, therefore, as a triumph for the more radical political forces in Woolwich, its existence was never secure. Soon after the depot appeared the Labour Party lost its majority on the borough council to the Municipal Reformers, one of whose aims was to shut down the depot. Echoing the feelings also expressed in Kensington, they argued that the depot was merely a form of 'municipal trading' which was too expensive to run and a waste of ratepayers' money. The depot was a costly business involving not only the purchasing of milk, but also the daily collection and cleansing of bottles. By 1909 the depot was costing between £400 and £500 a year. After attempts to have the depot taken over by a private firm failed the depot was finally closed in 1909.[18]

Such pressures from the Municipal Reformers also meant that during its existence the depot was forced to economize and to not be seen to be wasting ratepayers' money. This constraint had repercussions for the ways in which mothers were charged. Any mother who fell behind on her payments, even if only for a week, was denied supply from the depot. In 1908 the strict application of this rule had led to the withdrawal of milk to many infants.[19]

While the more conservative lobby had the final upper-hand in Woolwich both in restricting the extent to which the very poor could be provided with the service, and in shutting the depot, such pressures were subject to much contest within the borough. This tension can most clearly be seen in the struggle that ensued after its closure. The debates that took place over its closure illustrate the very different perceptions and demands that surrounded the provision of welfare services as a whole. Numerous letters of objection were sent to the Council from individual mothers as well as associations such as the Woolwich Workers' Union, the Woolwich and District Trades and Labour Council, the Labour Representation Association, and

Plumstead Radical Club. The Woolwich branch of the Women's Labour League also collected 129 signatures from mothers to register their objection. Such protests signified the widespread grassroots support for the depot and their concern for maternal and infant welfare provision.[20]

One of the results of this campaign was the setting up of an investigation into the utility of the depot. In summarizing the results of the investigation a report highlighted some of the justifications that proponents for the depot put forward. From this it was clear that they had a high degree of sympathy for the financial struggles poor mothers had in securing good milk. As they argued,

> The cost of baby's milk is a serious item in a poor family. The parents expect that the baby will cost nothing for food in the first year of life. When, owing to failure of nature's supply, the child has to be provided with cow's milk, the mother finds to her regret that the baby's milk costs as much, or more than the total food of his seven year old brother – say 1s.6d. to 2s.6d. a week. Frequently, to economise, less money is spent on the infant's milk, and the child is partially starved with disastrous effects in after life.[21]

It was for this reason that the milk depot had deliberately set low prices for the supply of its milk. This countered against any ideas put forward by the Municipal Reformers who argued that the depot should be a self-supporting institution.[22]

One of the arguments put forward by the Municipal Reformers for the closure of the depot was that it covered only a small proportion of infants and was therefore an inefficient use of the council's resources.[23] Others claimed, however, that the depot had been a popular service, and had provided for nearly half of the infant population in the borough who were hand-fed.[24] Indeed, they stressed that such a service was important even if it had saved only one infant life within the borough. This view was not only put forward by the mothers themselves, but also the Labour Party, the chief medical officer of health, and Alice Gregory the honorary secretary of the British Hospital for Mothers and Babies.[25] For these campaigners the question was not one of saving the ratepayers' money, but rather one of long-term investment for the health of the whole borough and ultimately the future of the nation. Its importance was highlighted by the medical officer of health who in concluding the investigation argued,

> The results of the Depot on the health of the infant population having been so particularly satisfactory, obviously the closure of the

Depot must be prejudicial to the health of the Borough. A lowered
mortality always means an improvement in the health of the sur-
vivors. Illness which kills a few, injures many, and .... I have shown
that a reduced infant mortality has been accompanied by a reduction
in the mortality at nearly all ages under 65, showing that children
who survive the perils of infancy are stronger to resist the diseases of
adolescence and early manhood.[26]

Kensington Baby Clinic and the Need for Municipally Funded Comprehensive Services, 1912–36

Much of the debate over the provision of milk depots centred on the
degree to which municipal authorities should have responsibility for
welfare provision as well as the degree to which services could be
judged to be the most effective in combating infant mortality. These
issues dominated other areas of maternal and child welfare work,
such as the provision of municipal baby clinics.

The provision of such clinics was particularly contentious in
Kensington, where in 1912 the Women's Labour League under the
auspices of the Labour Party set up the first baby clinic in the country.
Based in Telford Road in North Kensington, an area housing some of
the poorest residents and with one of the highest rates of infant mortality in the borough, this clinic differed from other maternal and
infant welfare services in these years in that it explicitly provided free
medical treatment alongside preventative and educational measures.[27]
Mothers bringing their infants to the centre could not only consult a
doctor, but also had access to a dentist once a month, a resident nurse,
and a dispenser. Minor operations were performed on a monthly basis
and children could also have dressings and syringing from a nurse
daily. In 1919 the range of medical treatments offered was extended
by the establishment of a baby hospital, which was directly linked to
the clinic. From the start both the clinic and hospital catered not just
for babies, but for all children under five, and aimed to provide a full
medical service for a child.[28] Other infant welfare centres only began
to provide facilities for toddlers in the late 1920s.

The medical facilities as provided by the baby clinic were vital
given that the majority of the poor infants and young children did not
have easy access to such medical facilities in the years between 1902
and 1936. Most infant welfare centres only provided educational
advice and referred any patients needing medical treatment elsewhere.[29]
In addition, children were not covered by the National Insurance
scheme of 1911 which ensured free medical treatment for men in
regular employment but not their families. Any medical treatment

infants received was dependent either on engaging a local doctor which could be very expensive, or being treated as charitable cases by medical missions, voluntary hospitals or Poor Law infirmaries, which could cause embarrassment and even shame among parents. One of the aims of the founders of the clinic was that it 'would give to working women that great advantage, which richer women always have at hand – skilled care and advice in order to prevent as well as cure illness'.[30]

The importance of the clinic not only lay in its provision of free medical treatment, but that it was provided alongside educational and preventative activities under the same roof thus enabling mothers and their infants to receive a comprehensive service. One of the criticisms made by campaigners of the baby clinic of the infant welfare services, was that educational and preventative work tended to be divided from medical treatment. This division of services involved mothers travelling long distances between institutions and forking out unnecessary and costly expenses on transport; often resulting in medical treatment being delayed. The advantage of the baby clinic was that mothers attending for advice did not have to be referred elsewhere and could get medical treatment immediately, which meant infants were attended at the first sign of disease, rather than waiting until the last possible moment.[31]

Much of the campaign waged over the Kensington Baby Clinic was not only that infant welfare services should be providing medical treatment, but that baby clinics should be a municipally funded service. While established as a result of the voluntary efforts and funding of the Labour Party, many within the Labour Party saw this clinic as a model for those campaigning for all local authorities to initiate and fund baby clinics for the medical treatment of children under school age.

Arguments were couched in terms of the needs of mothers, and also what it would cost the whole nation. Ethel Bentham (a Labour councillor and key organizer of the Baby Clinic) pointed out that municipal funding of curative care alongside preventive measures from early on would help the mothers and their infants, and also promote healthier infants who would not be a burden on the state in later life.[32] For both her and the others involved in the clinic, the health of the infants and ultimately that of the community, was something which could only be guaranteed by municipal funding.

Yet this attitude was not universal within Kensington, as can be seen by the many fierce debates that took place over the issue within the council chamber.[33] For the more conservative councillors such a municipally funded scheme was a waste of public funds when such services were already being adequately provided by voluntary agencies within the area.[34] Labour councillors, however, pointed out that the service was scanty and not comprehensive because it was divided between many different institutions and reliant on voluntary subscription.

Much of the debate over the need for municipally funded baby clinics in Kensington was also linked to arguments about the need for greater state intervention to ameliorate wider social and economic conditions, such as the provision of better accommodation and higher wages. Without this, Labour councillors claimed, other measures such as the educational advice offered by an infant welfare centre would be ineffective. This view was not only expressed by those running the Kensington clinic, and nor was it confined to Kensington. Indeed, it formed a core demand for other Labour Party activists and women's organizations such as the Women's Co-operative Guild outside the borough as well as a number of progressive doctors such as Arthur Newsholme both before and after the First World War.[35]

This demand, however, was much more far-reaching and required more extensive state intervention than the majority of councillors in Kensington were willing to advocate. Reticence in state intervention was not only apparent in the discussions concerning baby clinics. In the years immediately before the First World War, Kensington Poor Law Guardians and borough councillors in debating whether to give outdoor relief to women who had either been deserted by their husbands or were the wives of imprisoned men, or whether support should be given to the extension of state provision for the feeding of schoolchildren, revealed similar attitudes highlighting the need to protect the ratepayer. Many of their objections were that such measures relieved parents of their true responsibilities in the care of their children and undermined the independence of the working class.[36]

Milk and Nourishment for Necessitous Mothers and Children, 1914–36

Some of the most interesting discussions over the degree to which municipal funds were to be used in the provision of welfare emerged in the struggles over expenditure on milk and nourishment for necessitous mothers and babies. Originating from the free milk order issued by the Local Government Board during the First World War, such provision had become a vital component in the maternal and child welfare budgets of local authorities by the early 1920s. Under this order the Local Government Board covered 50 per cent of the cost of milk distributed by local authorities to mothers and infants.

Nevertheless, while expenditure on such provision was seen as a national necessity in wartime, its importance rapidly diminished with the onset of the post-war economic depression. In 1921 the Ministry of Health cut its expenditure on milk to mothers and babies on the grounds of national economy. Such a measure sparked outcry all over the country, and generated much condemnation among groups from a wide political spectrum. It was particularly contentious in the light of the post-war slump and the very high unemployment prevailing in these years.

Some of the most outspoken protests came from the Labour Party's women's organizations and a number of Labour-run borough councils who saw that such reductions would cause great hardship and lead to a rise in infant mortality which would ultimately impair the efficiency of the whole country.[37] For many Labour women what was at stake was the kind of priority the government allotted to protecting the future of the nation. As an article in *Labour Woman* declared the choice was between 'Milk v. Warships':

> The Treasury's contribution for the present year will be near £200,000 and we are seriously told that milk for mothers and babies must be cut down because this is too large a sum for the country to afford. If we go on feeding the babies we are informed that we must spend less in the provision of hospital, medical, and nursing care. Apparently the nation has only a few hundred thousand pounds to spend on securing the healthy birth of its children, but what is the use of maternity and child welfare work amongst hungry mothers and babies? Why should we make such drastic economies here when we still spend some £300,000,000 on armaments? Our Government can still spend £20,000,000 for new warships... and yet it cannot pay the dairy bill for its infants.[38]

Such protests were not confined to women nor to the Labour movement. In 1921 the Hampstead medical officer of health decried the fact that the cuts meant that a mother had to be 'very necessitous' before she could receive the daily pint of free milk and that 'a class of very hard working and deserving mothers', who were 'just struggling along at poverty level on the small weekly but regular wage earned by their husbands' had to go without milk. Indeed, it seemed that it was those people, whom the Milk (Mothers and Children) order was designed to help, who were now going without.[39]

Table 4.1: Different scales of income set by Stepney and Kensington Councils and the MH for the provision of milk

Number in family	Ministry of Health scale 1922		Hampstead Council's Scale				Stepney Council's Scale 1922 & 1927	
			1921		1925			
	Free	Half cost	Free	Half cost	Free	Half cost	Free	Half cost
1	13s.	15s.	16s.	18s.	13s.	15s.	16s.	18s.
2	10s. 6d.	12s. 6d.	13s.	14s. 6d.	10s. 6d.	12s. 6d.	13s.	14s. 6d.
3	8s. 6d.	10s.	10s. 6d.	11s. 6d.	8s. 6d.	10s.	10s. 6d.	11s.
4	7s. 6d.	8s. 6d.	9s. 6d.	10s. 6d.	7s. 6d.	8s. 6d.	9s. 6d.	10s. 6d.
5	7s.	8s.	8s. 6d.	9s. 6d.	7s.	8s.	8s.	9s. 6d.
6	6s. 6d.	7s. 6d.	8s.	9s.	6s. 6d.	7s. 6d.	8s.	9s.
7	–	–	8s.	9s.	6s. 6d.	7s. 6d.	7s. 6d.	8s. 6d.
8	–	–	8s.	9s.	6s. 6d.	7s. 6d.	7s.	8s.
9	–	–	–	–	–	–	6s. 6d.	7s. 6d.
10	–	–	–	–	–	–	6s.	7s.
11	–	–	–	–	–	–	5s. 6d.	6s. 6d.
12	–	–	–	–	–	–	5s.	6s.
13	–	–	–	–	–	–	4s. 6d.	5s. 6d.

All charges were assessed per head and were calculated once rent had been deducted.

The difference in the scales set by the MH and Stepney Council remained more or less the same. Note that Stepney and Hampstead (before 1925) set a higher income level under which mothers were eligible. After 1925 Hampstead seems to have conformed to the scale set by the MH.

Sources: Stepney MCW Committee Minutes, 10 October 1922, 130–1; 14 June 1927; Hampstead MOH, *A/R* (1921, 1925).

Condemnation of the cuts by the Ministry was widespread, but the degree of resistance was highly variable and greatly dependent on the political composition of each borough as well as their social and economic conditions. The degree of resistance was intricately connected to the financial relationship between the central government and the local authorities. While local authorities could draw on ratepayers' money to provide their services, under the Maternal and Child Welfare Act of 1918 they could also claim up to 50 per cent of expenditure on such services from the national government. Thus while the local authorities had some financial autonomy, their budgets were still dependent on central government decisions.[40]

The power that the central government had over local authorities can be seen from the limits that were imposed on them in setting the scale of income which would entitle mothers and infants to milk. Table 4.1 shows that the level of income whereby mothers could receive free or cheap milk set by the councils in Hampstead and Stepney in 1921 and 1922. In both cases the boroughs set a higher limit than that of the Ministry of Health. Of the two boroughs, however, Stepney took longer to conform to the scale set by the Ministry. While Hampstead appears to have complied by 1925, Stepney only did so in 1927.

Table 4.2: Total expenditure on milk by Hampstead and Kensington councils and per child aged 0–4 years, 1921–38

Date	Hampstead		Kensington		Woolwich	
	Total	Per child	Total	Per child	Total	Per child
	expenditure	0–4 years	expenditure	0–4 years	expenditure	0–4 years
1921	£1,545**	6s. 3d.	£619	1s.	£2,477	3s. 8d.
1922	£309*	1s. 3d.	£143	2d.	£2,134	3s. 3d.
1923	£190	7d.	£226	4d.	£1,588	2s. 4d.
1924	£456	1s. 9d.	£155	3d.	£1,261	1s. 9d.
1925	£427	1s. 7d.	£202	3d.	£1,093	1s. 6d.
1926	£367	1s. 5d.	£196	3d.	£1,294	1s. 9d.
1927	£327	1s. 3d.	£202	3d.	£1,198	1s. 8d.
1928	£353	1s. 4d.	£153	3d.	£1,248	1s. 9d.
1929	£283	1s. 1d.	£174	3d.	£1,177	1s. 8d.
1930	£373	1s. 5d.	£222	4d.	£1,256	1s. 9d.
1931	£616	2s. 5d.	£360	6d.	£1,449	2s. 2d.
1932	–	–	£700	1s. 4d.†	£2,124	4s. 4d.†
1933	–	–	£1,015	1s. 9d.†	£2,298	4s. 8d.†
1934	–	–	£1,429	2s. 7d.†	£1,956	4s. 1d.†
1935	–	–	£2,309	4s. 4d.†	£2,003	4s. 2d.†
1936	–	–	£2,605	5s.†	£1,651	3s. 4d.†
1937	–	–	£3,631	6s. 9d.†	£1,157	2s. 4d.†
1938	–	–	£3,679	7s.†	£1,161	2s. 4d.†

* Price of milk was as high as 11d per quart during 1921.
** Does not include administration costs.
† Measured by children aged 0–5 years.

All figures are rounded up.
Kensington and Woolwich figures are based on expenditure for fresh and dried milk.

Source: Hampstead, Kensington and Woolwich MOH, *A/Rs* (1922–38).

Such a delay in the case of Stepney can partly be explained by its greater number of Labour councillors who were more opposed to the Ministry's limitations. Indeed, Stepney was among those boroughs which were at the forefront of the battle against the cuts imposed by the Ministry of Health. This opposition contrasted with Hampstead where the Municipal Reform Party ruled the council and were generally more reticent about state-funded services. Unfortunately no figures of the scales of income remain for the other two boroughs, but the pressure to resist the Ministry of Health was much less in Kensington where the Labour Party only had six councillors on the council, than in Woolwich, where the council was dominated by the Labour Party.

Table 4.2 indicates that in three of the boroughs the total expenditure on milk dropped greatly after 1921. While it is difficult to gather the exact expenditure each council made on milk in these years, material from three of the boroughs indicates a decline in expenditure after 1921 indicating the power that the central government had in determining expenditure on milk and food on a local level. From Table 4.2 we can see that even the more radical borough of Woolwich was forced to halve its expenditure in the early 1920s.

During the 1920s local authorities all over the country reduced their milk and nourishment bills. While milk and food accounted for 17.3 per cent of the national maternity and child welfare budgets between 1919 and 1920, by 1929–30 this had declined to 13.4 per cent.[41] Table 4.2 indicates that on a local level the cuts were even more drastic. Despite this, however, it would seem that such provision did not totally disappear. Indeed, during the depression years of the 1930s Hampstead and Kensington, which tended to be less forthcoming with municipally funded welfare provision, greatly increased their expenditure on milk and food along with the more progressive councils such as Woolwich.

Such spending patterns were not necessarily the result of policies from the Ministry of Health, who in these years did not reflect the general concern over the status of nutrition and maternal and infant health.[42] The growth in expenditure in these three boroughs reflected the increasing concern among local medical experts and campaigners within these neighbourhoods, especially in the face of the economic depression. While ignored nationally, their voice was more likely to be heeded on a local level where the realities of starvation and mortality were much more apparent. In Stepney, for instance, the council received numerous protest letters from local voluntary committees pointing to an increase in the number of children being fed on condensed milk and cheap brands of tinned milk, and a deterioration in health as a result of the cuts imposed by the Ministry of Health.[43] Such anxiety was not confined to the poor borough of Stepney but also appeared in the rich borough of Hampstead.[44]

Yet despite the concern expressed over the cuts and the detrimental effects they were having on the health of mothers and their infants, opinions still varied over the degree to which the state and local authorities were to fund such provision. What was most at stake was whose interests were to be given priority. This can be seen from a statement made in 1931 by Mrs R. Carnegie, the chairman of the Hampstead Maternal and Child Welfare Committee when commenting on the very large rise in expenditure that had occurred during that year on milk. While she shared the concern over the need for extra nutrition for mothers and children, she was also acutely aware of the need to restrict the burden imposed on the ratepayers. As she stated, 'We have to see in a time like this [of economic depression] that no mother or child suffers, but we also have an equal duty to the ratepayers of the borough to see that none of the money is wasted.'[45] Table 4.2, however, shows that, although aware of the need to protect the ratepayer, the Hampstead Council doubled its expenditure on milk between 1930 and 1931 indicating some appreciation of the need of the mothers within the borough. None the less, how far such provision helped mothers on an individual basis is less clear.

Birth Control in the Inter-war Years

The struggle over milk and food expenditure for mothers and their infants indicates the tension between interest-parties that was inherent in the politics and policies surrounding maternal and child welfare provision in these years. Such a conflict of interests not only emerged between the poor who paid no rates and the ratepayer. One matter which attracted more controversy than any other area in maternal and child welfare in the inter-war years and which shows the complexity of interests involved in welfare provision, was the supply of birth control.[46] Unlike other forms of maternal and infant welfare provision which was directed towards saving the health of infants already born, contraception touched upon the health and welfare of the unborn. What is most interesting about the struggle over such provision, was that both the protagonists and antagonists of birth control justified their stand on the grounds of protecting the future and the health of the nation.[47] Many of these debates also cut across class and gender interests, and were highly dependent on religious affiliations.

Some of the earliest advocates of birth control in the twentieth century were the Eugenicists. Their support for birth control was rooted in the belief that the quality of a population was a crucial factor in determining the power of a nation, and that deterioration in physical health was a sign of genetic weakness caused by too much breeding on the part of what was seen as the inferior races and social classes. For them birth control was seen as the means of limiting reproduction among these unsuitable groups. Their advocation of birth control, however, did not extend to the wealthier classes who they wanted to encourage to multiply. Indeed, they were the ones the Eugenicists classified as genetically and socially superior and thus the ones on whom the future of the nation rested. Another group who campaigned for birth control were the Neo-Malthusians. While sharing the Eugenicists' fears over the deterioration of the race, they rooted this not in inferior genes but rather in the social and economic devastation that had resulted from the rapidly growing population. For them the most effective way of combating this problem was in providing greater access to birth control for the working class. One of the most instrumental groups in promoting this idea was the Malthusian League, which from the late nineteenth century began to distribute literature on contraception and by the 1920s, with the aid of the Society for the Provision of Birth Control, to establish birth control clinics. Yet while the Malthusian League advocated birth control on the grounds that it would also eliminate the poverty of the working class by enabling working-class families to limit their families, their efforts did not meet with universal approval.[48]

One of the strongest opponents to birth control provision was the Church. In 1908 the Lambeth Conference of Bishops of the Anglican Communion unanimously opposed birth control, and only renounced its decision 22 years later. The strength of feeling on the subject was exemplified by the famous court battle between Marie Stopes and the Catholic Church in the 1920s. On a state level there was also great resistance to such provision because of the fears in these years about the decline in the national birth rate and the need for pronatalist measures. In this context birth control was seen as countering rather than defending the interests of the nation.[49]

Within the Labour Party and among other socialist circles, birth control proved a particularly thorny issue, and was not clearly delineated by class or gender. Some of the strongest advocates of birth control came from a number of working-class women's groups and the Workers' Birth Control Group (established 1924). Much of their campaign was aimed at continuing the momentum generated within the Women's Sections of the Labour Party to pressurize the Minister of Health to allow for the provision of birth control within maternal and infant welfare centres. This they justified on the grounds that birth control was already widely available to those who could afford to pay for it. In this context birth control was viewed as a right and something which should not be left to be provided through voluntary private clinics.[50] Many of their arguments also reiterated those made by the Eugenicists, stressing state provision of birth control as a matter which affected the 'physical and mental constitution of the community'.[51] Many women in the Labour movement saw contraception as a class issue and something which should be free to all women, and a means of ending the oppression of motherhood and the high maternal mortality caused by the high rates of abortion that resulted from the absence of access to birth control.[52]

Not all Labour women, however, were so enthusiastic about birth control. Ethel Bentham, for instance, opposed such provision on the grounds that it would subject women to more oppression by husbands.[53] Similarly some Labour women, alongside other male Labour supporters, saw birth control as a 'side issue' which did not tackle the more important need to redistribute wealth and 'the means of life'.[54] Many within the Labour Party also rejected such provision because of the connections it had to the Malthusian League, and the perceived discrimination towards the working class.

Birth control was, therefore, a controversial issue and a matter which generated conflict which not only traversed lines of class and gender, but also raised questions of promiscuity and religion. At the centre of the debate was whether state funding for contraception would enhance or undermine the welfare of the nation. Opponents of state-funded birth control argued that such a measure would prompt an even faster decline in the national birth rate, hence depleting a population that was seen as so crucial to maintain for the nation's military and economic strength in the rest of the world. Much of their concern was drawn from the fact that the birth rate had halved from slightly over 36 per 1,000 population in 1876, when the birth rate stood at its peak, to 17 in 1927, and was predicted to be falling even more.[55]

By contrast, advocates of birth control saw such provision as a means of securing better health for women and their infants and hence enhance the future of the nation. Many promoters of contraception including Marie Stopes and Margery Spring Rice, stressed that birth control was about enabling women to space their families, and thus improving the quality of women's health and their capacity for reproduction and hence increasing fertility. This priority was summed up in an annual report from the North Kensington Women's Welfare Centre in 1935, when it stated,

> We feel a special responsibility both to the public and to the hundreds of young women who come or may come to the Clinic for advice, to emphasize that our work is directed to the improvement of family life and therefore to a healthier and happier population.

We believe that this consideration is of greater importance than mere numbers, and that the control of conception is essential to the achievement of this end; this does not imply a small family for those parents who can give their children a reasonable chance of health and independence.[56]

Following in a similar vein the National Birth Control Association argued,

As is widely known, the population of Great Britain will shortly become stationary and will then begin to decline. The question whether or not this decline is regrettable is one which must be answered by economists and other experts. The practical and humane way of checking this decline is, not by *substituting illegal abortion for legal contraception, but by reducing the mortality rates of infants and of mothers (and here birth control clinics play an important part), and by making parenthood easier for all classes of the community.* The positive side of Planned Parenthood will predominate in proportion as the number of unwanted children born to overburdened or unhealthy parents is reduced.[57]

The provision of birth control within state-funded maternal and child welfare centres not only raised questions of how best to preserve the population and the strength of the nation, but also the extent to which the state could intervene in areas which were seen as purely private matters. Central to this was also the degree to which such provision conflicted with religious beliefs. Should birth control be encouraged by the state in the interests of safeguarding the health of the wider community regardless of religious considerations? Of the four boroughs, Stepney and Kensington are particularly good for examining these questions and highlight the complexities involved in the provision of birth control clinics and the different approaches that were adopted. Central to the policies taken were the social relations of each borough.

Advocates of birth control were especially powerful in Kensington, where the third birth control clinic in the country was established under the auspices of the Society for the Provision of Birth Control Clinics.[58] Known as the North Kensington Women's Welfare Centre, this clinic was founded on the premises evacuated by the mother and baby clinic established by the Women's Labour League.[59] Yet the provision of birth control in Kensington was not linked to the activities of the Labour women.[60] Those who were most active in pushing for such provision came not from Labour women who as we have seen were not universally in favour of birth control, but from those who mixed in more politically conservative circles. The founding

members of the North Kensington Women's Welfare Centre, for
instance, included Margery Spring Rice who had ties with the Liberal
Party, and Stanley Owen Buckmaster, former lord chancellor in
Asquith's wartime government, and his daughter the Honorable Mrs
Dighton Pollock, and Lady Sprigg, wife of Sir Squire Sprigg the editor
of *The Lancet*.[61] Beyond the clinic other supporters of birth control
included Miss Pennefather, chairman of the maternal and child
welfare Committee in the 1930s and a key spokesman on such
provision. She was a Municipal Reform councillor from 1922 through
to the 1930s.[62]

Much of the pressure within Kensington from these women and
those involved in the North Kensington Women's Welfare Centre
stemmed from the strong tradition of the women's movement in
Kensington which put the rights of women high on the agenda. Yet it
would be a mistake to see such efforts as solely the result of the strong
suffragette movement within Kensington. During the inter-war years
many birth control groups found little sympathy nationally from
middle-class and upper-class membership of feminist organizations to
make contraception accessible.[63] As we shall see below one of the
motivations of these individuals undoubtedly stemmed from the dire
poverty within the borough and the need to resolve this problem.

The degree to which Margery Spring Rice and others succeeded
in prioritizing birth control within the borough can be seen from
the fact that in 1926 Kensington became the first council in
London, and the second in the country, to campaign for changes in
the laws governing contraception so as to enable it to be provided
through infant welfare centres run by local authorities. This policy
was justified on the grounds that it would guarantee greater con-
tinuity of care and enable women to be served by those who knew
their backgrounds.[64]

The Ministry of Health, however, opposed such a measure on the
grounds that birth control advice was not in the remit of the infant
welfare centre. Those women needing contraceptive advice for
medical reasons it argued were to be referred to a private practitioner
or hospital. When in 1930 the Ministry finally allowed local councils
to provide birth control information for the first time, Kensington
Council was quick to point out the limitations of the Ministry's
guidelines. Provision was restricted to cases where further childbearing would be dangerous to the health of the mother and to
married women only.[65] Such stringencies meant that the number of
maternal and infant welfare clinics who offered birth control advice
remained small. By 1937 only 95 of 423 of these centres had opened

birth control clinics.[66] Many within the Kensington borough council felt provision should be available to all women, and that it should be provided on social and economic grounds as well as medical ones.[67]

A deputation from the council and the North Kensington clinic to the Ministry of Health in 1934 (consisting of Sir Allan Powell, Miss Pennefather, and Lady Limerick), illustrates the ways in which many within the borough felt about such provision. One of the premises of the campaign for greater access to birth control was that it was an issue which affected the whole life of the borough and the future of the nation. For those leading the deputation, birth control was not only a matter of preventing the unnecessary deaths of mothers and infants, who were the key to the next generation, but was a means of limiting state intervention on a grander economic scale. Many of the arguments they used were reminiscent of those used by the Eugenicists and Malthusian League. This reasoning can be seen most clearly in Sir Allan Powell's statement to the Ministry in which he argued

> Kensington was a progressive borough and they were not making any exaggerated claim. The main issue, whether there should be birth control or not was...over, but the conditions under which birth control advice could be given were hedged about. Kensington was a borough consisting of quite distinct classes. In North Kensington people were living in a warren, and he felt that if some movement were not made in the direction of freer birth control advice, the Government would be faced with other alternatives such as family allowances, rent allowances, and increased unemployment pay.[68]

Birth control was seen, therefore, as a much cheaper option than other social welfare options. Those leading the deputation saw birth control as an issue that was intertwined with the conditions prevailing in North Kensington, which Powell and many others not only feared would undermine the reputation of Kensington but also fuel revolutionary fervour for greater state intervention. Powell's remarks contrasted with the demands made by those involved in the Labour Party who saw the provision of free contraception as something which should supplement, rather than be an alternative to, state help in areas such as family allowances and cheaper housing.[69]

In this way the rhetoric around health and the future of the nation were intricately bound up with state intervention and policy decisions which were tied to perceptions of the needs of the local neighbourhood. What also lay behind the demands of Powell and others was the need to help improve the quality of the race. Birth control was seen as one of the answers to Kensington's very high rate of infant mortality.[70]

In Stepney the debate around birth control was very different and more heavily influenced by religious considerations. The strong presence of Irish Catholic immigrants and their children within the borough especially on the council, made the municipal provision of birth control a particularly contentious issue. During the 1920s grassroots Catholic organizations within Stepney, as well as elsewhere, were particularly active in opposing birth control.[71] Fearing that public institutions were about to be given public money to offer contraceptive advice, the Catholic community with the support of Catholic residents in East London sent a circular to the Ministry of Health in 1925 calling on them not to do so.[72]

Not all in Stepney, however, were Catholic, nor were they all opposed to the provision of birth control. In 1927 a voluntary birth control clinic was established in Stepney, prompting a heated discussion within the council chamber. Some councillors such as Miriam Moses, who was Jewish, called for municipal provision of contraceptive information for poor mothers, arguing that they should have it available in the same way as rich people. Although Miriam Moses saw this as a question which should not be determined by a question of religion, those who opposed municipal provision saw it as paramount to the issue and regarded it as a question which should not even be discussed by the council.[73] The strength of such opposition within the council and in the borough can be measured by the resolution that was passed in 1929, which forbade any council workers to provide information on birth control, arguing that the practice was not only 'probably illegal' and against the public policy of the Ministry of Health, but also 'highly offensive to the religious beliefs and conscientious opinions of many inhabitants of the borough'.[74]

Yet while the resolution in 1929 showed the council to have a certain consideration of the residents it was serving, this changed in 1931 when the council accepted the Ministry of Health's new ruling that contraceptive information should be made available through maternal and child welfare centres to those women for whom childbearing would be dangerous.[75] Clearly what was at stake was not only the type of resident the council saw itself as serving, but also the degree to which it was bound by central policy from outside the borough.

Political Influence on the Structure and Funding of Services

Many of the differences of opinion expressed over the services explored above reveal the ways in which political affiliations affected the rhetoric and the priority various groups within each borough accorded to different maternal and child welfare services. Little,

151

however, has been revealed about the impact such politics had on the overall structure and funding of services within each borough. By the early twentieth century, maternal and child welfare services were increasingly funded by the state, most notably in the form of municipal health visitors. State sponsorship of services increased under the Maternal and Child Welfare Act of 1918 which enabled local councils and voluntary institutions to apply for grants to cover up to 50 per cent of the expenditure on maternal and child welfare services such as paid midwives, health visitors, infant welfare centres, day nurseries, and milk and food for necessitous mothers and infants. However, such provision was not made mandatory by the act, which meant that these services varied enormously between councils and regions.[76] Some new schemes were developed under the act, but many of those which did emerge stemmed from voluntary activities of the nineteenth century.[77] Voluntary organizations, often supported by local government grants continued to play a vital role in the provision of maternal and child welfare well into the inter-war period. The degree to which voluntary organizations played a part in the provision of such services, was, however, highly dependent on the precedent for such work in each individual borough, and shaped by their political outlook.

Significantly municipal provision of maternal and child welfare services, particularly infant welfare centres appeared earliest in Woolwich. Part of the strength of municipal services within Woolwich was attributable to the strong representation of the Labour Party on its council from early on. Such services were also essential in an area where very few middle-class residents resided to undertake philanthropic work. Woolwich only had one voluntary maternal and child welfare centre which emerged at the relatively late date of 1914.

By contrast with Woolwich, Stepney had an abundance of voluntary agencies working in the field of maternal and child welfare. This can partly be explained by the weakness of the Labour Party in Stepney in the years before the war, but was more strongly linked to the abundance of voluntary institutions in Stepney which had grown up as a result of the focus of social concern on the East End as a whole. The large presence of Irish and Jewish immigrants also made the area a fertile place for medical missions who offered infant and maternal health care facilities. Added to this were the charitable Jewish and Irish Catholic organizations who provided for their respective poor, such as the Jewish infant welfare centre, the Jewish Maternity Home, and the different Catholic district nursing associations.[78] Equally important in the area was the presence of the large teaching voluntary hospitals such as the London Hospital and the East End Maternity Home. Such an abundance of voluntary agencies rendered the importance of council initiative far less important in Stepney than in Woolwich. These charitable enterprises did not disappear with the rise of the Labour Party in the 1920s, rather they were incorporated into municipal provision. When members of the Carnegie Trust visited Stepney in 1930 with the intention of establishing a large centre for maternal and child welfare, they declared that such an institution was not needed because voluntary and municipal bodies already catered so well for the area.[79]

Table 4.3: Number of women of childbearing age and children 0–4 years as proportion of population in four London boroughs

Borough	Years	Women aged 15–44		Children aged 0–4 years	
		Number	%	Number	%
Hampstead	1901	31,042	38	6,448	7.9
	1911	31,736	37	5,771	6.8
	1921	28,875	33	4,889	5.7
	1935	29,059	32	4,000•	4.4
Kensington	1901	63,628	36	14,148	8.0
	1911	60,921	35	13,105	7.6
	1921	57,081	32	11,572	6.5
	1935	56,859	32	10,414•	5.8
Stepney	1901	71,500	24	39,804	13.3
	1911	66,519	24	35,706	12.7
	1921	61,269	25	24,835	9.9
	1935	58,019	27	16,041•	7.5
Woolwich	1901	26,940	23	13,823	11.8
	1911	28,549	24	12,861	10.6
	1921	34,417	24	13,021	9.2
	1935	35,316	24	9,528•	6.5

• Children aged 0–5 years

Sources: Census for England and Wales (London: 1901–21); 'Before School Age', 1937, Appendix 1, London Council of Social Service Early Publication Box.

As in Stepney, voluntary organizations tended to dominate maternal and child welfare services in both Hampstead and Kensington. The abundance of such voluntary services was largely due to the presence of a large upper and middle class in these boroughs who could sponsor and work for such ventures. In Hampstead the Hampstead Council for Social Welfare was a major promoter of voluntary work in this field. Originally established as the Hampstead Associated Agencies in 1902, and renamed the Hampstead Council for Social Welfare in 1907, this organization provided an administrative body for bringing together independent societies and parish relief programmes, and in later years initiated cooperation between voluntary and state activities. Its aims were to provide representation through standing committees of different agencies involved in the provision of social services through an administrative body, and to coordinate policy. Among the schemes it pioneered were the School Care Committee and in 1913 the first tuberculosis sanatorium in London. In 1911 the Council set up a borough health institute based in Kilburn, which provided an infant welfare centre and a range of other services such as antenatal sessions and the provision of milk for poor mothers and babies.[80] Much of the work of this organization was due to the energy of Thomas Hancock Nunn who actively campaigned for an extension of the council to other parts of the country and helped to establish the National Council for Social Welfare.

Table 4.4: Rateable value per head and rate poundage spent for borough purposes in four London boroughs, 1936–7

Borough	Rateable value per head £	Rate poundage spent for borough purposes £ d
Woolwich	8.0	6 0.3
Stepney	8.3	7 0.3
Hampstead	1 6.8	2 7.0
Kensington	1 8.9	2 3.6

The actual rateable value of the borough is the aggregated sum of the rateable values of each separately rated piece of property. The rateable value is therefore an index to the economic wealth of a borough.

Source: E. C. R. Hadfield and J. E. MacColl, *Pilot Guide to Political London* (London: 1945), 131–2.

No comparable body existed in Kensington, but in 1921 voluntary maternal and child welfare organizations were linked up through the establishment of an Advisory Body, which constituted all the representatives of the voluntary infant welfare centres in the borough. Their task was to coordinate all the different activities undertaken by the infant welfare centres and to advise the borough council of any particular gaps in the provision. Under this body the infant welfare centre came largely to be seen as an extension of the borough council, although they were run by voluntary bodies. Within Kensington it would seem that overall the strength of the Labour Party in North Kensington together with the influence of the suffragette movement in the early years of the twentieth century and the campaigns of individual women such as Ethel Bentham and Margery Spring Rice, gave the borough a different outlook on maternal and child welfare services than might be expected for such a traditionally conservative area.

Table 4.5: Annual expenditure on MCW, shown as a percentage of total expenditure by the borough council

	Hampstead		Kensington		Stepney		Woolwich	
	MCW Expenditure	%	MCW Expenditure	%	MCW Expenditure	%	MCW Expenditure	%
1919/20	£1,880	0.32	£1,960	0.17	£10,658	1.09	£6,325	1.14
1931/2	£5,879	0.73	£12,784	0.78	£19,420	1.42	£17,236	1.87

Source: Local Taxation Returns in Parliamentary Papers.

Table 4.6: Percentage of change in annual expenditure on MCW by four borough councils, 1919–31

	% change 1919–31
Hampstead	+2.13
Kensington	+5.52
Stepney	+0.82
Woolwich	+1.7

Source: Local Taxation Returns in Parliamentary Papers.

Table 4.7: Annual expenditure per child aged 0–4 years in four London boroughs, 1919/20 and 1931/2

	1919/20	1931/2*	% change 1919–32
Hampstead	7s. 6d.	27s. 7d.	+3
Kensington	3s. 3d.	24s. 5d.	+7
Stepney	8s. 5d.	24s. 2d.	+2
Woolwich	9s.	36s. 17d.	+3

* Children aged 0–5 years
Source: Local Taxation Returns in Parliamentary Papers.

It would seem, therefore, that while Woolwich was unusual in its early municipal provision of services, this was counteracted in the other three boroughs by their prolific voluntary services. What differentiated the boroughs more was the level of money each of them committed to services. One difficulty in assessing this question is that much of the information on expenditure ignores the contribution voluntary agencies made in each borough. Such voluntary contributions, however, especially in the case of Stepney, Hampstead and Woolwich played a crucial role in the provision of welfare. Any accurate assessment of the expenditure levels in each borough would need, therefore, to take this into account. Much of this expenditure was locally determined and highly variable and cannot be estimated easily.[81] All that remains is the expenditure accounts left by the municipal authorities. These, however, are important for understanding the level of commitment each borough was willing to make in the form of municipal funding of services.

Table 4.8: Expenditure on MCW and on provision of milk and dinners per child 0–4 years old by 11 London borough councils, 1922–3. List in order of highest estimate set for MCW by each council

Borough Council	MCW		Milk and Dinners	
	Council's estimate	Expenditure approved by MH	Council's estimate	Expenditure approved by MH
1. Shoreditch	£2 1s. 4d.	14s.	£1 8s. 4d.	5s. 4d.
2. Poplar	£1 2s. 4d.	10s. 4d.	15s. 6d.	3s. 8d.
3. St Pancras	£1 2s.	£1 8d.	4s. 2d.	1s. 8d.
4. Woolwich	£1 4d.	12s 6d.	8s. 6d.	2s. 6d.
5. Stepney	17s.	10s. 2d.	9s. 6d.	3s. 2d.
6. Chelsea	16s. 6d.	15s.	4s. 4d.	4s. 4d.
7. Hampstead	13s. 2d.	12s. 6d.	1s. 2d.	1s. 2d.
8. Fulham	13s. 2d.	13s. 2d.	1s. 8d.	1s. 8d.
9. Southwark	10s. 2d.	5s.	4s.	1s. 6d.
10. Hackney	8s. 4d.	8s. 6d.	3s. 4d.	3s. 4d.
11. Kensington	7s.	6s. 8d.	1s. 7d.	1s. 7d.

All sums are based on the total estimates divided by population 0–4 years old.

Sources: Summary of replies received by Shoreditch borough council for the Financial Year 1922–3 to assess the provision of milk supplies. In Stepney MCW Committee, Minutes, 12 June 1922, 75; *Census for England and Wales* (London: 1921), Table 13.

One of the vital determinants of expenditure was the different levels of need that existed in each borough. Stepney which was the poorest of the boroughs, for instance, would be expected to have had a greater demand for services and therefore a higher burden on its expenditure than the more prosperous borough of Hampstead. Similarly we would also anticipate that those areas with a higher number of mothers and children to have had greater expenditure. Table 4.3 indicates that Hampstead and Kensington had more women aged 15 to 44 than the other two boroughs, partly reflecting their very high number of domestic servants. Such a large proportion of women who were of childbearing age, however, did not necessarily result in a high demand for maternal and child welfare services as not all of these women fell pregnant. Children aged between 0 and 4 are a more reliable index of demand for maternal and child welfare. Within this context we can see that Stepney and Woolwich, which had a larger proportion of children aged between 0 and 4 years within their population, reflecting their high birth rates, had a greater demand for maternal and child welfare services than the two other boroughs. Overall, it would seem, therefore, that Stepney had the highest burden on its budget both in terms of its social and economic conditions and its demographic profile, while Hampstead had the least. Added to this was the fact that Stepney also had fewer ratepayers who could afford to subsidize the services. Table 4.4 shows the rateable value per head in Hampstead was double that of Stepney in 1936–7. Thus, while Stepney had a greater demand on its services it had less resources to cope with it.

The level of expenditure was not only determined by the level of need in each area and the resources available, but also by the politics and the policy of the council in each borough, as well as the degree to which voluntary agencies sponsored services. Table 4.4 shows that Woolwich and Stepney, although having a lower rateable value and therefore fewer resources, spent more of their rates on borough services than the richer boroughs of Hampstead and Kensington, indicating a high commitment to municipally funded services.

Such differences were also important within the context of maternal and child welfare. Table 4.5 reveals that while the annual expenditure on maternal and child welfare was increasing in all areas in the years 1919 to 1931, Stepney and Woolwich appear to have spent slightly more of their total budgets on maternal and child welfare from early on than the councils of the two other boroughs. None the less, when viewed over time, the greatest increase in expenditure occurred in Kensington (Table 4.6) and not the poorest boroughs.

The same was true when the expenditure is calculated per child aged 0–4 years (Table 4.7). Such low increases in Stepney and Woolwich, might reflect the fact that expenditure on maternal and child welfare in these two boroughs had started off high in the early 1920s, and Kensington was merely catching up. Other figures from 1922–3 illustrated in Table 4.8 suggest that of 11 councils in London Kensington ranked as the lowest in terms of the expenditure it was willing to spend per head of child not only for maternal and child welfare provision but also for the provision of milk and dinners. Table 4.8 also shows that Kensington had the smallest disparity in the estimated sum put forward by the council and that approved by the Ministry of Health. This discrepancy is difficult to explain, but it might be a reflection of political inertia on the part of the council in these years.

By 1932, however, there had been a very high increase in expenditure within Kensington, which suggests a shift in the attitudes within the borough. Part of the change might have stemmed from the pressure that was mounting in the borough to resolve its very high levels of infant mortality which galvanized many within the borough, whether from conservative or more radical circles, to provide better services. Added to this was the influence of the Labour Party in the north of the borough which was beginning to grow in strength during the years 1902 to 1936 as well as the pressure from particular individuals such as Margery Spring Rice whose campaign for the provision of birth control and establishment of the North Kensington Women's Welfare Centre was important in raising the level of health services in the borough.

A particularly striking feature of the expenditure patterns in the four boroughs, is the remarkably small rise in expenditure within Stepney in the years 1919 and 1932. This phenomenon is puzzling given the inflation in these years as well as the high degree of political commitment within the borough for maternal and child welfare provision. Indeed, as Chapters 5 and 6 show, the provision of services in Stepney was very high in these years. Stepney was also among those boroughs in London who were at the forefront of the campaign against the Ministry of Health's cuts in expenditure on milk and nourishment in the 1920s. Similarly, as Table 4.4 reveals, in 1936 Stepney was spending much more of its rates on borough services than the other boroughs.

One reason for the relative lack of increase in expenditure in Stepney could have been due to the very good voluntary services in the area, which while not accounted for in expenditure tabulations, would have reduced the costs of the Council in providing maternal and child welfare services. Another explanation might be the lack of resources in Stepney which limited its ability to increase spending despite its political commitment to maternal and child welfare. Added to this was the financial hardship many residents in Stepney faced as a result of the economic depression in the late 1920s and early 1930s. To some extent the same was true within Woolwich where the level of expenditure also did not increase substantially. In the case of Woolwich, however, it would seem that the borough apportioned a much greater sum per child than was possible in Stepney, reflecting the smaller proportion of its residents living in poverty, the fewer number of voluntary agencies providing care, and the greater strength of the Labour Party within the council chamber.

Conclusion

As we have seen the political composition of each borough was an important element not only in shaping the perceptions and the values attached to maternal and child welfare provision, but also in determining both the structure and the funding of services. While a sense of national urgency over the military and economic strength of the British nation fuelled a growing demand for greater state provision in health care services in these years, particularly for mothers and their infants, what direction these services were to take and who was to fund them remained a burning question. What was mostly at stake was whose interests were to be preserved. Such an issue was continually being challenged, and was largely determined by the class, gender, and in the case of birth control provision, religious affiliation of those campaigning and providing for welfare provision.

The priority given by each interest-group changed over time, yet there were some perceptible trends between the boroughs. In Hampstead and Kensington the dominance of conservative forces meant that it was the ratepayer rather than the poor who was prioritized. This policy was reflected in the fact that services in these boroughs tended to be dominated by the voluntary sector. By contrast, services in Woolwich were predominantly provided by the local council, reflecting the strength of the Labour Party and the strong trade union movement within the borough. Of all the boroughs it was Stepney which showed the most mixed picture, having a high degree of voluntary and municipally funded services, reflecting the historical tradition of both philanthropy in its area as well as the growing strength of the local Labour Party.

Within the context of expenditure it was those boroughs who were more prosperous and politically conservative who initially showed the most reluctance in spending money on maternal and child welfare services. By the 1930s, however, this seemed to have changed, with these boroughs, particularly Kensington, showing the greatest increase in expenditure. Part of this was merely a phenomenon of these boroughs catching up with the poorer boroughs who had started off with a higher level of expenditure. It also reflected the growing acceptance of municipal provision and the need for greater maternal and child welfare services in the inter-war years. The change in attitude is particularly apparent in the case of Kensington, where persistently high rates of infant mortality pushed residents within the borough to pursue measures they were initially reluctant to undertake. Even so, political will was not the only determinant of expenditure patterns. Much depended on the local resources and need of an area. As the expenditure patterns of Stepney illustrates for the 1930s, the budget apportioned to maternal and child welfare could be severely limited by a lack of resources and a high demand on services.

While the political outlook and social and economic conditions of each area influenced the structure and the funding of services greatly, what this chapter has not revealed is the degree to which this affected the quality and comprehensiveness of the services provided in each area. This is particularly important when considering the effect that such provision had on the standards of health in each borough. What is particularly surprising is that Stepney experienced the greatest decline in infant and maternal mortality. Yet this was the borough which experienced the worst socio-economic conditions and had the scarcest resources to commit to maternal and child welfare. By contrast infant and maternal mortality did not decline as substantially in Kensington, which had more resources and by the 1930s had substantially increased its expenditure on maternal and child welfare. As the following two chapters show, part of the difference between these two boroughs lies in the types of services that were provided and the degree to which such services reached those who were in most need.

Notes

1. *Hampstead and Highgate Advertiser,* 16 June 1917, 3.
2. See for example the speech by Ethel Bentham. When standing as a Labour candidate for the 1910 LCC election, she declared the election to be a struggle between the Labour Party who favoured 'London being governed in the interests of the people generally' and the Municipal Reformers who saw 'the government in the interests of one select class'. She argued that 'the electors had to decide whether they would support those working for the good of a limited class, leaving the others to take their chance'. (*Kensington News and West London Times*, 25 February 1910, 2.)
3. This is a theme also explored in G. Rose, 'Imagining Poplar in the 1920s: Contested Concepts of Community', *J. Hist. Geog.,* 16/4 (1990), 425–37.
4. See Ch. 3.
5. *Kensington News and West London Times,* 17 October 1902, 5.
6. *Kensington News and West London Times,* 24 June 1904, 5; 28 November 1913, 6. Just as the high infant mortality in Kensington was regarded as an anathema to the reputation of the borough, similar feelings arose over the higher death rates found in Kilburn, the poorer part of Hampstead. Hampstead MOH, *A/R* (1906), 36; *Hampstead and Highgate Advertiser,* 5 December 1912, 3.
7. *Kensington News and West London Times,* 4 July 1902, 5; 17 October 1902, 5; 5 November 1907, 6; 9 May 1913, 6. Similar tension emerged over the question of more housing in Kensington just after

the First World War (15 February 1918 and 17 May 1918, 5).

8. Hampstead MOH, *A/R* (1906), 49.

9. D. Dwork, *War is Good for Babies and Other Young Children: A History of the Infant and Child Welfare Movement in England 1898–1918* (London: 1987), 105–7.

10. Milk depots originated from the Goutte de Lait system established in France in the 1890s and had spread to Britain by the turn of the century, the earliest being the St Helens milk depot created in 1899. For more details on milk depots see Dwork, *op. cit.* (note 9), 101–23.

11. Woolwich MOH, *A/R* (1906), 82–3.

12. Woolwich MOH, *A/R* (1908), 149.

13. Woolwich Council Minutes, 23 November 1906, 101.

14. Woolwich MOH, *A/R* (1908), 149.

15. Woolwich Council Minutes, 17 June 1910, 577.

16. This stemmed from the size of the borough, which had made it necessary to either provide several distributing stations or to deliver the milk from house to house. The second option was chosen, because more stations were seen as unsatisfactory. Woolwich MOH, *A/R* (1906), 84–5.

17. Woolwich Council Minutes, 5 July 1905; 23 November 1906, 101; 11 October 1907, 897–8; 9 October 1908, 822–3; 17 June 1910, 576–7; Woolwich MOH, *A/R* (1906), 82–95; (1907), 87–8; (1908), 149–50; (1909), 114–15.

18. R. B. Stucke (ed.), *Fifty Years History of the Woolwich Labour Party 1903–1953* (London: 1953), 14; Woolwich MOH, *A/R* (1910), 108; Woolwich Council Minutes, 15 March 1910, 378.

19. Woolwich MOH, *A/R* (1908), 150.

20. Woolwich Council Minutes, 20 April 1910, 426; 23 May 1910, 454.

21. Woolwich Council Minutes, 17 June 1910, 577–8. The lowest wage found among parents receiving milk from the depot was 21s. a week.

22. In 1907 the medical officer for Woolwich had also stressed the need for a municipally funded and run service, arguing that voluntary depots abroad were far less well organized than the municipally run British ones. (Woolwich Council Minutes, 11 October 1907, 897).

23. Milk depots had also closed in many other areas and this action was justified on similar grounds. Many of the arguments for their closure were reinforced by the fact that the provision of cheap clean milk was increasing on a private basis. Conflicts also arose over whether milk depots were an effective measure. Part of this stemmed from the difficulty of quantifying the effectiveness of the scheme, which was made worse by the fact that only a small proportion of babies were bottle-fed and therefore required such a service. The price that depots charged for milk was also often beyond the pocket of many mothers. (Dwork, *op. cit.* (note 9), 116– 22).

24. Woolwich Council Minutes, 17 June 1910, 582.

25. *The Pioneer,* 2 November 1906. For more information on Alice

Gregory see Ch. 2.

26. Woolwich Council Minutes, 17 June 1910, 582–3.
27. *The Labour Woman,* September 1913, 85; March 1914, 177. The clinic is also discussed in detail in Ch. 8.
28. *Ibid.,* March 1914, 177; March 1915, 1.
29. For more information on this policy see Ch. 5.
30. *The Labour Woman,* September 1913, 1/5, 85.
31. *Ibid.,* March 1914, 177; *Kensington News and West London Times,* 28 November 1913, 6; 20 February 1914, 6.
32. For more information of Bentham see Ch. 2.
33. *The Labour Woman,* March 1914, 177; *Kensington News and West London Times,* 28 November 1913, 6; and 20 February 1914, 6.
34. This consisted of five infant welfare centres as well as hospital provision. For more information on such voluntary provision within Kensington see Ch. 5.
35. M. Llewelyn Davies, *Maternity, Letters from Working Women* (London: 1915, repr. 1978); P. Thane, 'Visions of Gender in the Making of the Welfare State: The Case of Women in the British Labour Party and Social Policy, 1906–45', in G. Bock and P. Thane (eds), *Maternity and Gender Policies: Women and the Rise of European Welfare States, 1880s–1950s* (London: 1991); Dwork, *op. cit.* (note 9), 215.
36. *Kensington News and West London Times,* 5 November 1907, 6; 4 July 1902 5; 9 May 1913, 6.
37. *The Labour Woman,* November 1921, 171; J. Lewis, *The Politics of Motherhood: Child and Maternal Welfare in England, 1900–1939* (London: 1980), 173.
38. *The Labour Woman,* 1 January 1922, 3. A similar argument surfaced in the Co-operative Societies local newspapers in 1934, in an article declaring the National Government to be robbing poor mothers and infants of vital food, while squandering money on defence. Referring to the high rates of maternal mortality, the article claimed, 'the lives of our mothers are being sacrificed to "economy"'. (*Hampstead Citizen,* December 1934, 3). See also C. Kenner, 'The Politics of Married Working Class Women's Health Care in Britain, 1918– 39', unpub. M.Phil, Sussex, 1979, 91. Traditionally historians have argued that the inter-war years were a period which witnessed a national cut and not an increase in military expenditure. Part of this can be attributed to the inflated figures in defence expenditure in the years immediately following the First World War, which stood in contrast to the lower sums spent in the inter-war years. Yet while anger on the part of the Labour movement at the cuts in milk expenditure and the rise in finance for defence would appear to be more of a propaganda exercise than based in reality, recent research has shown that rather than cutting down on defence, the government was making the highest investment in military technology and defence in the world during the inter-war years. See D. Edgerton,

'Liberal Militarism and the British State', *New Left Review,* 185 (1991), 138–69, 149–50. One example of this increase can be seen from the total naval expenditure on armaments and other warlike items such as new warships in the 1920s which rose from £11.8 million in 1923–4 to £16 million in 1926–7. See A. Peacock and J. Wiseman, *The Growth of Public Expenditure in the UK* (Oxford: 1961), 170. This contrasts with what was going on in expenditure for maternal and infant welfare.

39. Hampstead MOH, *A/R* (1921), 75; *Hampstead and Highgate Advertiser,* 20 September 1922, 5.

40. For an analysis of the financial relationship between central and local government funding of maternal and infant welfare and the tight rein that the central government kept on local councils see Kenner, *op. cit.* (note 38), 91–2.

41. Lewis, *op. cit.* (note 37), 173.

42. *Ibid.,* 174–7; C. Webster, 'The Healthy or Hungry Thirties?', *Hist. Workshop. J.,* 13 (1982), 110–29.

43. Limited by what it could do the council turned to the Boards of Guardians to cooperate in a scheme which would enable necessitous mothers with children under 5 years of age to claim dried milk from welfare centres in the borough alongside parish relief. Stepney MCW Committee Minutes, 2 October 1928, 48, 58 (THL file 1086).

44. See for instance Dr Mary Kidd's comments in Hampstead MOH, *A/R* (1933), 3.

45. *Hampstead and Highgate Advertiser,* 26 December 1931, 5.

46. C. Collins, 'Women and Labour Politics in Britain, 1893– 32', unpub. Ph.D., LSE, 1991, 281–2.

47. *The Labour Woman,* 1 March 1924, 34.

48. For a more detailed description of the aims and motives of Eugenicists and Neo-Malthusians and the work of the Malthusian League see C. Usborne, *The Politics of the Body in Weimar Germany: Women's Reproductive Rights and Duties* (London: 1992), 4–8; and R. A. Soloway, *Birth Control and the Population Question in England, 1877–1930* (London: 1982).

49. R. Hall (ed.), *Dear Dr Stopes, Sex in the 1920s* (London: 1978, 1981), 59; R. Hall, *Marie Stopes: A Biography* (London: 1978), 193, 197–241; and B. Brookes, *Abortion in England 1900–1967* (Oxford: 1988), 63.

50. *Report of the Conference on the Giving of Information by Public Health Authorities* (April 1930), (Fawcett Library File: 362.82).

51. Many within the Labour Party blamed the government's reluctance to make such provision on their fear that it would create a shortage of soldiers. (*The Labour Woman,* 1 July 1925, 123; 1 March 1926, 88).

52. Soloway, *op. cit.* (note 48), 284, 296. The risks associated with abortion and the lack of birth control were not only espoused by Labour women, but also men. See *Kensington Citizen,* July 1937, 1.

Health professionals were also making these arguments. In 1928 the County MOH for the LCC reported, 'If no woman had borne children after the age of 35 in the period 1911–21 the total births would have been lessened by 20.3%, but the maternal deaths would have been reduced by as much as 34%. Thus birth control may have a considerable effect upon maternal mortality rates.' (NKWWC, *A/R* (1928–9), 5). For more information on the maternal mortality and abortion see Ch. 3.

53. Collins, *op. cit.* (note 46), 281–2; J. Lewis, *Women in England 1870–1950* (Brighton: 1984; 1986), 32; Lewis, *op. cit.* (note 37), 196–200; A. McClaren, *Birth Control in 19th Century England* (London: 1978), 61, 215–18; Letter from Isabel Peterkin to Lucy, 15 October 1976, in papers relating to Mary Middleton and Margaret MacDonald Baby Clinic and Hospital (National Museum of Labour History, Box BAB 429).

54. *The Labour Woman,* 1 May 1924; 1 October 1926, 151. For a fuller discussion of the conflict over birth control within the Labour Party see Collins, *op. cit.* (note 46), 281–90. One of the key issues that was at stake within the party was how much importance the party should attach to decisions made by its organized women.

55. N. E. Himes, 'The Present Status of Birth Control in England', unpub. MSS., 4, Countway Library, BMS C77 Box 85 fo. 903.

56. NKWWC, *A/R* (1935–6). For similar arguments made by Stopes see D. A. Cohen, 'Private Lives and Public Spaces: Marie Stopes, The Mothers' Clinics and the Practice of Contraception', *Hist. Workshop J.,* 35 (1993), 95–116.

57. National Birth Control Association, *A/R* (1936–7), 4.

58. Although initially tied to the Malthusian League, the Society quickly broke away and became an autonomous organization which was able to adopt more popular measures in promoting birth control than the Malthusian League had achieved. The Society was more committed to solving practical problems in family limitation and less tied to the Neo-Malthusian ideology than the League. The first clinic established by the Society for the Provision of Birth Control was the Walworth Centre in South London in 1921. Although initially conducted like a maternal and child welfare centre, in the absence of state funding, the Walworth Centre was forced to rely on voluntary contributions and concentrated its efforts on birth control provision. By 1929 the Society had ten clinics around the country, three of which were in London. In 1926 a clinic had been opened in Burdett Road in Stepney. See Society for the Provision of Birth Control Clinics, *A/R* (1928–9), 5; E. H. Martyn and M. Bird, *The Birth Control Movement* (London: 1930), 18; Soloway, *op. cit.* (note 48), 192–5.

59. For more detail on this clinic see Ch. 7.

60. Ethel Bentham, for instance, opposed such provision on the grounds that it was oppressive to women, and argued that it should not be

included within the remit of MCW centres. See Letter from Isabel Peterkin to Lucy, 15 October 1976, in papers relating to Mary Middleton and Margaret MacDonald Baby Clinic and Hospital (National Museum of Labour History, Box BAB 429). See also Collins, *op. cit.* (note 46), 283.

61. Soloway, *op. cit.* (note 48), 259, 291.

62. *Kensington News and West London Times,* 3 November 1922, 3; 23 October 23 1925, 5; *North Kensington Citizen,* December 1931. Pennefather was elected in Pembridge Ward in 1922.

63. Soloway, *op. cit.* (note 48), 298.

64. Kensington Council Minutes, 27 July 1926, 359; 6 March 1934, 164.

65. Stepney MCW Committee Minutes, 14 April 1931, 38.

66. Lewis, *op. cit.* (note 53), 33.

67. 'Kensington Public Health Survey', 1932; letters between Kensington Council and MH, 25 February 1931; 17 March 1931; 24 February 1931; 15 April 1931; 13 February 1934 (PRO file MH 52/177); Kensington Council Minutes, MCW Committee, 24 February 1931, 183; 6 March 1934, 165–6; 24 July 1934, 346–7.

68. Notes from Deputation to MH from NKWWC, 1 June 1934 (PRO file: MH 52/177).

69. *North Kensington Citizen,* July 1937, 1.

70. Notes from Deputation to MH from NKWWC, 1 June 1934 (PRO file: MH 52/177).

71. The Union of Catholic Mothers organized classes on a local level to explain the evils of birth control to mothers as well as health professionals such as nurses, midwives, nuns and lay-folk who visited mothers in their homes and in hospitals. (M. M. Thornely, 'A Record of the Catholic Women's League. Union of Catholic Mothers', 19 May 1935, 19 (WDA file: Hi 2/95)).

72. *Magazine of the Sacred Heart,* September 1925, v–vi. See also *The Tablet,* 9 April 1921, 475; 5 August 1922, 187; 28 October 1922, 579; 29 November 1924, 701; 13 December 1924, 812–13.

73. Stepney MCW Committee Minutes, 15 March 1927, 308.

74. *Ibid.,* 19 February 1929, 63.

75. *Ibid.,* 14 April 1931, 38.

76. For more information on the development of the Maternity and Child Welfare Act and what it provided for see F. Honigsbaum, *The Struggle for the Ministry of Health* (London: 1970) and *The Division in British Medicine* (London: 1979); and Lewis, *op. cit.* (note 37), 34;

77. F. Prochaska, 'A Mother's Country: Mothers' Meetings and Family Welfare in Britain, 1850–1950', *Hist.,* 74 (1989), 379– 99; A. Summers, 'A Home from Home – Women's Philanthropic Work in the Nineteenth Century', in S. Burman (ed.), *Fit Work for Women* (London: 1979).

78. L. Marks, 'Irish and Jewish Women's Experience of Childbirth and

Infant Care', D.Phil., Oxford, 1990, especially Chs 4 and 8.

79. Stepney MOH, *A/R* (1930), 85.

80. M. Moore, 'Social Work and Social Welfare: The Organization of Philanthropic Resources in Britain, 1900–1914', *J. Br. Stud.*, 16 (1977), 85–104, 98–102; *Hampstead and Highgate Advertiser*, 26 June 1937; COS *A/R of Councils and District Committees:* HCSW 1917 (GLRO file: A/FWA/B2/47), 36; HCSW, *Biannual Report of the Executive* 1921–2 (NCVO archive).

81. This difficulty is highlighted by Lee in his analysis of local authority expenditure patterns in the inter-war years. His article provides crucial information on municipal expenditure patterns in welfare provision for this period. See R. Lee, 'Uneven Zenith: Towards a Geography of the High Period of Municipal Medicine in England and Wales', *J. Hist. Geog.*, 14/3 (1988), 260–80, 275.

5

Infant Health and Welfare Services

Today politicians constantly argue about the efficiency and quality of the National Health Service, questioning the degree to which it reaches those most in need and the effect it has on their overall health. Much of the controversy has been shaped by arguments about how we can measure the effectiveness of such care. All too often the outcome of treatment and its overall impact on the health of the population are lost in struggles over the length of waiting lists and the measures needed to ensure economy and efficiency.

Similarly fierce battles raged over maternal and child welfare services in the earlier part of the century, and have continued to be the subject of much historical debate. Some historians see these facilities as influential in the decline of infant mortality. Others argue such measures were largely ineffective in coping with the greater problems of social and economic deprivation that were the real ravagers of health.[1] While historians may not agree on the relative importance of the maternal and child welfare services, their work has shown the complexities involved in assessing the facilities provided and the need for caution in singling out one factor as an explanation for the decline in infant and maternal mortality. In this and the next chapter I examine these complexities, firstly exploring the range of services that were provided for infants and mothers in the years 1902–36, and then the impact that they had on health standards.

By the 1930s many medical experts and politicians were proudly trumpeting the achievements that had been undertaken in the facilities they had helped to establish. They argued these services had improved infant and maternal health. This chapter concentrates on those facilities which were available for the care of the infant, the physical location of which can be seen alongside other services in each borough in Appendices 1 to 4. A wide range of services were provided, but in this chapter I focus on health visiting and infant welfare centres, which were among the first and most prominent services provided for infants in these years. Both of these services had their origins in the early twentieth century, but experienced an unprecedented increase in the First World War. Between 1914 and 1918 the number of health visitors employed by local authorities more than quadrupled, and the number of infant welfare centres doubled, and similar expansions had also happened in the voluntary sector. By 1936 health visiting was the one service which was uniformly provided all over the country, with infant welfare centres being the next most widely provided service.

The health visiting service and infant welfare centres shared the common aim of curbing infant mortality, but they differed greatly in the nature of their work. Infant welfare centres, for instance, tended to be more reliant on mothers and infants coming to them for their services, while health visitors, because they paid visits to people in their own homes could be seen as much more involved with the local community as well as potentially more invasive. While Chapter 7 considers what impact this had on the perceptions of those who came into contact with these two different services, this chapter looks at the type of services offered by them and their overall effectiveness.

One of the key questions asked in this chapter and the next one is to whom the services were directed and how far they met their target. In all the boroughs maternal and child welfare services were primarily directed towards those who could not afford to purchase their own health care. Part of this stemmed from a compassionate desire to help the more unfortunate, but it was also bound up with national concerns about infant and maternal mortality. One of the reasons that the poor were targeted for maternal and child welfare provision was the fact that they experienced the highest rates of infant mortality. While many politicians and reformers acknowledged that such mortality could be attributed to socio-economic deprivation, others were quick to place the blame on the poor themselves. Ignorance, apathy, alcoholism and wilful neglect were often cited as the reasons for the high infant mortality among the poor.[2]

Infant mortality, therefore, was closely tied to particular assumptions about the poor and to the idea that it was the fault of the parents, particularly the mother. The only remedy was to inculcate self-help and eradicate ignorance. For this reason many of the maternal and child welfare services, particularly infant welfare centres and health visitors, were aimed at educating poor mothers in good child-rearing practices, domestic skills and thrift. This emphasis often took precedence over providing actual medical treatment. Many medical professionals argued that wealthy mothers needed just as much instruction as poor mothers, but it was generally assumed that these mothers could not be imposed upon in the same way as their poorer sisters, for fear of causing offence. What was at stake was the degree to which the state and its officials could interfere in what were seen as primarily private family matters.

Middle-class mothers, however, did not escape scrutiny. As infant mortality declined and increasing attention turned to maternal mortality, which was shown to be high among all social classes of women, maternal and child welfare began to be directed towards a larger proportion of the population. This is not to say comprehensive free medical and welfare provision was available to all women and their children by 1936. Means tests continued to play an important part in all the services provided, whether it be to purchase food supplements at a maternal and child welfare clinic or to gain access to a maternity hospital bed.

The Comprehensiveness of Maternal and Child Welfare Services

The continuance of means tests in the provision of services raises important questions about the degree to which maternal and child welfare services were provided on a comprehensive basis. By the 1930s it had become common for many politicians and medical experts to highlight maternal and child welfare services as among the most comprehensive and widely spread of the health services in the country. The Maternal and Child Welfare Act of 1918, for instance, was viewed, as one medical expert George McCleary put it, as 'the most important landmarks' in the development of maternal and child welfare services. Under this act the Local Government Board could cover up to 50 per cent of the expenditure incurred by local authorities in providing health services for expectant and nursing mothers, and children up to the age of five. The model the Local Government Board envisaged for maternal and child welfare services covered 12 main areas ranging from the provision of food and milk, to nursing and medical care (see Table 5.1). From this it would indeed seem that a comprehensive maternal and child welfare service had come into being. Expenditure on maternal and child welfare by the Local Government Board also grew phenomenally in these years, rising from £11,000 in 1915 to £218,000 in 1919.[3] Such a growth in expenditure continued into the inter-war years and as Chapter 4 has shown was occurring on a local as well as a national level.[4]

169

It would be a mistake, however, to herald the Maternal and Child Welfare Act as a watershed in the history of maternal and child welfare provision. Under the Act local authorities were not compelled to provide such services, with the result that some authorities made better provision than others. As Peretz has shown in the case of Tottenham, Oxford, Oxfordshire, and Merthyr Tydfil, the degree to which the Maternal and Child Welfare Act was put into action was highly dependent on local interpretation and policy making.[5]

Table 5.1: LGB model of MCW services to be provided by local authorities, 1918

1. Health visiting
2. Infant welfare centres
3. Food and milk for expectant mothers, and infants and young children
4. Service of trained midwives
5. Doctor to assist midwives in cases of emergency
6. Nurses to cater for illnesses of pregnancy and confinement and diseases suffered by infants and children
7. Hospital accommodation for acute illness connected with pregnancy, confinement and infancy
8. Maternity homes and homes for infants suffering from malnutrition and other comparable complaints not usually admitted to hospital
9. Convalescent homes for women after confinement and for infants and young children and rest homes for expectant mothers in certain cases
10. Accommodation and assistance for children of widowed, deserted or unmarried mothers
11. Day nurseries for children of women forced to go out to work
12. Home helps to undertake housework and childcare for women during their confinement

Source: G. F. McCleary, *The Maternity and Child Welfare Movement* (London: 1935), 21–2.

Years after the Maternal and Child Welfare Act was put into effect, a committee, set up in 1934 to investigate the persisting problem of maternal mortality, indicated wide variation in the types of services provided by local authorities around the country. The Committee's findings included county councils in rural areas, county boroughs in urban places, and the metropolitan boroughs of London. When viewing the services overall, the councils in London appear to have provided a greater range of services than elsewhere. According to the Committee, 22 out of 28, or 79 per cent of the metropolitan boroughs had put 'into force half or more of the services they have power to provide'. This compared with 72 per cent of the county boroughs and only 47 per cent of county councils. The Committee concluded that while some local authorities were utilizing their powers to a very large degree, usually to provide the more important and fundamental services, none of them were using them entirely.[6] Summing up their findings the Committee indicated that there had been a definite improvement in the services in most parts of the country since 1918, but that further advances were needed in the quality and comprehensiveness of the care offered.

It is the quality and comprehensiveness of the services provided in the four boroughs of Hampstead, Kensington, Stepney and Woolwich that is the focus of this and the next chapter. While metropolitan councils tended to provide more maternal and child welfare facilities than councils in other parts of the country, these services were not uniform. Much of this variation was due to their differing needs and the priorities of their local authorities, as well as the historical development of voluntary services in each area.

Health Visiting, 1890s–1930s

One of the first measures undertaken in maternal and child welfare was the provision of health visitors. The original appointment of health visitors grew out of the voluntary sanitary visiting schemes initiated by the Manchester and Salford Sanitary Reform Association in 1862. In 1892 Buckinghamshire County Council became the first local authority to employ a full-time health visitor. This move caught on quickly and by 1905 health visitors were working in at least 50 towns or rural districts in Britain.[7] By 1914 there were 470 salaried health visitors at work in 195 different localities; of these 350 were paid entirely out of the rates, 38 partly out of the rates, and 82 drew their salary from a philanthropic organization cooperating with the local authority.[8] Health visitors continued to be the 'bedrock' of maternal and child welfare services after the war. Of the grants for maternal and child welfare made by the Minister of Health in 1919–20 31 per cent was allocated to health visiting.[9]

Like everywhere else, health visiting in Hampstead, Kensington, Stepney and Woolwich grew out of sanitary inspection schemes which had been developed in these boroughs in the 1890s.[10] Of the four boroughs, Hampstead was the earliest to appoint a health visitor, who started work in 1902. Woolwich and Kensington followed suit in 1904 and 1905 respectively. In all three boroughs these health visitors were employed by the council, but their work was supplemented by voluntary workers. By contrast, Stepney Council provided a health visitor relatively late despite numerous attempts by the Public Health Committee to have them appointed from 1902. Instead the employment of health visitors in Stepney was left to a voluntary organization which sponsored a health visitor for five years.[11] Only in 1909 was the first council health visitor appointed. Such a move partly stemmed from the fact that in 1908 the London County Council (General Powers) Act empowered London authorities to appoint health visitors through the financial support of the Local Government Board.[12] Although slow to provide municipal health visitors, Stepney rapidly developed a large network of health visitors, both voluntary and municipal. By 1935 Stepney had 11 municipal and 15 voluntary health visitors, which was a much larger number than the other boroughs (Table 5.2).

Table 5.2: Number of health visitors and number of births and children 0–4 years per health visitor, 1911–35

Borough	Date	Number of health visitors	Births		Children 0–4yrs	
			Total	per health visitor[1]	Total	per health visitor
Hampstead	1911	2	1,276	638	5,771	3,244
	1921	3	1,342	447	4,899	1,633
	1935	4·	911	228	4,000	1,000
Kensington	1911	2	3,223	1,612	14,148	6,552
	1921	7*	3,237	462	13,105	1,653
	1935	8	2,241	280	11,572	1,301
Stepney	1911	1	8,464	8,464	39,804	39,804
	1921	12	6,169	514	35,706	2,069
	1935	26·[2]	3,027	116	24,835	616
Woolwich	1911	3†	2,814	938	12,861	4,287
	1921	7	3,197	456	13,021	1,860
	1935	11	2,053	186	9,528	866

• In addition to the 4 health visitors, a woman sanitary inspector also did health visiting 40% of her time. This meant that each health visitor had less than 250 births to cover.

* 9 health visitors were employed by the council, but only 7 were directly concerned with visiting mothers and infants.

† This included 2 women sanitary inspectors and 1 unpaid health visitor.

•1 Births per health visitor is used to indicate the potential number of young infants visited by the health visitor.

•2 This included 11 municipal health visitors and 15 voluntary ones.

Sources: Hampstead, Kensington, Stepney and Woolwich MOH, *A/Rs* (1911–35); 'Kensington Public Health Survey', 1932, 12 (MH66/359); *Census for England and Wales* (London: 1911 and 1921); London Council for Social Services, Early Publications Box, Leaflet 'Before School Age', 1937, Appendix.

The increasing number of health visitors in the four boroughs as shown in Table 5.2 indicates the growing acceptance in the voluntary and municipal sectors of the importance of maternal and child welfare work, of which health visiting formed a vital component. The duties expected of the health visitors covered three main areas. Firstly, they were to visit the homes of the poor and give advice on matters of home hygiene, proper feeding and the clothing of infants. Secondly, they were to visit houses in districts where infectious diseases were prevalent and to educate the relatives on how to care for them. Finally, they were expected to report any insanitary conditions to the medical officer of health.[13] In later years, health visitors increasingly became linked to the work of infant welfare centres, acting as crucial liaison figures between the centre and mothers at home. After 1918 health visitors also began to visit and supervise antenatal cases. Whether caring for infants, toddlers, or mothers, the primary role of the health visitor was an educative one.

The extent to which health visitors could achieve all these aims depended on their case load. According to the Local Government Board in 1917 every borough was to have one health visitor for every 500 births occurring annually (reduced to 400 in 1918).[14] From Table 5.2 it would appear that by 1921 in all the boroughs the number of cases per health visitor was just above the maximum set by the Local Government Board in 1918, with Stepney having the highest load. In all four boroughs each health visitor had to cover a very large number of births and children between the ages of 0–4 years old, especially in the years before the 1920s. The number of births and toddlers per health visitor went down as the number of total births decreased over the years and the number of children aged 0–4 declined. It was this reduction in the number of births and children, rather than the appointment of extra health visitors which lessened the load on each health visitor, particularly in the years 1921 to 1935. The one exception to this was in Stepney where the number of health visitors more than doubled, corresponding with a sharp drop in the number of births and children per health visitor. Whatever the reasons the reduction in the case load per health visitor suggests that the number of hours a health visitor could spend with each person increased between 1911 and 1935. This contraction in cases potentially allowed the health visitor more time to chat and find out the needs of each mother and her child, and indicate where to go for help.

Table 5.3: Number and percentage of all infants under 1 year receiving at least one visit from a health visitor in four London boroughs, 1908–38

Borough	Date	Number of infants visited once by a health visitor	Number of infants receiving a visit by the health visitor as % of total births in borough
Hampstead	1921–2	2,012	77
	1924–5	1,659	73
	1926–30	3,975	78
	1931–5	4,144	87
	1936–8	2,480	79
Kensington•	1921–5	10,638	69
	1926–30	9,084	69
	1931–5	8,679	76
	1936–8	4,831	73
Stepney	1912–15	8,914	28
	1921–5	21,036	89
	1926–30	20,717	92
	1931–5	17,611	101
Woolwich*	1908–10	8,863	60
	1911–15	6,392	45••
	1918–20	5,563	62
	1921–5	12,651	89
	1926–9	8,451	91
	1931–5	9,786	97

Figures for Hampstead and Kensington for 1911–15 are unavailable.

• Up to 1930 all numbers of infants receiving at least 1 visit from the health visitor in Kensington refer to infants under 21 days. These included after 1930 all infants under 1 years old.

* All births visited by the health visitor in Woolwich were those classified as notified births.

•• The drop in the number for this period might be a reflection of World War I which interrupted services and displaced many residents.

Sources: Hampstead, Kensington, Stepney and Woolwich MOH, *A/Rs* (1906–38).

Health visitors were not expected to attend all young infants and children within the borough. In all the boroughs the work of health visitors was directed primarily towards the poorest mothers and children. In Kensington in 1909, health visitors tended to visit those families whose incomes were less than 40s. a week, which covered a large proportion of its poor residents.[15] Those mothers who had the financial means to purchase the care of a general practitioner, a monthly nurse, or a nanny, were not seen as needing the advice and help of a health visitor.[16] We might, therefore, expect, that a larger number of infants were covered by health visitors in an area where there was a high level of poverty. Table 5.3 indicates that by the 1920s the percentage of infants visited by a health visitor out of the total number of births was higher in poorer boroughs like Woolwich and Stepney, than in Kensington and Hampstead where there were larger numbers of rich residents. In 1926–30, for instance, the percentage of infants visited in Woolwich was 91 per cent while in Kensington it was 69 per cent.

From Table 5.3 we can see that the proportion of infants visited by health visitors increased substantially in the years following the First World War. This increase was most perceptible in the case of Stepney which jumped from 28 to 89 per cent. None the less, while the overall proportion of infants was growing in all the boroughs, such evidence tells us little about the success of the health visitors in reaching those they most wanted to target. It is difficult to measure the degree to which this was achieved because maternal and child welfare workers usually did not separate out the numbers of infants and mothers that they regarded as suitable for attention from the overall births within the borough.

Only in Kensington were the figures for the targeted population recorded, but this is unusual. These figures were drawn together to gauge the number of births that were suitable for attention by infant welfare centres in different parts of the borough, and give us some idea of the extent to which mothers and infants were seen as in need of help within a particular area. This is especially interesting in the case of Kensington, which, as already highlighted in previous chapters, had a very high level of poverty as well as prosperity, resulting in differing levels of need. From Table 5.4 we can see that despite the prosperity of the borough, between 75 and 80 per cent of the total births in Kensington were seen as suitable for welfare attention.[17] Of these births, a very large proportion received attention from a health visitor. Indeed, while the overall percentage of infants visited by a health visitor never reached more than 76 per cent of the total births in the borough in 1931–5, among the targeted births the percentage was much greater at 97 (Tables 5.3 and 5.4). The difference in the proportion of births visited by health visitors between the total births and those designated for welfare attention is not surprising, but it does indicate that in the case of Kensington, health visitors reached a high number of infants and mothers they specifically targeted. One of the most interesting aspects to Table 5.4 is the very high escalation in the percentage of mothers visited by health visitors in the early 1930s. This increase might be a reflection of the growth in poverty in Kensington in these years resulting from the economic recession, which made many mothers and infants more reliant on municipal services. The absence of similar material from elsewhere unfortunately makes it difficult to see how the procedure of targeting within Kensington compared with the other boroughs.

Table 5.4: Number and percentage of births designated as suitable for welfare attention in Kensington, with the number of expectant mothers and infants visited once by a health visitor and attending an infant welfare centre shown as a percentage of births designated as suitable for welfare attention, 1921–38

Date	Births designated as suitable for welfare attention		Number visited by health visitor as % of births suitable for welfare attention		Number attending an IWC as % of births suitable for welfare attention	
	Number	% of total borough births	Infants	Expectant mothers	Infants	Expectant mothers
1921–5	11,654	76	91	14	78	17
1926–30	9,831	75	92	31	90	25
1931–5	8,989	78	97	91	126•	40
1936–8	5,276	80	92	–	–	72

• The proportion being more than a 100 per cent might be a reflection of multiple births, or of individual infants who were recorded more than once. This is also true for the other percentages over a 100 recorded in other tables.

Source: Kensington MOH, *A/Rs*, (1921–38).

The success of a health visitor's work, however, was not only dependent on paying a call. As Chapter 7 shows the degree to which a mother could absorb the health visitor's advice depended greatly not only on the attitude of the health visitor towards her client, but also on the material circumstances of the mother. Another of the most important determinants was the time a health visitor could spend with a mother and whether any subsequent calls were made. As the Local Government Board pointed out in 1916 to the Woolwich council, improvements in 'home conditions and infant care' could only 'be secured by repeated and frequent visits'.[18]

Health visitors made return visits in all the boroughs, paying particular attention to those they saw in most need of help. In 1909 health visitors in Kensington tended to pay their visits to infants between 10 and 20 days after the birth. The mother was left with an instruction card and a second follow-up visit was made 3 months later to ascertain whether the mother had carried out the instructions.[19] Those revisited tended to be those who were regarded as more ignorant and inexperienced, and where homes were seen to be more dirty and neglected.[20] The number of visits increased over the years. By 1926 the health visitor called upon those infants who were seen as suitable for revisiting (usually between 25 and 50 per cent of those initially visited) at least three times within the first 4 months. Another visit was paid as soon as the child was 6 months old and another at 12 months. After this follow-up visits were left to the discretion of the health visitor.[21] Such policies were also followed in other boroughs. In addition to attending infants, health visitors in Kensington also visited a child three times during his or her second year, and where practical, two visits were made during the third and fourth years and one in the fifth year.[22]

Nevertheless, despite the increasing number of visits a child received over the years there was no guarantee that this had a significant impact on the health of those that were visited. One problem in North Kensington, for instance, which hampered the work of the health visitors was the 'large floating or migrant population' which was 'continually moving in and out of the borough' and which 'rendered it difficult for the health visitors to keep all families under adequate supervision'. In order to catch those who had moved the health visitors had to allot a 'certain time to the systematic house-to-house visiting of the streets in their area in search for children who were unknown to them'. This process was often time-consuming and not always rewarding. In 1937, 102 streets were visited with 3,574 houses investigated; resulting in 27 infants and 223 toddlers being added to the list for supervision, a success rate of about 7 per cent per household.[23]

Infant Welfare Centres, 1906–36

Initially health visitors were the backbone of maternal and child welfare services, but their supervision and teaching of mothers was soon supplemented by the establishment of infant welfare centres. Originally known as Babies' Welcomes and Schools for Mothers, many of these centres derived their activities from the mothers' meetings held in the nineteenth century. The first centre appeared in St Marylebone in 1906 under the direction of Dr Eric Pritchard. A year later the St Pancras School for Mothers was created. By 1911 there were a hundred such centres, and the following year a National Association of Maternal and Child Welfare Centres was created. The majority of centres were voluntary, but by 1913, 27 of them were supplementing their income by grants from the Board of Education. When in 1914 the government began to fund maternal and child welfare on a national basis, infant welfare centres also began to receive financial support from the Local Government Board.[24] Between 1915 and 1918 the number of infant welfare centres grew from 650 to 12,787, most of the increase being attributable to institutions established by local authorities.[25]

Table 5.5: Number of infant welfare centres and number of births covered by each centre in four London boroughs, 1915 and 1935

| | Number of infant welfare centres | | | | Number of births per IWC* | |
| | 1915 | | 1935 | | 1915 | 1935 |
	Council	Voluntary	Council	Voluntary		
Hampstead	–	3	–	8	442	114
Kensington	–	5	1	7	615	280
Stepney	–	6	7	9	1,251	189
Woolwich	1	–	8	–	2,815	256

* Calculated by dividing the total number of births in the borough by the number of infant welfare centres.

Source:s E. W. Hope and J. Campbell, *Report on the Physical Welfare of Mothers and Children: England and Wales*, 1 (London: 1917), 290, 300, 378 and 424: Hampstead, Kensington, Stepney and Woolwich MOH, *A/Rs* (1935); London Council for Social Services, Early Publications Box, Leaflet 'Before School Age', 1937, Appendix 1.

Table 5.5 reveals that by 1935, with the exception of Hampstead, all of the boroughs in the study had experienced a large growth in municipally funded infant welfare centres. This contrasted with the situation in 1915 when nearly all of the infant welfare centres in the boroughs, except in the case of Woolwich, were voluntary. Such a growth in municipally run centres reflects the increasing recognition that the success of maternal and child welfare could not rest on voluntary funds alone. This attitude, however, was not universally shared.[26] By 1935, for instance, Stepney and Woolwich had a far greater number of municipal centres than the two other boroughs, partly reflecting the existence of Labour Councils in these two boroughs. As discussed in the previous chapter, Labour Councils were more willing to endorse public expenditure on maternal and child welfare than the more conservative councils in Kensington and Hampstead. By 1935 all of the infant welfare centres in Hampstead were organized by the voluntary body, the Hampstead Council of Social Welfare. Similarly, all but one of the centres in Kensington were voluntary.

It is difficult to judge whether the source of income, whether it be voluntary or municipal, affected the quality of the service provided. Much depended on the coordination of the infant welfare centres with other bodies in the borough. In Kensington, the strength of the voluntary sector does not seem to have undermined the efficiency of the service, partly because a centralized voluntary advisory committee was set up to coordinate maternal and child welfare provision under the auspices of the borough council. A survey of the maternal and child welfare services in Kensington in the 1930s indicated very good coordination between the voluntary centres and other services run by the council, particularly health visitors.[27]

By contrast, in Hampstead where the Hampstead Council for Social Welfare kept a tight hold on particular maternal and child welfare services such as infant welfare centres, cooperation with the borough council was poor. This policy partly stemmed from the fact that Hancock Nunn, the leader of the Hampstead Council for Social Welfare, was opposed to the municipalization of such services. In 1933 a report revealed that there was practically no coordination between the work of infant welfare centres run by the Hampstead Council for Social Welfare and health visitors. Until 1920 health visitors were not even allowed into infant welfare centres.[28] Although they were let into the centres in that year they were forbidden to receive mothers at the infant welfare centres (run by Hampstead Council for Social Welfare) and were not allowed to advise them, or to select particular cases for the doctor. All they were expected to do was sit at the doctor's table to take note on every serious case, which, as the report pointed out, 'was a serious waste of time'.[29] While no explicit reason was given for why health visitors were so restricted in their contact with such centres, it might have stemmed from the fact they were a municipally funded service which Hancock Nunn and the Hampstead Council for Social Welfare adamantly opposed.

In Stepney and Woolwich, relations between the council and voluntary initiatives were more harmonious. While in all the boroughs the degree to which infant welfare centres were integrated with other maternal and child welfare services depended on co-operation between voluntary and municipal agencies, individual centres usually ran their own services. Even in Hampstead it was pointed out that the centres in themselves were well organized.[30]

Whether run on a voluntary basis or by the local council, the overall purpose of the centres was the same. Unlike the health visitors, whose objective was to go out into the homes of mothers, the very nature of infant welfare centres made it a less invasive institution and more of a resource to be used when and how mothers chose. Although these two services differed in this respect, they shared the objective of educating mothers in the fundamentals of good childcare and household work. Accordingly the centres offered not only lessons in infant management, but also sewing classes alongside other facilities such as savings clubs.[31] They also sold cod liver oil and malt, and in later years vitamins, as well as materials for making babies' clothes. All these items were sold at lower prices than in shops, and were sometimes half-price. Ordinarily these items were very costly and often outside the reach of those mothers operating on a very tight budget.[32] In addition some centres also provided free or cheap milk, and dinners to necessitous mothers and children.

Such nutritional aid, however, was not uniform, and was largely dependent on the provision made by the local authority which, as discussed in the previous chapter, tended to be more generous in the poorer and more politically radical boroughs of Woolwich and Stepney than in the other two. For many medical and social welfare experts the provision of such nourishment was seen as detrimental to the educational function of the centre. As the British Medical Association argued in 1921,

> the gratuitous supply of artificial food and dried milk has proved detrimental to the best interests and influence of the centres. The people who go to them mainly for what they can get very cheaply or for nothing are not as a rule people who value or will benefit from the educational work of the centre.[33]

The stress on educational work also prevented infant welfare centres from providing any medical treatment.[34] This emphasis was not only true for those infants seen in these centres, but also for the mothers who after 1918 began to attend such centres for antenatal supervision; and, from the late 1920s, toddlers for whom special clinics were provided. Those running the toddlers' clinics in Woolwich, for instance, stressed,

> The clinic is not intended to be a purely inspection clinic for note-taking purposes; it is intended to be of constructive benefit to the health and progress of the child. For this reason, though it includes a routine examination (like school medical inspections), it attempts to touch much more generally the questions of home management in the pre-school child and to supply what may be wanting, or can be corrected in each case through domestic means, ie diet, exercise, hygiene, sleep, disciplinary training, etc., without impinging on the sphere of medical treatment.[35]

180

At most centres mothers and children were usually examined by a nurse and a doctor, and referred on to their own general practitioner or another medical agency if any problems were detected. Part of the reasoning behind this was firstly the idea that the services provided by such a centre should not compete with general practitioners, and secondly the belief that infant mortality was primarily the result of maternal ignorance. Such attitudes were not confined to those centres organized by voluntary bodies, but also those run by borough councils.[36]

In later years sunlight treatment, massage and dental care for children and pregnant and nursing mothers began to be provided by infant welfare centres, but no surgery or drugs were available. Even the facilities that were offered varied greatly and were introduced at different times. By 1935, for instance, sunlight treatment, which was used to help those suffering rickets and tuberculosis, was available in all four of the boroughs, but massage in only three. Dental treatment was also much more widely accessible in Kensington and Stepney where there were eight and five dental centres respectively by 1935, while only two such centres existed in Woolwich and one in Hampstead.[37] The greater number of dental centres in Kensington and Stepney partly reflected the larger population in these boroughs than in Woolwich or Hampstead.

While the number of amenities the centres provided increased over the years, their existence tells us nothing about the level of attention they provided for mothers and their children. The level of care they provided was not only dependent on the types of services offered, but, as in the case of health visitors, also on the number of clients each centre had to see. In 1918 the Local Government Board specified that there should be at least one infant welfare centre per 400 births.[38] Table 5.5 shows that in 1915 only Hampstead was near this target, with Stepney and Woolwich lagging far behind. By 1935, however, as the table indicates, these two latter boroughs had caught up. In Woolwich such centres began to appear immediately after the passing of the Maternal and Child Welfare Act of 1918, and by 1919 there were five such centres.

Overall, it would appear from Table 5.6 that by 1935 infant welfare centres in all four boroughs had many fewer births to cover. As in the case of health visitors this partly reflected the decline in the birth rate as well as the increase in the number of centres established. This pattern was again most apparent in Stepney where the total number of centres more than doubled between 1915 and 1935 at a time when the number of births in the borough halved. Much of the increase stemmed from municipal sponsorship (Table 5.5). By 1935 all four boroughs appear, therefore, to have had an adequate number of centres to cater to the needs of their populations.

The accessibility of services within each centre was greatly dependent on the frequency of the sessions that it held. Table 5.6 indicates that in all the boroughs the centres held a number of sessions each week, thus affording their clients greater possibility to attend and not confront long waiting times. This policy was especially important for those women with very limited time and resources. In the case of Kensington and Woolwich, for instance, the number of sessions appears to have reduced the case load on each centre by more than half (compare the final columns of Table 5.5 with Table 5.6). Overall infant welfare centres in the poorer boroughs seem to have had a greater number of sessions and therefore slightly lighter case loads, reflecting again the stronger political and financial commitment of the councils in these boroughs to maternal and child welfare than in Hampstead and Kensington.

Table 5.6: Number of infant welfare sessions at infant welfare centres and proportion of births covered in four London boroughs, 1935

	Number of sessions per week in all the centres	Number of births covered by each session
Hampstead	7	130
Kensington	13*	172
Stepney	26	116
Woolwich	22	93

* 1932 refers to infant consultations only.

Sources: 'MCW Provisions Made or Provided in Metropolitan Boroughs', in LCC, *Maternal Mortality: Hospital and Medical Services (Hospital Management Sub-Committee), Report by MOH*, 10 May 1935, Appendix A (GLRO file: Ph/Gen/3/7/7); 'Kensington Public Health Survey', 1932, (PRO file: MH66/360).

Whatever the case load per centre or the number of sessions, such statistics give no indication of the uptake of the services. Unfortunately, this is difficult to gauge because there was no uniform or set procedure for recording attendance, which hinders the comparison of different centres. Numbers were also often recorded as a means of proving the importance of the service in a bid for more funding from government and voluntary sources, and therefore do not necessarily reflect the extent to which women liked or disliked a service. No details remain of how many mothers returned to a clinic after their first visit or were never seen again. Such material also makes no distinction as to whether a mother and her infant received an hour of patient advice, or whether she was dismissed within five minutes of being seen without any real treatment or support.[39] Of the boroughs, Stepney has the least information on this issue. In all the boroughs the numbers recorded are confusing because they do not always reveal the number of visits of any individual. Nevertheless, while it is impossible to accurately assess the degree to which mothers and their children attended infant welfare centres, of the evidence that remains it would seem that in all the boroughs the attendance numbers did increase over the years, as did the average numbers of visits made.

Table 5.7: Number and percentage of infants under 1 year attending an infant welfare centre, with attendance numbers in Hampstead, Kensington and Stepney

Borough	Date	Total Number of infants under 1 year attending an IWC	Number of infants attending an IWC as % of total boroughs births	Total Number of attendances	Average number of attendances per infant attending an IWC
Hampstead	1915–18	2,470	55	17,972	7.2
	1934–8	2,931	58	47,507	16.2
Kensington	1921–5	9,093	59	–	–
	1926–30	8,841	68	–	–
	1931–5	11,369	99	126,053	11.0
Stepney	1914–15	2,379	16	15,136	6.4
	1921–5	–	–	35,562	–
	1931–5	–	–	67,430	–

Hampstead – the number of infants visiting the infant welfare centres in Hampstead in 1915–18 are calculated from the number of infants weighed at the infant consultations. The number for 1935 and 1938 refer to all the infants who attended the centres.

Kensington – the percentage of infants attending infant welfare centres is much smaller when calculated on the basis of overall borough births designated as suitable for welfare attention. For comparison with the number of births designated as suitable for welfare relief see Table 5.4.

Sources: Hampstead, Kensington and Stepney MOH, *A/Rs* (1915–38).

The case loads outlined in Tables 5.7 and 5.8 did not necessarily bear any relation to the attendance rates as can be seen from Table 5.9. Centres in Kensington, for example, which had heavier case loads than centres in other boroughs, had a very high percentage of its infants attending, particularly by the early 1930s. By this time the number of infants attending such centres had reached 99 per cent of the total births. When measured by the number of births suitable for welfare attention the percentage of infants seen by the centre was even higher, climbing from 78 per cent in 1921–5 to 126 per cent in

183

1931–5 (Table 5.4 above). In Hampstead, however, where centres had a lighter case load than those in Kensington, a much smaller proportion of the infant population were visiting infant welfare centres. Moreover, unlike centres in Kensington, which doubled its percentage of attenders between 1921 and 1931, centres in Hampstead experienced no significant rise in the percentage of overall infant population attending a centre. Although Hampstead appeared inferior to Kensington in this respect, the average number of visits an infant made to a centre in Hampstead doubled between 1915 and 1938 and was greater than the visits paid by infants in Kensington. Thus, while the proportion of infants reached by centres in Kensington increased, those in Hampstead saw their infants more often. Part of the frequency of the visits in Hampstead might be attributed to the high number of middle-class residents in the borough who could have been more enthusiastic to utilize the opportunities offered by the centres.

Table 5.8: Number of toddlers' clinics and children 0–4 years covered by each centre in four London boroughs, 1935

Borough	Number of toddlers' clinics	Number of children 0–4 years per centre*
Hampstead	6	667
Kensington	8	1,302
Stepney	16	1,003
Woolwich	8	1,191

* Calculation based on the total population aged 0–4 years in the borough by the number of toddlers' clinics.

Sources: Hampstead, Kensington, Stepney and Woolwich MOH, *A/Rs* (1935); London Council for Social Services, Early Publications Box, Leaflet 'Before School Age,' 1937, Appendix 1.

A similar pattern also prevailed among toddlers. Tables 5.7 and 5.8 show that toddlers' clinics in Hampstead had a lighter case load than in other boroughs, and reached a smaller proportion of toddlers overall. None the less, the average number of visits each child paid to the clinic was high. Of the boroughs, Woolwich had one of the heaviest case loads and the largest percentage of children under five years attending infant welfare centres, reaching 53 per cent in 1937. By comparison in Kensington the percentage in 1937 was 48 and in Hampstead it was 20 in 1938. The greater proportion of children cared for in Woolwich might be linked to the widespread number of toddler facilities in the borough. From the 1920s infant welfare centres in Woolwich and Stepney looked after children aged up to five years old, but specialist clinics for toddlers were only set up in the very late 1920s. Woolwich was in fact one of the first boroughs in the country to include such clinics within the remit of maternal and child welfare work. By 1933 three such clinics were being held on a weekly basis in each of the three districts within Woolwich and the service was considered to be very efficient.[40] Indeed, Woolwich became renowned for its work with toddlers.[41]

Table 5.9: Number of total children under five years and their number of attendances at infant welfare centres

Borough	Date	Number of children		Attendances	
		Total attending IWC	As % of population aged 0–4 years in borough	Number	Average number paid by each child
Hampstead	1934	661	17	13,629	22.5
	1938	813	20	18,334	20.6
Kensington	1921	3,585	31	33,695	9.4
	1925	3,827	33	41,312	10.8
	1930	3,711	36	43,677	11.8
	1935	4,602	44	51,563	11.2
	1937	4,985	48	42,484	8.5
Woolwich	1920	3,122	24	21,613	6.9
	1925	4,318	33	24,834	5.7
	1930	4,728	50	35,220	7.4
	1935	5,259	55	41,323	7.9
	1937	5,074	53	39,383	7.8

Sources: Hampstead, Kensington, Stepney, and Woolwich MOH, *A/Rs* (1920–37); *Census* (London: 1921); London Council for Social Services, Early Publications Box, Leaflet 'Before School Age', 1937, Appendix 1.

As we have seen all the boroughs had extensive infant welfare provision for their population by the 1920s, but the services they provided varied, as did the burden of clients each centre had to deal with. Hampstead although having the lightest case load of the four boroughs, partly reflecting its low number of poor residents, overall made the least coverage for its infants and toddlers both in terms of health visitors and infant welfare centres. The coverage in Kensington was better than in Hampstead, but even here the services were not as extensive as those found in the poorer boroughs of Stepney and Woolwich. What impact these variations in the services had on the health of those they catered to is considered in the next section.

Effectiveness of the Services Provided

A major problem in evaluating the influence that the facilities had on health standards is the fact that the areas where mortality was recorded did not always correspond with the districts served by specific medical agencies. Even in cases where it is possible to match mortality rates with particular services, such evidence cannot be disentangled from the wider socio-economic circumstances and weather conditions. Similarly it is critical to distinguish between those services directed towards neonatal and post-neonatal mortality. This distinction is essential given the different determinants involved in each. As shown in Chapter 3 in the late nineteenth and early twentieth century post-neonatal mortality was more closely associated with socio-economic conditions than with medical provision. This factor, however, was less important in the case of neonatal mortality.

Health visiting and infant welfare centres were frequently championed as the reason for the decline in infant mortality at the turn of the century. This claim was widely asserted by medical experts and social reformers during this period and in later years. Their ammunition was gained from the coincidence in the reduction of infant mortality with the emergence of such provision. One of the clearest examples of this can be seen in the case of the appointment of the health visitor in Limehouse within the borough of Stepney in the years 1890–1913. During these years infant mortality overall dropped in the borough, but the most striking change occurred in Limehouse where the health visitor was deployed. In the years immediately preceding her appointment the rate of infant mortality was just over 200 per 1,000 births (1895–1904), but within a couple of years of her appointment it had fallen to 153 (1905–9). In the 1920s reductions in infant mortality in Woolwich and Stepney were similarly attributed to the intensive maternal and child welfare work carried out in the boroughs.[42]

One of the most noticeable features of the fall in infant mortality rates was the reduction in diarrhoeal deaths, the biggest killer of infants in this period. In these years this remained a disease for which there was virtually no effective medical treatment. The most that could be offered was kaolin, but this remained largely ineffectual against infantile diarrhoea. Educating mothers in preventative measures such as lengthy breast-feeding and the need for cleanliness in food preparation and storage as offered by health visitors and the infant welfare centres was, therefore, one of the most effective forms of care that could be offered.[43]

It would, however, be wrong to conclude that such educational advice was the sole explanation for the fall in infant mortality during this period. Part of the decline in infant mortality in these particular areas was due to the wider falls in infant mortality overall which can be attributed to the cooler and wetter summers and improvements in sanitation in these years which reduced the possibilities of epidemic diarrhoea usually brought on by hot weather.[44]

In addition, it is impossible to understand what degree of educational involvement and advice was necessary to prevent deaths. Evidence suggests that the changes in childcare and nursing practices that the health visitors and later the infant welfare centres promoted, particularly in relation to the need for fresh air and exercise, together with changes in diet might have contributed to the fall in rickets which lowered an infant's resistance to whooping cough and measles.[45] Yet while an infant's chance of survival might have been enhanced by the attendance of a health visitor or by visiting an infant welfare centre, as Peretz has pointed out, the benefits to the infant from such a visit did not necessarily increase with a greater number of attendances.[46]

Equally, the mere presence of an infant welfare centre did not guarantee better health. In North Kensington, for instance, infant mortality remained high despite an abundance of maternal and child welfare provision. In 1924 it was estimated that 50,000 of the 94,000 population were 'the poorest of the poor', for which six infant welfare centres and eight health visitors were provided. Table 5.10 indicates that the case load for infant welfare centres, whether measured by total births in the whole of North Kensington, or by those designated as suitable for attention, was large. Indeed, it was much higher when considered in relation to the average for the centres in the borough as a whole (Tables 5.6 and 5.5). None the less, in South Kensington only one infant welfare centre was provided to cover a population of 84,000 in 1924.[47] Table 5.10 also shows that South Kensington had a much larger potential case load when measured by total births in the area. Yet despite the higher number of facilities per head in North Kensington, infant mortality was much worse here than in the southern part of the borough. Throughout the inter-war years North Kensington had one of the highest rates of infant mortality in London while South Kensington had one of the lowest. Thus it could be argued that the large provision of infant welfare centres and health visitors in North Kensington had little impact.

**Table 5.10: Number of infant welfare centres in North
and South Kensington, with IMR and case load per centre
as measured by total births and those designated as
suitable for welfare attention, 1921–38**

Area	Date	IMR	Total IWCs	Number of total births per IWC	Number of births seen as suitable for welfare attention per IWC
North	1921–5	93	6	1,767	1,664
Kensington	1926–30	81	6	1,492	1,423
	1931–5	95	7	1,169	1,109
	1936–8	83	7	681	654
South	1921–5	61	1	4,113	1,672
Kensington	1926–30	60	1	3,423	1,288
	1931–5	58	1	3,023	1,222
	1936–8	67	1	1,763	93

Source: Kensington MOH, *A/Rs* (1921–38).

**Table 5.11: Percentage of births designated as suitable for
welfare attention and percentage of infants receiving care from
an infant welfare centre in North and South Kensington**

Area	Date	Births designated as suitable for welfare attention as % of total births	Infants attending an IWC	
			As % of births designated as suitable for welfare attention	As % of total births
North	1921–5	94	83	78
Kensington	1926–30	95	103	98
	1931–5	95	131	124
	1936–8	96	144	138
South	1921–5	41	50	20
Kensington	1926–30	38	68	26
	1931–5	41	98	39
	1936–8	40	125	49

Source: Kensington MOH, *A/Rs* (1921–38).

Part of the differential in mortality rates can be explained by the
disparity in socio-economic conditions in each area. It is clear from
Table 5.11 that a very high proportion of those born in North
Kensington, averaging between 94 and 96 per cent in the years 1921
to 1938, were regarded as suitable for welfare attention because of

their poor economic status. This percentage was much higher than South Kensington where it never rose above 41. The percentage of infants attending infant welfare centres whether measured by total births or by those deemed in need of care, was also much greater in the north than in the south. Overall the level of need and demand on services, therefore, was higher in the north. Potentially this disparity could have been countered by the fact that more facilities were provided in the north, but the high rates of infant mortality indicate that this was not the case and is particularly striking when compared with the scarcity of such centres in South Kensington and its low rates of infant mortality. From this evidence it would seem that the deprivation in North Kensington and the wealth of South Kensington were more important in determining the health of infants than the lessons in hygiene and infant care offered in the infant welfare centres.

The advice and attention health visitors and infant welfare centres gave, however, was not totally ineffectual. As Dr Fenton observed in Kensington in 1926, the work of infant welfare centres had resulted in many working-class mothers and their children being 'in better health than was the case 25 years' previously, and that many of these mothers were 'better educated in mother craft than many of the women of the middle classes'. Students of the Kings College for Women visiting working-class mothers in Kensington were also particularly impressed by 'the depth of knowledge of food values, vitamins, domestic hygiene and mothercraft' such women possessed. From this Dr Fenton concluded that infant welfare centres had a far-reaching impact on the women they helped and on health standards. As he noted,

> Attendance at the centre brighten up the women in many ways. They are more self-respecting, and they and their children are cleaner. The health visitors note that they take pride in having their homes clean and tidy. These women are intolerant of unsanitary conditions in and around their homes. Indeed the whole environment has improved and this is a great factor, not only in reducing the death rate, but in the prevention of those diseases which, whilst not killing and adding to the death rate, hamper and handicap young children through life.[48]

While it might be true that the educational policies undertaken by health visitors and infant welfare centres raised health standards among infants and mothers, the impact they had was largely governed by the socio-economic and environmental conditions individual families faced. Indeed, as will be seen in Chapter 8, many of the instructions were impossible to follow where there was no running water, poor sanitation, inadequate heating and cooking facilities, and limited resources to spend on warm clothing and adequate nourishment.

Similarly, as many contemporary women campaigners and Labour Party activists pointed out, more substantial provision of food and money and greater improvements to living conditions were needed if the advice of infant welfare centres and health visitors was to have any impact. While food and milk supplements and vitamins were offered at the infant welfare centres in the four boroughs of London in the earlier part of this century, as we have seen in the previous chapter this was severely restricted by the cuts imposed by the Ministry of Health after 1921. Such provision, as in the case of Stepney, also required much greater finance than the borough council had at its disposal, or, as in the case of Kensington, the council was willing to spend. Even if provided, however, it is difficult to know the extent to which this could have ameliorated the problem of infant mortality. While some research in developing countries has shown that nutritional status is a significant factor in curbing infant and child deaths, particularly in relation to measles, others have suggested this is outweighed by factors such as the intensity and duration of exposure to the disease.[49]

It is similarly difficult to judge the degree to which medical provision would have benefited infants. As already stated medical treatment was largely ineffective for infantile diseases in this period. Even so, as Hardy has pointed out in relation to her study of infectious diseases among young children, good nursing care and medical advice could make a difference between life and death. While infant welfare centres and health visitors attempted to educate mothers in the elements of such care, mothers did not have direct access to medical treatment or nursing care through these centres, which, as we shall see in Chapter 8, they regarded as their major disadvantage. The greater popularity of clinics, which provided medical treatment, over the infant welfare centres, suggests that while medical intervention may have been limited in the extent to which it could cure ailing infants, it was clearly held as valuable.

Conclusion

This survey of infant health services in the four boroughs indicates that while maternal and child welfare provision expanded tremendously in these years, it was never as comprehensive nor so complete as contemporaries such as McCleary asserted. Overall maternal and child welfare services tended to be better provided in the more centralized metropolis of London than in the provinces, but even here it was subject to the political will of particular councils and the economic resources in their hands.

Of the four boroughs Stepney and Woolwich appear to have provided more health visitors and infant welfare centres to care for their infants and covered a larger proportion of its population under the age of 5 than the other two boroughs. The greater provision in Stepney and Woolwich partly reflected the greater poverty and need of their residents, as well as the higher political commitment of their councils to make such provision possible.[50] This impetus is most clearly seen in the context of the larger number of municipal infant welfare centres in the two boroughs than in Hampstead and Kensington where voluntary impulse remained the stalwart of maternal and child welfare provision.

Despite these differences in the provision, it is clear that even in the richer boroughs, it was the poor who were the focus of the services provided. This policy, however, did not guarantee that those who were most disadvantaged were covered, and that the services raised their levels of health. Even where an abundance of services was provided, poor social and economic conditions could undermine the valuable benefits they yielded as can be seen in the context of North Kensington where infant mortality remained extremely high despite numerous services and efforts to curb the problem.

Notes

1. Those who see the MCW services as having some impact on mortality levels include D. Dwork, *War is Good for Babies and other Young Children: A History of the Infant and Child Welfare Movement in England 1898–1918* ((London: 1987); S. Szreter, 'The Importance of Social Intervention in Britain's Mortality Decline c.1850–1914: A Re–interpretation of the Role of Public Health', *Soc. Hist. Med.* 1/1 (1988), 1–39; and A. Hardy, 'Rickets and the Rest: Childcare, Diet and Infectious Children's Diseases, 1850–1914', *Soc. Hist. Med.* 5/3 (1992), 389–412. For some opposite views see A. Davin, 'Imperialism and Motherhood', *Hist. Workshop J.* (1978), 9–65; C. Dyhouse, 'Working-class Mothers and Infant Mortality in England 1895–1914', *J. Soc. Hist.* 12 (1978), 248–67; H. Marland, 'A Pioneer in Infant Welfare: The Huddersfield Scheme 1903–1920', *Soc. Hist. Med.*, 6/1 (1993), 25–50; and E. P. Peretz, 'Maternal and Child Welfare in England and Wales Between the Wars: A Comparative Regional Study', unpub. Ph.D., Middlesex University, 1992, Ch. 2.
2. See for instance Stepney MOH, *A/R* (1913), 66.
3. G. F. McCleary, *The Maternity and Child Welfare Movement* (London: 1935), 17–18 and 21–3. McCleary was MOH for Hampstead from 1906 to 1912.
4. See particularly Tables 4.5 and 4.6

5. Peretz, *op. cit.* (note 1).
6. Maternal Mortality Committee, *Maternal Mortality Report* (London: 1934), 4–11, 16. This report is examined in more detail in the next chapter.
7. R. Hale, 'The History of Health Visiting', in R. Hale, M. Loveland and G. M. Owen (eds), *The Principles and Practice of Health Visiting*, (Oxford: 1968), 10; C. Davies, 'The Health Visitor as Mother's Friend: A Woman's Place in Public Health, 1900–14', *Soc. Hist. Med.*, 1/1 (1991), 39–59, 42.
8. Stepney MOH, *A/R* (1914), 72.
9. Between 1918 and 1929 the amount of grants allotted to such work halved, but the overall proportion designated for such work was 16 per cent, which was higher than for many other MCW services. J. Lewis, *The Politics of Motherhood: Child and Maternal Welfare in England, 1900–1939*, (London: 1980), 105.
10. McCleary, *op. cit.* (note 3), 30; Kensington MOH, *A/R* (1900), 52.
11. Stepney MOH, *A/R* (1913), 65–6.
12. McCleary, *op. cit.* (note 3), 30.
13. Stepney MOH, *A/Rs* (1902) 85 and (1910), 38. Davies, *op. cit.* (note 7); Peretz, *op. cit.* (note 1), 107–13.
14. 'Kensington Borough Council Survey: MCW Report' – letter from acting MOH to MCW Committee, 5 July 1917 (PRO file: MH 48/164). See also, Woolwich Council Minutes, 26 January 1916, 139, and 16 October 1918. It is unclear on what basis this figure was calculated.
15. Kensington MOH, *A/R* (1909), 13. See also Woolwich MOH, A/R (1907), 87–8.
16. In 1913, for instance, the Hampstead MOH noted only 89% of the total births were visited by a health visitor, 'the other 11% being considered outside the scope of our facilities for sundry reasons, chiefly economic'. (Hampstead MOH, *A/R* (1931), 34; see also Peretz, *op. cit.* (note 1), 107).
17. It is not clear from the records who is deciding which mothers were suitable for welfare relief, but it was probably dependent on the local MOH and his staff. What criteria they used and how adequate this was in relation to the conditions mothers were living in is unclear.
18. Woolwich Council Minutes, 26 January 1916, 139.
19. Kensington MOH, *A/R* (1909), 13.
20. Stepney MOH, *A/R* (1911), 52; Woolwich MOH, *A/R* (1906), 91–2 and Woolwich Council Minutes, 23 November 1906, 102. For many mothers such revisits could feel very invasive. See Ch. 7.
21. Kensington MOH, *A/R* (1937), 28–9; and Kensington Council Minutes, 29 September 1936, 391.
22. 'Kensington Public Health Survey', 1932, 12 (PRO file: MH 66/359).
23. Kensington MOH, *A/R* (1937), 28–9; and Kensington Council Minutes, 29 September 1936, 391.

24. The different sources of funding of infant welfare centres partly stemmed from the struggle between voluntary associations and municipal authorities over who should have jurisdiction over such provision and the battle for the establishment of the MH. See F. Honigsbaum, *The Struggle for the Ministry of Health* (London: 1970), 20–2.

25. McCleary, *op. cit.* (note 3), 11–18; E. W. Hope and J. Campbell, *Report on the Physical Welfare of Mother and Child*, 1 (London: 1917), 84–6.

26. For the struggle in the years leading up to 1919 see Honigsbaum, *op. cit.* (note 24), 20–2.

27. 'Kensington Public Health Survey', 1935, (PRO files: MH 52/177 and MH 66/360).

28. 'Hampstead Public Health Survey', 1933, 10, and 12 (PRO file: MH 66/347).

29. *Ibid.,* (1933), 2.

30. *Ibid.*

31. Such activities were reminiscent of those undertaken by the mothers' meetings in the nineteenth century. F. Prochaska, 'A Mothers' Country: Mothers' Meetings and Family Welfare in Britain, 1850–1950', *Hist.,* 74 (1989), 379–99.

32. E. P. Peretz, 'The Costs of Modern Motherhood to Low Income Families in Inter-war Britain', in V. Fildes, L. Marks and H. Marland (eds.), *Women and Children First: International Maternal and Infant Welfare, 1870–1945,* (London: 1992), 261; Lewis, *op. cit.* (note 9), 96–104.

33. 'The Value of Maternity and Child Welfare Work in Relation to the Reduction of Infant Mortality: Report of the Medico-Sociological Committee of the British Medical Association', BMA pamphlet, 1921; cited in Peretz, *op. cit.* (note 32), 259.

34. 'MCW Report', in 'Woolwich Public Health Survey', 1934, (PRO file: MH 66/404).

35. Woolwich MOH, *A/R* (1931), 100.

36. Lewis, *op. cit.* (note 9), 102–5.

37. 'MCW Provision Made or Provided in Metropolitan Boroughs in 1935', in LCC, *Maternal Mortality: Hospital and Medical Services (Hospital management sub-committee) Report by the MOH,* Appendix A (GLRO file: Ph/Gen/3/7/7).

38. Woolwich Council Minutes, 16 October 1918.

39. It is also difficult to measure the degree to which such attendance had an impact on a mother's awareness and education. Peretz, *op. cit.* (note 1), 64–5.

40. 'MCW Report', in 'Woolwich Public Health Survey', 1934.

41. *Ibid.*

42. Stepney MOH, *A/Rs* (1921), 4–5 and (1922), 30–1; Woolwich MOH, *A/R* (1922), 27.

43. This is an argument forcefully put in Dwork, *op. cit.* (note 1), Ch. 5.

See also Szreter, *op. cit.* (note 1), 30–3. The importance of breast-feeding and hygiene in preventing diarrhoeal deaths can most clearly be seen in the case of Jewish immigrants in East London, who although living in equal poverty and poor sanitation to their neighbours, none the less had remarkably low rates of infant mortality due to the intricate Jewish rituals in cleanliness and food preparations which protected infants from an environment which was otherwise very hazardous. L. Marks, *Model Mothers: Jewish Mothers and Maternity Provision in East London, 1870–1939* (Oxford: 1994), Ch. 2.

44. This is a point also made by Marland in her assessment of the health visitors' scheme established in Huddersfield *op. cit.* (note 1). For an in depth study of the effect of sanitation and meteorological conditions and their interaction with socio-economic factors on rates of infant mortality see N. Williams, 'Death in its Season: Class, Environment and the Mortality of Infants in Nineteenth Century Sheffield', *Soc. Hist. Med.,* 5/1 (1992), 71–94. A wide exploration of the reasons for the overall fall in infant mortality also appears in R. I. Woods, P. A. Watterson and J. Woodward, 'The Causes of Rapid Infant Mortality Decline in England and Wales, 1861–1921', *Pop. Stud.,* Part I, 42 (1988), 343–66 and Part II, 43 (1989), 113–32.

45. Hardy, *op. cit.* (note 1), 389–412.

46. Peretz, *op. cit.* (note 1), 64–5.

47. Dr Fenton, speech in *Third English-Speaking Conference on Infant Welfare* (London: 1924), 143–4.

48. Dr Fenton, speech in *Fourth English-Speaking Conference on Infant Welfare* (London: 1926), 61.

49. For a discussion of this and how it relates to historical trends of infectious disease among infants and young children see Hardy, *op. cit.* (note 1), 395–7.

50. The influence of Labour-controlled Councils on the provision of services and the benefits this bestowed on infant health seems to have been stronger in London than elsewhere. See J. M. Winter, 'Infant Mortality, Maternal Mortality, and Public Health in Britain in the 1930s', *J. Eur. Econ. Hist.,* 8 (1979), 439–62, 451–3.

6

Maternal Health Services

Just as it is difficult to pin-point the degree to which infant welfare centres and health visitors affected the levels of infant mortality in each borough, so it is hard to judge the influence of maternity facilities on maternal mortality. None the less, in the case of maternal mortality a closer association can be made between provision and outcome. In 1932 the Departmental Committee on Maternal Mortality estimated that at least 48 per cent of all the deaths they investigated in 1930 to 1932 could have been prevented. Of these deaths 17 per cent had resulted from errors of judgement in practice or treatment by doctors or midwives, 5 per cent from the lack of reasonable medical facilities, and 17 per cent from the absence of antenatal care. Negligence on the part of the patient or friends to adopt medical advice accounted for the remaining 9 per cent of the preventable deaths.[1] In their opinion, therefore, poor medical supervision before and during the birth were the main cause of preventable deaths.

In this chapter I consider what types of care were available to mothers in the early twentieth century and what impact this had on maternal health. Much of the focus of the maternal and child welfare provision established in the first two decades of the twentieth century, such as health visiting and infant welfare centres, was on the well-being of the infant. While mothers were also held to be important, their health was generally viewed in relation to the welfare of the infant and not for their own sakes. By the early 1920s, however, mothers increasingly became the subject of concern.[2] Part of this stemmed from the fact that despite the noticeable fall in the overall rates of mortality and infant mortality, maternal mortality continued to be high and appeared to be rising in these years. This chapter considers what effect this growing interest in the health of the mother had on the provision of maternity care. As in the case of infant welfare centres and health visitors, these services proliferated tremendously in the inter-war years and covered a wide range of areas, but were divided between many different authorities and varied greatly from borough to borough. Each borough was, therefore, distinctive in the quality and kind of care available; in the level of institutional and domiciliary care provided; and in the degree to which antenatal care was available. Such differences were greatly influenced by the social and economic conditions in each area, as well as the historical development of certain services, such as voluntary teaching hospitals.

This chapter firstly examines the different types of services that were available to mothers during their deliveries, and then the provision that was made for the ante- and postnatal period. As we shall see these services were all expanding greatly in the early twentieth century, much of them driven by the growing concern over maternal mortality in these years. In the final part of the chapter I consider the impact such services had on mothers' health and whether the disparities in maternal mortality noted for the four boroughs in Chapter 3 can be attributed to the different services provided in each area.

Costs and Unevenness of Maternity Care

In 1934 a committee reporting on the problem of maternal mortality highlighted the diversity and incompleteness of the maternity services provided. Their conclusions are summarized in Table 6.1, which shows that overall services tended to be better provided by the Metropolitan councils in London and by the urban county councils than by the rural county boroughs.[3] In the case of London and other urban councils antenatal care and maternity beds tended to be the most common services provided. By contrast the appointment of municipal midwives was rare everywhere, and poor provision was made for skilled district nursing of mothers who had experienced a complicated birth. Similarly, financial coverage for patients who could not afford the full fee of a midwife was infrequent, and assistance for unmarried mothers and their children was rare. The provision of home helps, convalescent homes, and other services more concerned with domestic than with direct medical problems were given least priority.

Table 6.1: Type and extent of MCW provision among 28 Metropolitan Boroughs in London compared with other councils nationally, 1932

	Percentage of Councils investigated providing services		
	Metropolitan Councils	County Councils	County Boroughs
Total number of authorities	28	61	84
Antenatal clinics	90	65	98
Midwifery provisions:			
a) sterilized maternity outfits free/cost price	57	26	26
b) municipal midwives	21	3	11
c) payment to midwife if patient cannot pay	39	10	37
Maternity beds in maternity home or hospital:			
a) for complicated cases	82	75	85
b) for patients with unsuitable housing	79	60	79
c) for antenatal observation	71	43	70
d) for treatment of puerperal sepsis	85	62	81
Complicated midwifery:			
a) payment to doctor to attend••	89	57	44
b) skilled nursing at patient's home	46	20	14
c) bacteriological examination in case of puerperal infection	32	30	26
Home helps	61	8	29
Provision of milk and food to expectant & nursing mothers	93	57	82
Convalescent Home treatment for mothers	61	7	13
Payment to District Nursing Association for midwifery & maternity nursing	71	67	36
Assistance for unmarried mothers and their children	32	21	29

• several authorities had insurance schemes for mothers who might need services of a doctor.

•• includes complicated cases and puerperal sepsis cases. All women in all boroughs could also get such provisions from the LCC.

Source: Maternal Mortality Committee, *Maternal Mortality Report* (London: 1934), 4–12.

Such an unevenness of services was particularly important when we consider the costs of maternity care in these years. Costs were a large determinant of the kind of attendant a woman received during her labour as well as before and after the event. As Table 6.2 shows, the most expensive options were to be a private patient in a hospital, to hire privately the care of a general practitioner, or to go into a maternity or nursing home. By contrast one of the cheapest forms of care at the turn of the century was the untrained midwife or handywoman. These midwives, however, became increasingly scarce after the Midwives Act of 1902 which outlawed their practice. The qualified midwives who replaced them were not always as cheap. In later years, however, their fees were usually more affordable than those of a doctor. Charitable maternity care offered by voluntary hospitals was also one of the more cost effective options, although the amount women were expected to pay for this service was dependent on an assessment of their family income. Free maternity care could be obtained from the parish, but like other forms of parish relief, the stigma attached to such care initially limited its use to only the most impoverished and destitute. By the 1920s, however, this stigma had diminished greatly and Poor Law institutions had become increasingly popular for women seeking in-patient maternity care.[4]

In 1911 the National Insurance Act introduced a maternity benefit of 30s. to cover some of the costs of midwifery care. This benefit, however, was restricted to the wives of men who were in regular employment. Given the prevalence of casual work and unemployment in Stepney and North Kensington, many women could not hope to claim the benefit. In 1913, and again in 1934, one hospital in Stepney reported that many mothers, whose husbands were involved in dock work and casual labour, could not 'even get work to keep their Insurance cards up to date' and were 'therefore ineligible even for Maternity benefit'. Even those who could claim maternity benefit found it insufficient.[5] In an area like Woolwich, where many husbands were able to keep up their insurance through regular employment, fewer mothers were ineligible for maternity benefit, but even here it was difficult. The British Hospital for Mothers and Babies in Woolwich, for instance, reported in 1913 that 24 per cent of their patients were unable to claim the benefit.[6]

In some cases the introduction of the maternity benefit also resulted in a rise in the cost of midwifery care. Doctors and midwives who knew their patients now had access to extra funding raised their charges, as did the hospitals. In 1913, for example, the British Hospital for Mothers and Babies added an extra 3s. to the services they offered to women receiving such benefits. Wives of unemployed men, however, were only expected to pay 3s. 6d. if attended by a district midwife.[7]

In addition to the costs of maternity care, women were also expected to fork out large sums of money to cover for equipment both for herself and the baby. As late as 1942 it was estimated that the average cost of a working-class mother's confinement in London was £17. This fee did not even include the charges incurred if she entered a hospital or a rest-home, the expenses of prenatal medical attendance, or additional dietary requirements during pregnancy. Maternity benefit only covered a fraction of these costs.[8]

Table 6.2: Range of fees for maternity care from different sources in London, 1902–36

		1902–5	1913	1917–22	1930s
Midwives					
(i) Untrained		5s.	–	–	–
(ii) Trained	1st birth	Between 2s. 6d. & 21s.	–	Between 15s. & 12s. 6d	Between 25s. & 50s.
	Multiparous	Between 2s. 6d. & 21s.	–	Between 12s. & 7s. 10d.	Between 21s. & 50s.
Hospitals					
(i) *British Hospital for Mothers and Babies*					
Charitable cases•	In-patient	1s. (day) 7s. (week)	1s. (day) 7s. (week)	Between £3 & £4 (fortnight)	–
	Out-patient	7s. 6d.	7s. 6d.	–	–
Receiving maternity	In-patient	–	4s. (day)	–	–
benefit	Out-patient	–	10s. 6d.	–	–
Unemployed	Out-patient	–	–	–	–
(ii) *The London Hospital*					
Private patient	–	£3 3s. (week)	–	–	£5 5s.
(iii) *Small Maternity Hospital in London–*		–	–	–	0 to £3 (average 30s.)
(iv) *Teaching Hospital in London*			–	–	15s. (£2 10s. weekly income)
		–	–	–	30s. (if maternity benefit received)
Nursing Home		–	–	–	>£5 5s. *
Doctor					
(i) Normal delivery	1st birth	£1 1s.	–	–	£3
	multiparous	£1 1s.	–	–	£2
(ii) Instrumental delivery	1st birth	£2 2s.	–	–	–
	multiparous	£2 2s.	–	–	–

• charged according to their income. * £5 5s. was the lowest fee charged for midwife's attendance. If a doctor attended the cost was much greater.
Sources: J. Lewis, *The Politics of Motherhood: Child and Maternal Welfare, 1900–1939* (London: 1980), 141: M. Chamberlain and R. Richardson, 'Life and Death', *Oral Hist. J.,* 11 (1983), 33; BMB, *A/R* (1905), 11; (1912); 14; LH, *A/R* (1913, 1925, 1937); Woolwich MOH, *A/R* (1922), 78; Letter from Miss Gregory in BMB Managing Committee, Minutes 31 March 1905 (GLRO file: H14/BMB/A9/2); LCC, *Maternity Services of London: Report by the County MOH to the Hospital and Services Committee* (London: 1934), 9 (GLRO Library: LP 26.8 LCC).

199

Many of the difficulties women experienced in financing their maternity care would have restricted their choice of attendant, especially among the poorer women. In addition to this many of the options open to them would have been governed by the kind of maternity provision within their own vicinity. The type of services provided within a particular locality was crucial in determining the type of care mothers received.

Hospital Attendance during Childbirth, 1902–36

At the turn of the century most women were delivered in their own homes. Yet by the 1930s many women were increasingly being confined in an institution. As Table 6.3 indicates this transformation was particularly noticeable in London, which contrasted with other urban areas such as Birmingham, Hull, Liverpool, Manchester, and England and Wales as a whole. Yet while women in London were much less likely to give birth at home than their sisters elsewhere in the country, the degree to which this occurred within London varied between boroughs. Table 6.4 indicates that by the 1930s boroughs in the East End had higher rates of institutional births than those in the West End. The rise in institutional births is particularly noticeable in the case of Stepney, where 73 per cent of all the births were taking place in an institution by 1935. The percentage in Stepney was much higher than the average for the county of London as a whole, and more than double that recorded for England and Wales (compare Tables 6.3 and 6.4). Although not quite as high as Stepney, Hampstead and Woolwich also had a high proportion of institutional births. In contrast to the other three boroughs, Kensington had much fewer institutional births, and while below the average for London, was more comparable to the national average in 1934.

One of the reasons for the high percentage of institutional births in London was the large dominance of hospital medicine within the capital. From early on London had become a major site for voluntary teaching hospitals, partly because it served as the headquarters for the medical profession.[9] London was also an attractive area for such hospitals because of its large number of poor who were ideal subjects for teaching students. Many of these hospitals tended to be sited in the poorest boroughs, such as Stepney.

London had also witnessed a proliferation of municipal hospitals, which was partly initiated by the Metropolitan Poor Law Amendment Act in 1867. This legislation had allowed London Poor Law unions to combine to build large district asylums and to build separate infirmaries. In later years special provision was also made for lunatics, and fever and smallpox patients. All these institutions were managed by the Metropolitan Asylums Board.[10] Such a centralized body of care was reinforced by the establishment of the London County Council in 1889. In the inter-war years this trend gathered momentum as a result of the 1929 Local Government Act which enabled local authorities such as the London County Council and metropolitan boroughs to take control of Poor Law hospitals.[11]

Table 6.3: Percentage of home and institutional confinements in London and other areas, 1915–46

Place	Year	% home confinements	% hospital confinements
County of London	1934	40	60
	1938	31	69
Birmingham	1915	>97	<3
	1935	67	33
	1915	>97	<3
	1935	88	22
Liverpool	1915	>97	<3
	1935	59	41
	1938	51	49
Manchester	1938	50	50
England and Wales	1927	85	15
	1933	76	24
	1937	75	25
	1946	46	54

Sources: Royal College of Obstetricians and Gynaecologists, *Report on a National Maternity Service* (London: 1944), 25; LCC, *Maternity Services of London, Report by the County MOH to the Hospital and Medical Services Committee* (London: 1934), (GLRO Library: P 26.8 LCC); J. Lewis, *The Politics of Motherhood: Child and Maternal Welfare, 1900–1939* (London: 1980), 120.

By 1925 London had nine voluntary hospitals with 443 maternity beds and was admitting 10,000 women annually.[12] These institutions were not only caring for in-patients, but also provided wide coverage for out-patients. In 1928 the Registrar General reported that 68 per cent of all domiciliary and hospital births in London were attended by voluntary hospitals. In the context of institutional births voluntary hospitals dominated the scene, accounting for 51 per cent of all such births in 1934 (Table 6.5). A very high percentage of women were also being cared for by London County Council hospitals (originally Poor Law institutions). In 1928 these institutions accounted for 21 per cent of the total births in London (in-patients and out-patients).[13] By 1934 births within London County Council hospitals constituted 34 per cent of all institutional births in London. The number of births taking place within borough maternity homes and private nursing homes in London was small by comparison with those occurring in voluntary or London County Council hospitals (Table 6.5).

Table 6.4: Percentage of home and institutional confinements in East London and other areas, 1915–46

Place	Year	% home confinements	% hospital confinements
East London:			
Bethnal Green•	1931	56.3	43.7
	1935	41.2	58.8
Poplar*	1915	88.7	12.3
	1920	87.8	10.2
	1925	75	23
	1930	62	38
	1935	38.72	58
Stepney*	1920	79	21
	1927	56	44
	1935†	26.6	73.4
3 East End boroughs**	1934	34	66
West London			
Kensington	1924	72	28
	1930	68	32
	1934	67	33
5 West End boroughs••	1934	49	45
Elsewhere in London:			
Hampstead	1926	60	40
	1932	41	59
	1938	33	67
St Pancras	1915	88	12
	1935	44	56
Woolwich	1925	67	33
	1930	53	47
	1933	41	59
	1936	33	67

• The figures are taken from hospital sources only which might account for the stress on hospital care. The figures cited are for home and hospital deliveries undertaken by the major hospitals in Bethnal Green.

•• Five boroughs include Chelsea, Fulham, Kensington, Paddington and Westminister. The figures also do not include 6% of the births that took place in nursing homes.

* These percentages are calculated from births notified by doctors, midwives and parents as home confinements and births notified by hospitals. Some births are

unaccounted for and therefore the percentages are approximates and do not add up to 100%.

** Three boroughs include Poplar, Shoreditch and Stepney.

† The figures for this year are calculated according to an investigation undertaken by the Stepney MOH in 1935 on the level of skilled midwifery in the area and are therefore more accurate than most statistics for the time.

Note: Hampstead figures are worked out on the basis of the number of births occurring at home.

Kensington figures are based on the numbers of mothers reported to be giving birth in various institutions – this might be an underestimate because it does not include all the institutional births.

Sources: LCC, *Maternity Services in London: Report by the County MOH to the Hospitals and Medical Services Committee* (London: 1934), 4 (GLRO Library P26.8 LCC); Poplar MOH, *A/Rs* (1915–35); Bethnal Green MOH, *A/Rs* (1930–9); Stepney MOH *A/Rs* (1920, 1927, 1935); Hampstead MOH, *A/Rs* (1926–36); Kensington MOH, *A/Rs* (1924–34); Woolwich MOH, *A/Rs* (1925–38); J. Lewis, *The Politics of Motherhood: Child and Maternal Welfare, 1900–1939* (London: 1980), 120.

Table 6.5: Type of carer attending births in London, 1934

Domiciliary Confinements	Number	% of domiciliary births
(i) *Midwife:*		
private	9,750	38
borough	350	1
voluntary agency	850	3
voluntary/general hospital•	5,650	22
Total	16,600	64
(ii) *Doctor:*		
private	6,600	25
voluntary hospital•	2,800	11
Total	9,400	36
Total domiciliary confinements	26,000	100

Institutional confinements		% of institutional births
Voluntary maternity/general hospital	20,250	51
LCC maternity home	13,250	34
Borough maternity home	2,320	6
Private nursing home: (i) midwife carer	855	2
(ii) doctor carer	2,625	7
Total	3,480	9
Total institutional confinements	39,300	100

Source: LCC *Maternity Services of London: Report by the County MOH to the Hospitals and Medical Services Committee* (London: 1934), 4 (GLRO Library: P26.8 LCC).

Within London the extent to which women used voluntary or London County Council hospitals, or another institution varied greatly between different areas. Much of this was dependent on the socio-economic status of the residents within particular boroughs, and the historical antecedents of the facilities provided in each area. Table 6.6 demonstrates that by 1934 in the working-class boroughs of Stepney and Woolwich, a high percentage of institutional births took place in large teaching voluntary hospitals in these boroughs.[14]

Maternity provision in Stepney was dominated by three voluntary teaching hospitals: The London Hospital (known also as The London and founded as a general hospital in 1740) which began to provide maternity care for out-patients from 1853 and in-patients from the early twentieth century; the East End Maternity Home, established in 1884, and the Jewish Maternity Home, set up in 1913.[15] All these hospitals were important training institutions and by 1931 were providing 108 beds out of the total 190 beds in the area, the largest number of beds being provided by the East End Maternity Home.[16]

Table 6.6: Percentage of institutional confinements in various institutions in different areas of London and Birmingham, 1934

| | Nursing Home | Hospitals | | |
		Voluntary	Borough	LCC
Hampstead	29%	43%	–	26%*
Kensington	4%	21%	–	75%
Stepney	0	73%	–	27%
Woolwich	0.5%	62%	–	37%
14 London Boroughs•	11%	38%	10%	40%
Birmingham	12%	36%	52%†	–
County of London 1938	5%	28%	4%	34%

• 14 Boroughs includes Battersea, Camberwell, Fulham, Hackney, Hampstead, Holborn, Islington, Lambeth, Lewisham, Paddington, Poplar, Wandsworth, Woolwich, and the City of London.
* This includes some cases which were classified as borough hospital cases, but gave birth in a maternity ward in an LCC hospital.
† This relates to births in the city hospitals and maternity homes.

Sources: LCC, *Maternity Services in London: Report by the County MOH to the Hospital and Medical Services Committee* (London: 1934), 17 (GLRO Library: P26.8 LCC); V. Cox, 'Team Work and Post-natal Care', *Mother and Child* 5/9 (1934), 348 (in L. Fairfield's papers, GLRO file: Ph/Gen/3/6).

Table 6.7 shows the numbers of patients The London and the East End Maternity Home cared for between 1900 and 1939. The East End Maternity Home had a large intake of in-patients, constituting the majority of its maternity work from the late 1920s. By contrast

The London primarily catered for out-patients until the 1930s. Mothers in Stepney could also seek care from other voluntary teaching hospitals located just outside the borough boundaries, such as the City of London Maternity Hospital in the City, and the Salvation Army Mothers Home in Bethnal Green.[17]

Table 6.7: Number of in-patients and out-patients in the EEMH and The London Hospital, 1901–39

Year	EEMH		London Hospital	
	In-patients	Out-patients	In-patients	Out-patients
1901–5	1,614	2,081	–	14,298*
1906–11	2,492	3,600	–	24,478
1911–15	2,696	5,084	–	20,590
1915–20	3,868	5,332		8,863•
1921–5	5,154	6,134	1,257	13,226
1926–30	6,496	3,727	2,930	8,802†
1931–5	7,470	2,074	–	3,047
1936–8	4,558	849	2,191	1,327

* Figures missing for 1901

• Figures missing for 1918 and 1920

† Figures missing for 1929

Sources: EEMH and London Hospital, *A/Rs* (1901–39).

In Woolwich the voluntary teaching hospital, the British Hospital for Mothers and Babies, established in 1905, dominated maternity services. Initially the hospital had 12 beds, but this increased to 42 by 1927. By 1936 42 per cent of all institutional births in Woolwich were taking place at the British Hospital for Mothers and Babies. In 1928 the War Memorial Hospital also began to cater for maternity patients in Woolwich, but it took in a smaller proportion of mothers (Table 6.8). By the late 1930s these hospitals were catering for 78 per cent of the births within Woolwich taking place at home and in an institution.

Apart from the large voluntary teaching hospitals in Stepney and Woolwich, mothers also had access to maternity beds in these boroughs through Poor Law (later London County Council) hospitals. As Table 6.5 indicates 37 per cent of the institutional births in Woolwich, and 27 per cent in Stepney were occurring within a London County Council hospital by 1934, either within or outside the borough. In Stepney mothers had access to a large number of beds at Mile End Hospital, St George's-in-the-East Hospital and St Peter's Hospital, while those in Woolwich could seek the care of St Nicholas Hospital. Table 6.9 shows how many

beds each of these hospitals provided and how many patients were
cared for by them. In Stepney the proportion of births taking place
in such an institution was much smaller than in voluntary hospitals
in the early twentieth century. By the 1930s, however, the number
of mothers receiving care was equally divided between the voluntary
and London County Council hospitals (Table 6.10).

Table 6.8: Total number of patients cared for by the BMB and the War Memorial Hospital

Year	BMB	War Memorial Hospital
1925–7	1,945	–
1928–30	1,970	368
1931–5	3,759	880
1936–7	1,761	404

Source: Woolwich MOH, *A/Rs* (1925–38).

Table 6.9: Number of beds and patients in various LCC hospitals in the four boroughs, 1929–34

	Number of beds 1931	Total number of in-patients	
		1929–31	1932–4
Hampstead: New End Hospital	19	618	1,261
Kensington: St Mary Abbot's Hospital	20	1,363	2,325
Stepney: Mile End Hospital	42	1,616	1,956
St George's-in-the-East Hospital	25	965	858
St Peter's Hospital	13	453	470
Woolwich: St Nicholas Hospital	19	373	979

Source: 'Accommodation in Maternity Wards', in L. Fairfield's papers GLRO file:
Ph/Gen/3/6.

Table 6.10: Percentage of total births in Stepney occurring in Poor Law/LCC institutions or in voluntary hospitals, 1905–38

Year	% Poor Law/LCC hospital births	% Voluntary hospital births
1905–9	2	3
1910–15	25	7
1922–5	6	23
1926–30	17	30
1931–5	27	33
1936–8	33	32

Source: Stepney MOH, *A/Rs* (1905–38).

In Hampstead and Kensington where a large proportion of patients
could afford to pay for their own maternity care, maternity services

206

were much more mixed than in Woolwich and Stepney. Many of the mothers in these two boroughs were private patients either of midwives or doctors who delivered them at their own homes or in small maternity homes. In Hampstead 29 per cent of all institutional births took place in a maternity or nursing home. No other area in London revealed such a high percentage (Table 6.6). In Kensington only 4 per cent of births occurred in such homes, although this was higher than that recorded for the more working-class boroughs.

The higher numbers seeking care within a maternity home in the two boroughs, especially Hampstead, partly reflected the prosperity of the residents as well as the relative absence of large voluntary teaching hospitals in these areas. As Table 6.6 shows the proportion of institutional births taking place within a voluntary hospital was much smaller in Kensington and Hampstead when compared with the other boroughs. One of the major providers of institutional maternity care in Hampstead and Kensington was Queen Charlotte's Hospital, which was based in the borough of St Marylebone. This Hospital catered for private patients as well as those funded by the borough council. Mothers in Kensington could also make their own private arrangements to be confined in the St George's and St Marylebone Hospitals, and Princess Beatrice Hospital in Redcliffe, South Kensington, from 1930.[18]

In Hampstead some charitable provision, not sponsored by the council, was available through Queen Mary's Maternity Home in Hampstead, a voluntary home set up for the wives of ex-servicemen in 1921. Some in-patient provision was also made by the Hampstead and Kensington councils for the poorer mothers in these boroughs through municipal hospitals (originally Poor Law institutions), such as New End Hospital and Hampstead General Hospital in Hampstead, and St Mary Abbot's Hospital in Kensington (Table 6.9 for the number of beds provided and patients covered). As Table 6.6 indicates, of the two boroughs, Kensington had a much greater number of its institutional births being confined in a London County Council hospital, partly reflecting the greater number of poor mothers within the vicinity.

Domiciliary Midwifery, 1902–36

While hospital provision was increasing during the inter-war years, domiciliary midwifery was given less priority. This policy is particularly striking when we consider the popularity of municipal health visitors who were universally provided in these years. It would seem that while the state and local authorities were keen to fund preventive care such as health visiting, this did not extend to a form of care which would guarantee safe delivery. In London very few borough councils provided municipally funded district midwives. As can be seen from Table 6.1 only six of the 28 metropolitan councils in 1932 made such provision. Councils outside London were also reluctant to fund such midwives.

Like councils elsewhere, those in Hampstead, Stepney and Woolwich preferred to subsidize district midwifery by grants to district nursing associations. In part there was no need to fund a municipal midwife in these areas because of the wide out-patient provision being made by the hospitals, particularly in Stepney and Woolwich. In Hampstead it was also not a viable option because there were too few poor mothers. Overall the number of mothers eligible for help from Hampstead Council for district midwifery care was small rising from 7 per cent of all births in 1921–5 to 13 per cent in 1935–7. Table 6.11 shows how many patients this covered and how it compared with the provision Hampstead Council made for institutional care. What is puzzling is that institutional cases outnumbered district cases in the late 1920s and then dropped in the 1930s contrary to the overall rise in hospital births in Hampstead as a whole. By the 1930s, however, the number of district cases was equal to those cared for within institutions.

Table 6.11: Maternity cases covered by Hampstead Council's Maternity Scheme, 1921–37

Year	Midwifery cases undertaken by District Nursing Associations		Institutional Births		Maternity cases eligible for council help as % of total births
	Number	% of total births	Number	% of total births	
1921–5	499	7	–	–	–
1926–30	597	9	1,175	18	27
1931–4	587	12	665	13	25
1935–7	404	13	415	13	26

Source: Hampstead MOH, *A/Rs* (1921–37).

Unlike the three other boroughs, Kensington gave higher priority to domiciliary midwifery, appointing a municipal midwife in 1934. Based in South Kensington, this midwife was intended to fill a particularly important gap in maternity provision in Kensington. Maternity care was much better provided for poor mothers in North Kensington, the most poverty stricken part of the borough, than in South Kensington where poverty was more invisible because rich residents vastly outnumbered the poor. In 1916 a number of voluntary agencies provided certified midwives to mothers in North Kensington, which included the Kensington Maternity Association (serving Norland, Pembridge and most of the Holland wards), the Kensal Medical and Gospel Mission (catering to Golborne ward); and the St Mary Abot's Maternity Society (covering the parishes of St Mary Abbots, St Philips, St Mathias and St Barnabas). All these agencies had a subscription fee and guaranteed funding for a doctor in cases of emergency, although the Kensal Medical and Gospel Mission excluded first confinements from their scheme. From 1916 pupil midwives from Queen Charlotte's Hospital were using district maternity cases in Kensington for their midwifery training, undertaking 700 cases in that year.[19] In 1921 Kensington Council began to finance this scheme.[20]

North Kensington also had good facilities for in-patient care. From 1924 Kensington Borough Council began to fund maternity beds for residents in North Kensington either in cases of emergency or with bad housing conditions. Known as the Kensington Maternity Home, this home was based originally in St Mary Abbot's Hospital, on the southern edge of North Kensington, and later moved to Queen Charlotte's Hospital in St Marylebone in 1931.

An equivalent service was not provided for poor mothers in South Kensington.[21] Similarly district midwifery was poor in South Kensington. In 1924 one infant welfare centre in South Kensington attempted to provide a charitable midwifery service, but this had trouble surviving. One difficulty in providing domiciliary midwifery in South Kensington was that the poor mothers were widely scattered and there was no area which could provide a sufficient number of cases to enable a midwife in private practice to earn a reasonable living. Only when the council finally appointed a municipal midwife attached to the South Kensington infant welfare centre in 1934 was the problem resolved.[22]

Popular and Local Forces in the Provision of Maternity Care

The disparity of maternity services between North and South Kensington indicates the ways in which social and economic deprivation of certain areas shaped the provision of maternity care. Because of their high levels of poverty and correspondingly acute need for cheap and effective midwifery care, North Kensington, Stepney and Woolwich were ideal locations for teaching institutions. In exchange for the provision of charitable midwifery, these places could be guaranteed cases for teaching. This tactic was used not only in the case of maternity care, but also for medical training in general. For many poor patients access to cheaper or free medical care as provided in the voluntary hospitals was vital.

One explanation for the popularity of the hospitals among maternity patients was also the overcrowding and poor housing conditions in these areas. This reason was particularly apparent in Stepney where few houses had running water, and most were poorly furnished and lacked even basic utilities such as blankets and facilities for boiling water. Cramped housing also meant there was no escape from the noise and arguments of families in the background.[23] Kensington faced comparable conditions.[24] Even in an area like Woolwich, which had a low density of population and the highest proportion of working-class householders in London, the pressures on housing were great, and were particularly strained as a result of the influx of munitions workers during the First World War.[25]

During the inter-war period both Stepney and Woolwich councils invested in large housing programmes, but this was not enough to cover the needs of the population in each borough. By the 1920s new blocks of flats were appearing in East London with bathrooms and electric lighting, but the rent charged for such accommodation was 'quite prohibitive', forcing many to continue living in over-crowded insanitary tenement houses.[26] In Woolwich the number of tenement houses was much smaller than in Stepney and there was more room space per person, but the increasing population in the borough in these years none the less caused problems of overcrowding in particular parts of the borough. In 1925 it was estimated that additional accommodation was needed in Woolwich for 6,000 persons.[27] The difficulties this caused are highlighted by the appeal the British Hospital for Mothers and Babies made to its subscribers to

> Think a little of the respectable hardworking women who have frequently *only one room* for themselves and their growing girls and boys, the said room being their only refuge for confinement and convalescence. For such a room, many families pay as much as 10s. 6d. a week, out of an income of £2 or under, and sometimes the affair is even worse than this. One nice woman pleaded with me, recently, for a bed, because she had to share her room with a night worker, and therefore she said: 'During the day I have nowhere to go I have to walk about all the time.' And this, when she was shortly expecting a baby![28]

In 1931 the British Hospital for Mothers and Babies reported that

> Nearly all young married couples in Woolwich have one room only to live in, and our patients have to conceal the fact that they are expecting a baby from their landlady, for fear of being turned out at a week's notice in consequence. If she does not actually put them in the street, she makes life difficult in every way for the young couple,

so that in addition to their other anxieties they must find fresh lodging – often an impossible task at such a moment.[29]

Given these conditions it is not surprising that as early as 1913 the East End Maternity Home in Stepney declared that 'without doubt, the best place for a poor woman to be confined is not her own home'. Indeed, in later years the hospital argued that because many of the houses lacked the 'common necessities of life' normal cases of birth were at serious risk.[30] It reported that twice in one year a ceiling had fallen down while an infant was being born at home, leaving the mother less perturbed than the nurses.[31] Similar conclusions were reached by other hospitals in East London and in Woolwich, and were part of a more general feeling among government officials who saw an increase in the number of maternity hospitals and homes as a means of coping with such housing problems.[32] The urgency of the housing problems in the poorer boroughs is contrasted by the experience of Hampstead, where the need for hospital maternity beds was less acute because accommodation was less strained and many residents were living in more than one room.[33] Table 6.12 shows that very few of the home births in Hampstead took place in tenements with just one room, most had two to three rooms.

Table 6.12: Number of births that took place at home and the size of the houses in which the births took place, Hampstead, 1905, 1925–38

Date	Total home births	Home births as % total births	% births in 1-room tenements	% births in 2-room tenements	% births in 3-room tenements	% births occurred at mother's place of residence	% of births at other addresses
1905	–	–	12	46	26	–	–
1925–9	704	11	2	32	50	27	–
1930–4	1,441	23	7	40	39	46	3
1935–8	1,496	36	12	37	37	55	3

1905 figures from inspection by lady sanitary inspector of births.

Source: Hampstead MOH, *A/R* (1905, 1925–38).

According to the medical reports women in Stepney and Woolwich by the late 1920s were themselves demanding hospital rather than home confinements.[34] In the mid 1920s The London Hospital claimed that there was 'an even greater desire for in-patient treatment than in former years, owing no doubt to the abominable home conditions which prevail in many quarters'.[35] In 1932 those running the British

Hospital for Mothers and Babies reported a similar increase which they attributed to 'the growing enlightenment of parents who begin to see that a crowded one or two room tenement is not the favourable spot for the arrival of a new baby'. This trend in Woolwich was reinforced by the upsurge in overcrowding as well as the high rates of unemployment in these years.[36] Reflecting the economic hardship of this time Tables 6.7 and 6.8 both show a substantial increase in the number of hospital in-patients in Woolwich and Stepney in the late 1920s and early 1930s.

Housing conditions and economic hardship were not the only factors pushing women into hospital, but also the fear of death. Mrs A. who had lost both of her married sisters through childbirth, was determined to be confined in hospital. When under anaesthetic at the British Hospital for Mothers and Babies in 1924 she had repeatedly cried out 'Oh, I can't stay at home! If only I could get in there! I'll work my fingers to the bone. I'll save every penny.'[37] Some women saw their stay in hospital as a holiday and a chance to get away from the pressure of housework and family.[38]

Adequate provision for home confinements was also impossible in such conditions and most women could not afford to hire handy-women or home helps who could aid them in the house and with childcare during their confinement. Before the war most handy-women were paid 10s. for 10 days with food, which increased to a minimum of 15s. per week after the war.[39] This was a large sum compared with the average working-class wage of 25s.[40] As can be seen from the instructions to mothers from the City of London Maternity Home in 1936, the housing conditions required for a home birth as laid down by the hospitals would also have been particularly difficult to achieve for many impoverished mothers.

> The room should be the best available in the house with as much sun and air as possible, and near the bathroom is advisable as it saves endless steps for the nurse. Do not have more furniture in it than is really needed. Good lighting should be considered. The carpet should be rolled up, or if this is not possible, it should be well protected with sheets. A single bed is preferable and with a foot end. Plenty of bed linen and some old sheets, also a small one, are needed.[41]

Whatever the reasons for a woman's decision to have her baby in a hospital, it is clear that by the 1920s pressures were mounting on maternity beds all over London, and hospitals were struggling to cope with the costs and the demands being made on their beds.[42] In 1922 40 per cent of the patients seeking in-patient care at The

London Hospital had to be referred elsewhere. This percentage was reduced in 1927 to 22 as a result of the creation of more beds in the hospital. Other hospitals in East London and elsewhere reported similar demands on beds. In 1927 the medical officer of health in Woolwich complained that the number of maternity beds in the borough was 'not yet equal to the demand' and 'the provision of further beds would mean a further increase in the number of women entering institutions for their confinements'.[43] While many mothers pleaded with the British Hospital for Mothers and Babies to be let into the hospital, by 1934 over 1,000 were being turned away each year for lack of beds.[44] Pressures were also felt on the beds provided by the council in North Kensington.[45]

While the demand for in-patient care, particularly during the late 1920s and early 1930s might have stemmed from the economic recession in these years which was preventing many mothers from being able to hire a midwife to care for them at home, such a move towards hospital care was also part of a more general public debate concerning the dangers of childbirth. Many policy makers and medical officers such as Janet Campbell and Janet Lane-Claypon, and other women campaigners such as Lady Rhys-Williams of the National Birthday Trust, advocated hospital births for emergency cases and first confinements. They nevertheless saw home births as much safer and cheaper.[46] This view was confirmed by the Department Committee on Maternal Mortality and Morbidity in their final report in 1932. Even the College (later Royal College) of Obstetricians and Gynaecologists, founded in 1929, with its emphasis on building up the specialty of obstetrics and gynaecology, endorsed the government policy for a national maternity service in the 1930s, which was based on home deliveries by midwives and general practitioners as the backbone of the service, with hospital deliveries reserved for 'social' admissions, high risk cases and emergencies.[47]

This was a policy which Dr Fenton, the medical officer for health in Kensington, was also keen to follow. While he felt more accommodation was needed in the borough for first confinements, cases of complication, and those patients whose home surroundings were unsuitable for confinement, he felt that every effort should be made to provide domiciliary midwifery for poor mothers. He showed that while there was adequate charitable district midwifery in North Kensington, the absence of such provision in South Kensington was pushing many poor mothers to seek the care of voluntary hospitals. He felt that 'this was inadvisable from the obstetric point of view' as it not only led 'to overcrowding of the maternity wards', but also

added to the risk of infection and was uneconomical.[48] His reluctance
to promote hospital provision might also explain the low rate of
hospital confinements in Kensington overall compared to the three
other boroughs. The low rate of institutional births is particularly
interesting given the acute housing problems that existed in the
north of the borough.

Just as some medical professionals had reservations about hospital
confinements, some women were also reluctant to go into hospital.
Their hesitancy was not necessarily linked to their perceptions about
the safety of births in hospital. A number of women who were
told by their doctor to go to into The London refused because they
'didn't trust their husbands, and wouldn't leave them'.[49] Many women
could not rely on family or neighbours to look after the children in
their absence, and financial constraints also limited the possibility of
employing someone to undertake such work. In Stepney arrangements could be made by the council to board out children in a large
family where there was no alternative, but this was not utilized on a
large scale.[50] Many hospitals although keen to promote hospital
births, continued to provide an out-patient service in recognition of
these problems.[51]

Antenatal Provision, 1914–36

Much of the move towards hospital provision for births was linked
to questions about the safety of childbirth. During the 1920s antenatal care became an increasingly regular part of maternity provision. Much of this stemmed from the increasing anxiety over
maternal mortality which persisted and even seemed to be rising
despite the tightened restrictions on midwifery training and practice, and the improvements in antiseptics and obstetric care. The
seriousness of the problem was made that much more pertinent by
the fact that infant mortality by contrast was falling. For many medical practitioners and politicians preventative measures during pregnancy was increasingly seen as the only answer.[52]

The importance attached to antenatal provision can be seen from
the upsurge in facilities in these years. Between 1915 and 1918 the
number of antenatal clinics sponsored by local health authorities and
voluntary organizations grew rapidly from 12 to 120 and had risen to
1,417 in 1933.[53] Table 6.1 indicates that by the early 1930s antenatal
provision was very widespread in London. By 1934 this included 99
antenatal clinics provided by borough councils and 23 hosted by
voluntary hospitals.[54] In addition to this, women had access to antenatal
provision from London County Council clinics or alternatively

could get private care from their general practitioner.

Such an abundance of facilities, however, meant that the responsibility and location of antenatal services tended to be split between many different institutions, clinics and general practitioners' surgeries with minimal communications between all parties. Effective antenatal supervision therefore relied on a high degree of cooperation between midwives, general practitioners and hospital consultants, which was rare in the inter-war period. Lack of coordination was not only prevalent in London, but in the country as a whole. In 1932 the Committee investigating maternal mortality highlighted this problem as the chief reason for the poor quality of antenatal supervision in these years.[55] Leticia Fairfield, the chief medical officer of health for the London County Council, also pointed out that within London the mixture of clinics and the informal character with which they had been set up made it difficult to classify the extent of antenatal work within the metropolis. As she admitted, this made it 'totally impossible to define which of the patients' had 'received "full" or "inadequate" antenatal care'.[56]

According to the Committee investigating maternal mortality the ideal antenatal care had two functions. The first was to educate women on their own and their infants' health and diet. The second entailed a full medical examination of women, which included measuring a woman's pelvis, her blood pressure, examining her breasts and testing her urine, as well as monitoring the foetal heart beat. Where necessary vaginal examinations and Wassermann tests were also to be carried out. All these procedures were to be done alongside taking the woman's full medical and obstetric history, and details of her home conditions. Such antenatal supervision was to begin at the 16th week of pregnancy and to be repeated at the 24th and 28th weeks, then every fortnight until the 36th week, and thereafter weekly until confinement. While the initial and final examinations were to be carried out by a medical officer, routine check-ups were to be in the hands of midwives and where necessary nursing care was also to be provided.[57]

In reality antenatal attention did not match up to this model. Those mothers who sought their antenatal attention from their general practitioner usually received less rigorous antenatal attention than if they visited a clinic organized by the London County Council, borough council, or voluntary hospital. By 1934 doctors would almost certainly do one full antenatal medical examination if they were booked in advance and paid the minimum fee. Some offered a second examination in the later months of pregnancy and undertook regular urinanalysis and tests of blood pressure. Any intermediate attention needed, however, was not usually covered by general practitioners, most women having instead to rely on the borough antenatal clinic or hospital. Overall, clinics hosted by hospitals and the borough council offered a more comprehensive service from the start to the finish of a woman's pregnancy, and this was closer to the ideal set by the Committee investigating maternal mortality.[58]

None the less, while most hospital and council clinics expected women to attend at least once, rules varied as to the number of sub-sequent visits they were expected to make as did the degree of medical attention they actually received. [59] Most voluntary hospitals insisted mothers start attending an antenatal clinic from four months into the pregnancy. This policy was enforced in the voluntary sector because the women could not secure a booking for a hospital confinement after that date.[60] By contrast, London County Council hospitals and maternity homes did not enforce this rule, which meant that many of their women received antenatal care at a much later stage in their pregnancy.[61]

Once attending a clinic the degree to which a woman received medical attention varied. In 1925, replies to a survey undertaken of antenatal care in 25 metropolitan boroughs showed that 68 per cent of them ensured that patients were seen by a doctor at each visit, 69 per cent made vaginal examinations where advisable but only 18 per cent did such examinations in all cases. In 8 per cent of the cases no vaginal examination was undertaken at all, the woman being referred instead to the doctor or midwife engaged to deliver her. Of the replies 53 per cent said that their clinic had a close link with the hospitals or institution with antenatal beds and out-patient departments where specialist obstetric care was available, but 23 per cent of the replies denied having such links. Only in 6 per cent of the cases were there special arrangements for urgent cases. Of the centres surveyed 46 per cent communicated directly with the doctor or midwife caring for the patient, but in 5 per cent of the cases this was only done where there was an abnormality.[62] By the 1930s most abnormalities were being referred back to their general practitioner or to a hospital.[63] It was understood that no medical treatment was to be carried out in council clinics. This measure inevitably meant that antenatal attention for many women was divided between a variety of competing agencies and individuals. Cooperation between the different bodies, therefore, was crucial if antenatal care was to be successful.

As was the case elsewhere, antenatal provision in Hampstead, Kensington, Stepney and Woolwich was divided between a number of institutions. In all the boroughs general practitioners not only offered antenatal support, but so did health visitors and a host of special clinics. As Table 6.13 shows, the percentage of expectant mothers visited by a health visitor grew substantially in all the boroughs between the 1920s and 1930s, and was particularly high in Kensington. Their task largely consisted of checking whether the mother was following the instructions set by the clinic and to assess whether her home was suitable for a home confinement. Much of the work that the health visitors undertook in this respect was tied to that being carried out either in the hospitals or special antenatal clinics.

Table 6.13: Number and percentage of all expectant mothers receiving at least one visit from a health visitor in four London boroughs, 1918–38

Borough	Date	Number of mothers visited once by a health visitor	Number of mothers visited by a health visitor as % of total births in the borough
Hampstead	1921–5	671	11
	1926–30	689	14
	1931–5	1,001	21
	1936–8	1,327	43
Kensington	1921–5	1,674	11
	1926–30	3,053	19
	1931–5	8,172	72
Stepney	1921–5	3,187	11
	1926–30	3,068	14
	1931–5	6,608	38
Woolwich	1918–20	313	3
	1921–5	1,820	13
	1926–30	2,486	22
	1931–5	3,669	36
	1936–8	2,948	48

Sources: Hampstead, Kensington, Stepney and Woolwich MOH, *A/Rs* (1918–38).

Many of the antenatal clinics, like the one founded by the Kensington Maternity Association, had begun as voluntary initiatives as early as 1914. They were followed by the establishment of antenatal facilities in various voluntary infant welfare centres in Kensington.[64] By 1915 Queen Charlotte's Hospital was also offering antenatal care for primiparae women and those with complicated medical histories sent in by the pupil midwives in North Kensington.[65] Antenatal clinics were also hosted by hospitals in the other boroughs, such as the British Hospital for Mothers and Babies in Woolwich in 1915, and the East End Maternity Home, The London Hospital, and the Jewish Maternity Home in Stepney from the early 1920s.[66] In addition to these hospitals, antenatal attention was available through Poor Law (later London County Council) hospitals. At most hospitals women who wanted to be sure of maternity care during their delivery could only do so by making regular visits to antenatal sessions.

Table 6.14: Antenatal provision made in four London boroughs, 1935

	No. of Centres	No. of births per centre	No. of sessions per week	No. of births per session
Hampstead	2(a)	456	3(a)	303
Kensington	11(c)	204	c.5	448
Stepney	1(a)3(b)3(d)	432	1(a)6(b)4(d)	275
Woolwich	4(a)	513	6(a)	342

(a) provided by the borough council.
(b) provided by a voluntary association.
(c) provided by the borough council's agreement with a voluntary association.
(d) provided by the borough council's agreement with the LCC.

Source: 'MCW Provision Made or Provided in Metropolitan Boroughs', in LCC, *Maternal Mortality: Hospital and Medical Services (Hospital Management Sub-Committee), Report by MOH,* 10 May 1935, Appendix A (GLRO file: Ph/Gen/3/7/7).

Alongside the voluntarily sponsored provision municipally funded schemes also developed. In 1915 one of the first municipally funded antenatal clinics in the country was founded in Woolwich.[67] Two years later a similar clinic was established in Hampstead. Municipally funded antenatal clinics were less forthcoming in Stepney and Kensington, partly reflecting the fact that antenatal services were adequately provided by other bodies such as hospitals and infant welfare centres. Table 6.14 shows that by 1935 antenatal centres in Hampstead and Woolwich mostly remained in the care of the borough council, while those in Kensington were dominated by voluntary associations. Stepney, by contrast, had a mixture of providers, including the London County Council.

Of the boroughs, Kensington had the most antenatal centres when measured against the number of births, but a limited number of sessions. Stepney had fewer centres per birth, but the largest number of sessions. As Table 6.14 indicates the average case load of patients was potentially much lower in Stepney (when measured by sessions), therefore allowing for greater time and perhaps better attention than in the other boroughs.

There is little information, however, on the actual extent of the provision that was made, and it is difficult to assess because of the number of agencies involved. In 1932 it was estimated that in London and in over 33 large towns the number of women attending an

antenatal clinic had reached over 50 per cent of the births notified. In
only 7 per cent of the towns surveyed were attendances less than 20 per
cent of the births notified.[68]

Table 6.15: Percentage of women receiving antenatal attention in four London boroughs, 1923–37

Date	Hampstead	Kensington	Stepney	Woolwich
1923	–	–	–	18
1925	25	–	–	26
1926	–	59•	–	30
1927	–	–	–	35
1928	26	68	–	40
1930	>40	66	–	56
1931	31	–	–	54
1932	>33	–	–	52
1933	–	–	–	53
1934	c.33	85	–	57
1935	–	–	93*	50
1936	31	82	–	53
1937	–	–	–	56

The percentage of mothers attending antenatal clinics for Hampstead is calculated according to the number of women attending council clinics. This might be an underestimate of the true figure as it does not include the number of mothers who were receiving antenatal care from private general practitioners and private midwives.

In Woolwich the percentage of mothers receiving antenatal care is calculated according to the number of expectant mothers attending various council clinics. The type of treatment these mothers received is not specified, but most of these women would have received antenatal care at these clinics.

• The percentage for this year was based on the number of women the MOH considered eligible for council welfare provision. When based on the total number of women giving birth during this year the percentage of women receiving antenatal care is 43%. Like Hampstead, the figures for antenatal attendance might be an underestimate, as mothers receiving antenatal care from their own doctors and private midwives were not always included in the overall estimate.

* This figure is based on the findings of a questionnaire filled in by health visitors for the Stepney MOH to ascertain the supervision each mother had received during her pregnancy. Of the 3,118 mothers confined for that year, 2,737 or 88% responded to the questionnaire.

Sources: MOH, *A/Rs* for Hampstead, Kensington, Stepney and Woolwich (1918–1937); Kensington Council Minutes, 28 July 1931, 343; Stepney MCW Committee Minutes, 16 January 1935 (THL file 1088).

In Stepney and Kensington the coverage was much greater than the estimates of the survey, and than that of Hampstead and Woolwich. In 1935 a questionnaire answered by 88 per cent of pregnant mothers in Stepney showed that 93 per cent of them had attended an antenatal clinic.[69] As Table 6.15 illustrates, this was much higher than the national average of 54 per cent recorded two years later, and than the rates recorded for the other boroughs. Kensington had the next greatest coverage, reaching 85 per cent in 1934. Closest to the national average was Woolwich. By contrast, Hampstead had the lowest proportion of mothers receiving antenatal attention.

One of the reasons for the smaller coverage in Hampstead was the very high number of rich residents in the area. Many of these residents attended a private doctor or midwife, which makes it difficult to monitor the degree to which they received antenatal supérvision and the quality of care bestowed upon them.[70] When these mothers are excluded from the calculations, and antenatal care is considered in respect to mothers on a low income, Hampstead's record on antenatal care appears better than Table 6.15 suggests.

The two municipal antenatal clinics established in Hampstead were significantly placed in the poorer parts of the borough. Together these clinics held three sessions a week. Twice as many clinics were held at the centre in Kilburn, indicating the higher number of births in this area, and the larger number of poor mothers who could not afford to go to a private practitioner for antenatal supervision. All mothers in Hampstead who were not being attended by a doctor who were thinking of entering a hospital or institution or being attended by a midwife were strongly advised by the Council to avail themselves of the facilities of the council's antenatal clinics.[71]

Table 6.16 shows how the number of mothers attending an antenatal session at one of the council's clinics in Hampstead rose in the years between 1922 and 1938, peaking to 43 per cent of all births in 1931–5. In addition to the attendances at these clinics, mothers were also receiving care at clinics attached to maternity hospitals. By the early 1930s the medical officer of health in Hampstead noted that mothers were showing a marked increase in their readiness to take advantage of the antenatal provision than they had 16 years previously, and that expectant mothers were attending clinics much earlier in their pregnancies.[72] He also claimed that the coordination between the antenatal clinics and the midwives and nursing associations in Hampstead was more than adequate.[73]

While Hampstead provided good access to antenatal provision for its poor mothers, Kensington had greater coverage, partly reflecting its higher level of poverty. As early as 1923 51 per cent of those women considered to have an income which made them eligible for the council's maternal and child welfare services were attending an antenatal clinic, which accounted for 41 per cent of the total notified births. By 1931 the number of women in this category obtaining antenatal care from infant welfare centres in Kensington had risen to 70 per cent.[74] This high percentage indicates that a very high proportion of women in Kensington who could not afford private antenatal attention had access to subsidized antenatal care. Many of these women obtained their antenatal care through clinics run by the voluntary infant welfare centres. As Table 6.17 shows 58 per cent of all expectant mothers in Kensington received antenatal care from centres in the years 1936–8.

Table 6.16: Number and percentage of all expectant mothers attending an antenatal clinic for antenatal care in Hampstead, 1922–38

Date	Total number of expectant mothers attending an antenatal session	Number of expectant amothers attending antenatal session as % of total borough births	Average number of attendances per session
1922–5	1,127	24	16
1926–30	1,720	34	20
1931–5	2,054	43	27
1936–8	1,163	37	25

Source: Hampstead MOH, *A/Rs* (1922–38).

When considered in relation to the model of antenatal care set by the Committee investigating maternal mortality, antenatal care in Kensington also appears to have been of a high standard. In most cases pregnant women received a visit by the borough council's health visitor and were invited to attend one of the antenatal clinics.[75] The number of attendances each women made was also relatively high. By the 1930s women were calling on the antenatal clinic hosted by an infant welfare centre on average between three to four times in their pregnancy. This attendance was higher than the average number of attendances made at similar clinics in Woolwich, where it was just over two visits per woman (Table 6.17). The average attendance in Kensington matched that for London and the country as a whole, where the average was 4 and 3.5 respectively.[76]

While Kensington had extensive coverage and a good record for attendance at antenatal clinics, its provision was not without faults. In 1933 an investigation discovered ten different doctors engaged in antenatal work in the infant welfare centres, and that coordination was poor. This problem was remedied in 1934 with the appointment of a municipally funded full-time medical officer for antenatal care. She was not only expected to attend all the antenatal sessions held in the borough's maternity home, the maternity ward at St Mary Abbot's Hospital and the different infant welfare centres, but to also have her own regular consultation hours for mothers who needed urgent advice.[77] In this year arrangements were also made to hold a weekly evening antenatal session to help those mothers who could not attend during the day.[78] By 1934 there were ten institutions where antenatal clinics were held and hospital treatment was available at Queen Charlotte's Hospital and St Mary Abbot's Hospital.[79] Most of the Kensington midwives were also cooperating and sending their patients for medical supervision at antenatal clinics.[80]

Table 6.17: Number and percentage of all expectant mothers attending an infant welfare centre for antenatal care in Kensington and Woolwich, 1919–38

Borough	Date	Total number of expectant mothers	Number of expectant mothers attending an antenatal session as % of total borough births	Total number of attendances	Average number of attendances per mother attending the antenatal session
Kensington	1921–5	1,986	13	4,992	2.5•
	1926–30	2,454	19	9,230	3.8•
	1931–5	3,504	30	12,587	3.6•
	1936–8	3,798	58	16,608	4.4•
Woolwich	1919–20	487	7	1,225	2.5
	1921–5	2,848	20	4,801	1,7
	1926–30	4,692	41	9,117	1.9
	1931–5	5,368	53	13,550	2.5
	1936–7	2,241	54	5,776	2.6

• These figures refer to the number of attendances mothers made to a doctor's antenatal consultation within the infant welfare centre, divided by the total number of expectant mothers attending ante-natal sessions at the centre not all of which had a doctor present.

Sources: Kensington and Woolwich MOH, *A/Rs* (1920–38).

By 1937 the organization of antenatal care in Kensington was said to have had excellent results and close cooperation existed between clinics, doctors, midwives and hospitals. Only on rare occasions were women unable to obtain antenatal care.[81] In cases of abnormality picked up by the antenatal clinics, the patients' husbands were interviewed by the 'medical officer to obtain their co-operation', and the council's services for boarding out the children were utilized to allow the mother's immediate admission to hospital. Hospital staff were also consulted personally about the case, and it was claimed that in each instance 'the woman's life was saved'.[82]

Antenatal provision was also extremely good in Stepney where there was close cooperation between the hospitals and the voluntary and municipal infant welfare centres.[83] Most women who booked for a hospital confinement at the hospitals in Stepney could only do so by attending the antenatal sessions. Like elsewhere, young women about to undergo their first confinement were expected to attend the antenatal clinics more often than those who had already had children. Hospitals such as The London kept a 'strict watch' on 'possible defaulters'. While many women could have experienced such policies as coercive, most women were reported as returning to the clinics and taking full advantage of their facilities.[84]

In addition to the good antenatal care on offer in the hospitals, there was a high degree of cooperation with midwives in Stepney. All midwives were invited to attend and bring their own cases to the antenatal clinics. Where a midwife could not attend she was supplied with printed forms to send with their cases to a doctor at the clinic which was filled in by the doctor and returned to the midwife. Close liaison also existed between the voluntary antenatal clinics, the municipal home visiting scheme, and the hospitals. Hospitals were immediately informed of any cases of unusual poverty or illness through this scheme.[85]

Although Table 6.15 suggests that antenatal provision in Woolwich was not as extensive as that in Stepney or Kensington, the borough does seem to have provided a more than ample service for the needs of its population. By 1934 Woolwich had four antenatal clinics which were held on the premises of the infant welfare centres, and clinics were also held in all the hospitals of the borough with maternity beds. Table 6.17 shows that the percentage of expectant mothers receiving antenatal care at infant welfare centres rose steadily in the years between 1919 and 1937, and was greater than that of mothers attending similar facilities in Kensington by the late 1920s. Like the other boroughs, antenatal services were considered to be well coordinated in Woolwich. Most of the midwives sent their cases to the Council's antenatal clinics. This action was encouraged by the council who paid their fees in necessitous cases and also provided compensation when the cases were to be confined in hospital. Beds were also available for antenatal cases at the British Hospital for Mothers and Babies and War Memorial Hospital, at a charge of 9s. a day to the council.[86]

Table 6.18: Number of cases and attendances at antenatal clinics run by six LCC hospitals, 1931–4

Borough	Hospital	Total cases	Total attendances	Average number of attendances per mother
Hampstead	New End	1,097	4,121	3.7
Kensington	St Mary Abbot's	2,173	9,198	4.2
Stepney	Mile End	2,904	15,696	5.4
	St George's-in-the-East	1,327	6,380	4.8
	St Peter's	763	3,601	4.
Woolwich	St Nicholas	1,424	8,425	5.9

Sources: LCC, *Maternal Mortality: Hospital and Medical Services (Hospital Management Sub-Committee) Report by MOH,* 10 May 1935, Appendix B (GLRO file: Ph/Gen/3/7/7).

In addition to the coverage of the various schemes run in each of the boroughs, from the 1920s mothers also had access to clinics run by Poor Law (later London County Council) hospitals (see Table 6.18 for those hospitals in the four boroughs and their number of patients). The cooperation between these institutions and the other facilities in the borough was dependent on local conditions. At nine London County Council hospitals there were definite arrangements with the borough medical officer of health that patients who wished to be confined in hospital could, if they preferred, attend antenatal clinics run by the borough either throughout the whole of their pregnancy except for one or two examinations at the hospital clinics, or until the 36th week, thereafter transferring to the hospital clinic. Where any abnormality was detected the patient was to be sent straight to the hospital's clinic. By 1933 nearly 84 per cent of the patients confined in London County Council lying-in wards had attended London County Council run antenatal clinics.[87]

On average the number of attendances a woman made to antenatal clinics run by London County Council hospitals was high, reaching five visits in 1933.[88] Table 6.18 shows that the average number of attendances women made to antenatal clinics organized by the different London County Council hospitals in the four boroughs varied between 3.7 at New End Hospital in Hampstead and 5.9 at St Nicholas Hospital in Woolwich. This attendance level compared well with a voluntary hospital such as the British Hospital for Mothers and Babies in Woolwich, where the average number of visits was 5.4 in the years 1931–5.[89] Overall the percentage of women attending London County Council clinics for more than one session was high throughout London. Table 6.19 indicates that at least 31 per cent of women attending such clinics were making between four and six visits each. In 1934 a report for the London County Council on maternity services highlighted the good attendance, stating

> The experience of the Council's hospitals shows that the mothers (even the poorest and most destitute and the unmarried girls) show a remarkable degree of appreciation of the importance of antenatal care and of willingness to cooperate. They attend as often as is asked, and travel long distances if required. 'Lapsed' cases are very few, and are now followed up by the almoners and health visitors. If a woman fails to receive antenatal care it is either (a) because she belongs to a small and recalcitrant group who think it is not worthwhile, (b) because she is a multipara who is bound by household ties and has lost her fear of the danger of childbirth, or (c) is a single girl deterred for obvious social reasons.[90]

Table 6.19: Number and percentage of antenatal attendances at LCC antenatal clinics, 1933

Number of attendances	Number of cases	Number of cases as % of total
0	1,823	16
1 – 3	2,690	24
4 – 6	3,513	31
7 – 9	2,317	20
Over 10	1,015	9
Not known	74	0.6
Total	11,432	

Sources: LCC, *Maternal Mortality: Hospital and Medical Services (Hospital Management Sub-Committee) Report by the MOH,* 10 May 1935, 2 (GLRO file: Ph/Gen/3/7/7).

In all London County Council hospitals and voluntary hospitals, beds were available for antenatal women who had complications.[91] Both the East End Maternity Home and the British Hospital for Mothers and Babies were unusual in that they were prepared to take women in a few days before their confinement so that they could catch up on some rest. Most hospitals required that a woman actually be in labour before they would admit her.[92]

It would seem, therefore, that in all the boroughs, antenatal services were generally well coordinated by health visitors, London County Council and voluntary hospitals, and the various infant welfare centres. Such coordination was vital where those attending the woman for antenatal care differed from those who delivered her during confinement. Coordination, however, was difficult given the host of agencies involved. None the less, it would seem that in all the boroughs efforts were made to overcome this problem. Such measures were probably the best that could be undertaken in antenatal care during this period, and was particularly important for selecting and monitoring those cases considered to be at a high risk of dying during childbirth. What effect this had on the overall health of mothers will be considered in relation to maternity care as a whole below.

Effectiveness of the Services Provided

While it would seem that the four boroughs had good coverage in a range of services, such provision tells us nothing about the effectiveness that it had on maternal health in each of the areas. In considering this issue it is important to distinguish between the different causes of maternal mortality in these years. As highlighted in Chapter 3, puerperal sepsis, toxaemia and haemorrhages were the three principal causes of maternal mortality. While medical treatment for these conditions remained largely ineffective before the 1930s, certain precautions could be taken to limit their onset. Prior to the introduction of sulphonamides in the 1930s and the development of blood transfusion in the 1940s, good quality midwifery care with minimal medical intervention was the best that could be done to limit their incidence. While antenatal care was largely ineffective against puerperal sepsis and haemorrhages, it was useful for screening women suffering from toxaemia, who stood a better chance of survival if delivered in a hospital than at home. Yet although many proposals were put forward for curing toxaemia, its treatment was limited and the only real means of solving the problem was terminating the pregnancy, which was a hazardous process in these years.[93] The different determinants of puerperal sepsis and haemorrhages with toxaemia are important to bear in mind when considering the overall impact of maternity services on maternal mortality.

Risk of Infection with Different Birth Attendants

As Chapter 3 has already highlighted, many of the precautions taken to guard against puerperal sepsis and haemorrhages was dependent on the training, skill and supervision of the medical attendant. In this respect the private general practitioner was probably the worst attendant to engage. As late as the 1920s the level of obstetric teaching for general practitioners was poor, and very few medical students were given any training before going out on to the district.[94] In 1919 a report from The London Hospital indicated that its medical students were receiving very little instruction or supervision.[95]

Unlike midwives, doctors were allowed to use instruments in

their deliveries thereby increasing the possibility of interference during childbirth. In these circumstances adherence to antisepsis by a private doctor was not guaranteed. Measures to tighten up the standards of midwifery practised by practitioners were continually opposed in these years by the British Medical Association, which asserted that every doctor had the right to practise midwifery if he so desired and prevented them from admitting to any incompetence on the part of doctors.[96] Some recognition of the need to standardize the training and examination of postgraduates specializing in obstetrics and gynaecology and for an improvement of care by medical practitioners came about through the establishment of the British College of Obstetricians in 1929 (later renamed the Royal College of Obstetricians in 1938).[97]

The very nature of a general practitioner's practice meant, however, that problems remained. As Edith Summerskill pointed out in 1932, a general practitioner was unable to devote his or her sole attention to midwifery; and that he or she was frequently interrupted by the needs of other patients during delivery, which raised the risk of infection. This problem was made worse by the fact that many poor homes did not have sufficient hot water facilities for doctors to clean themselves.[98] In addition to the greater risk of spreading infection, doctors usually offered much less vigorous and complete antenatal supervision and as a consequence, often missed detecting cases of toxaemia.[99]

The risk of infection was usually less with midwives. However, the number of midwives attending mothers in London was smaller than elsewhere. In 1908 it was estimated that only 25 per cent of all births in the Administrative County of London were attended by midwives, which was much lower than the national average of 50 per cent for this year, or other urban areas such as Manchester where midwives attended 61 per cent of the births.[100] During the First World War the number of midwives attending births in London increased due to the shortage of doctors and continued to increase between 1918 and 1927. By 1927 51 per cent of all births in London were attended by midwives, but this was still smaller than in the county boroughs where the percentage was 70, or in the counties where it was 61.[101]

The different levels of regulation governing the practice of midwives and doctors would have had an important bearing, therefore, on the level of maternal mortality. In an area where there was a greater number of doctors practising it might be expected that the level of maternal mortality would be higher than in an area where midwives dominated. In 1915 the Local Government Board reported that the highest rate of puerperal mortality in London was to be found in the rich borough of Hampstead. This rate contrasted with the lower rates for the poorer boroughs West Ham, Bermondsey, Woolwich, Islington, Bethnal Green, Stepney and Poplar. Many more certified midwives were working in these poorer neighbourhoods than in Hampstead.[102] In 1918 the Hampstead medical officer of health, Dr Scrase, reported that eight trained and certified midwives worked in his borough, but that 600 out of every thousand births in Hampstead were being attended by women with 'practically no training at all'.[103] No explanation was given for this very high number of untrained midwives in Hampstead, but it might have stemmed from the large presence of doctors in the borough, who proved too much competition for the trained midwives.

It would be wrong, however, to connect the higher rate of puerperal mortality in Hampstead solely with the high number of untrained midwives practising in the borough. While Table 6.20 shows that between 1915 and 1932 the number of births notified by midwives grew from 20 to 40 per cent, Table 6.21 indicates the percentage of domiciliary cases delivered exclusively by midwives in 1934 remained smaller in Hampstead than in other parts of London. This percentage contrasted with Stepney where in the late 1920s the number of deliveries by midwives accounted for 71 per cent. In Hampstead, however, the percentage was only 43. When a midwife did deliver a woman in Hampstead, it was usually done in coopera-tion with a doctor. As these two tables indicate, doctors appear to have cared for a much smaller number of mothers in Kensington, Stepney and Woolwich, than midwives, who were a cheaper and therefore more attractive option to poor women in these areas.[104]

While there are no reliable statistics for judging the standard of care received by well-to-do mothers who hired a doctor, and that available to poorer mothers through trained and untrained midwives, the difference in the overall rates of maternal mortality noted in Chapter 3 suggest that there was some disparity in the quality of attendance provided in each area. What is most striking about Stepney is that its rate of maternal mortality was not only lower than that of Hampstead, but than that of England and Wales as a whole.[105] Yet this was clearly an area of acute deprivation and poor health.

Such low rates of maternal mortality in Stepney raises questions not only about the quality of care offered by different attendants, but also the degree to which the socio-economic status of mothers affected the risk of death. The lower rate of maternal mortality found among the poor mothers of Stepney was also found in Kensington. In 1937, the rate among the 'well-to-do class' was 10 per 1,000 births, while it was only 1.8 among poor mothers,[106] which suggests that although rich mothers were better fed and housed, and had the finance to engage an attendant of their choice, they were not guaranteed better protection against the scourges of maternal mortality. It could be argued that their risk of death was related to their ability to employ a doctor.

Table 6.20: Number and percentage of births out of total births attended by doctors and midwives and others in the four boroughs

Borough	Date	Deliveries by doctor		Deliveries by midwife		Births notified by other sources	
		No.	%	No.	%	No.	%
Hampstead	1915–17	907	29	621	20	1,558	49
	1920–5	2,302	27	3,108	37	3,072	36
	1926–30	1,881	29	2,853	43	1,861	28
	1931–2	844	29	1,326	45	768	26
Kensington	1912–14	1,716	20	4,647	54	2,186	26
	1915–20	3,465	22	9,456	61	2,556	17
	1922–5	1,932	19	6,621	65	1,601	16
	1926–30	1,911	18	6,279	59	2,493	22
	1931–5	1,616	19	4,794	55	2,236	26
	1936–8	566	11	2,521	51	1,868	38
Stepney	1920	1,630	24	3,570	55	1,494	21
	1926–9	5,211	29	12,815	71	69	0.4
	1937*	–	–	2,685	91	–	–
Woolwich	1908–10	1,415	19	4,235	57	284	4
	1911–15	2,416	19	7,461	58	2,091	16
	1920–5	1,790	6	9,916	36	5,517	31
	1926–30	703	6	5,165	44	5,678	49
	1931–5	395	3	3,293	29	7,717	68
	1936–8	148	2	1,681	24	5,223	75

Other sources include those births notified by parents, institutions and others. In Hampstead the category 'other sources' also includes nurses notifying births.
• The percentage for this year for the notified births adds up to 98%, and does not include the 68 stillbirths, which accounts for the missing 2%.
* Figures for this year show the number of live births and stillbirths of all Stepney residents occurring inside and within institutions outside the borough. The number of births delivered for midwives might be an underestimate, as the total births of 2,958 is divided as follows: 2,685 midwives, and 273 as doctors and midwives.
Kensington births are the total births notified in the borough and do not include those notified of residents outside the borough. It is, therefore, not the total number of births registered. The births notified include stillbirths.
Woolwich – the percentages do not add up to 100% of all notified births. Some of the births are unaccounted for and could be covered by untrained midwives or other birth attendants.
Sources: Hampstead, Kensington and Stepney MOH, *A/Rs* (1915–38).

Table 6.21: Percentage of home confinements undertaken by different types of attendants in Birmingham and various parts of London, 1928 and 1934

	Midwife delivery	Doctor delivery	Midwife and doctor•	Medical students
Hampstead	37%	7%	56%	0.3%
Kensington (1928)	72%†	–	27%	–
Woolwich	74%	8%	17%	0%
14 London Boroughs*	61%	16%	13%	6%
Birmingham	92%	8%	–	–

• This is primarily doctor deliveries with the help of midwives or monthly nurses.
† This includes 2 midwives practising under the auspices of the Queen Charlotte's Midwives training Home who had close contact with doctors and 20 private midwives.
* 14 boroughs include Battersea, Camberwell, Fulham, Hackney, Hampstead, Holborn, Islington, Lambeth, Lewisham, Paddington, Poplar, Wandsworth, Woolwich and the City of London.
All figures quoted are for 1934, with the exception of Kensington which is 1928.

Sources: LCC, *Maternity Services in London: Report by the County MOH to the Hospitals and Medical Services Committee* (London: 1934), 17 (GLRO Library P 26.8 LCC); V. Cox, 'Team Work and Post-natal care', *Mother and Child* 5/9 (1934), 348 (in L. Fairfield's papers, GLRO file: Ph/Gen/3/6); J. Fenton, 'The Kensington Municipal Maternity Home', *Med. Offr.* 5 May 1928, 197–8.

Safety of Home and Institutional Births

The difference in maternal mortality between the boroughs cannot be solely confined, however, to the differences in the type of attenders in each borough, but must also be related to the type of institutional care available in each borough. Mothers were best protected from the hazards of infection if they gave birth at home. After home births the next safest option was to be delivered in a voluntary teaching or Poor Law institution. By the early twentieth century the risk of contracting puerperal sepsis through attendants from such institutions had been greatly diminished as a result of the introduction of antisepsis in the 1880s and improvements in medical training. Although an element of risk remained, the strict supervision of the attendants within these institutions assured mothers of a better standard of care than received elsewhere such as in maternity homes.

The variation in the safety of institutional care is partly illustrated in the case of an investigation that was carried out·of maternal deaths in Hampstead in the years 1926 to 1930. Although the figures are too small a number for an accurate measure of the true extent of maternal mortality in Hampstead during these years, Table

6.22 shows that overall mothers were best protected against puerperal fever if delivered at home. This contrasted those mothers who were giving birth within institutions in the borough, many of which were maternity homes where general practitioners tended to practise. In the years 1926 to 1930 ten mothers died out of 2,646 births as a result of puerperal sepsis either in hospitals or nursing homes in the borough, a rate of 3.78. Such a high rate of puerperal sepsis is particularly striking when compared with the rates recorded for in-patients at the East End Maternity Home for these years where there were two deaths from puerperal sepsis out of the total 6,496 in-patient births, a rate of 0.31. Within the borough as a whole Hampstead also recorded a high rate of puerperal sepsis. Of the 47 maternal deaths reported in 1921–30, 21 or 45 per cent died from puerperal sepsis. This was higher than among the number of maternal deaths investigated by the Departmental Committee on Maternal Mortality and Morbidity, where nearly one-third of the fatal cases were due to sepsis.[107]

Table 6.22: Number and cause of maternal deaths among district maternity cases and of in-patients in hospitals and institutions in Hampstead and the EEMH and BMB, 1926–30

Cause of death	Deaths of mothers giving birth at home						Deaths of in-patient mothers					
	Hampstead non-institutional births		EEMH		BMB		Hampstead hospitals & institutions		EEMH in-patients		BMB	
	No.	MMR	No.	MMR	No.	MMR	No.	MMR	No.	MMR	No.	MMR
puerperal sepsis	0	0	0	0	0	0	10	3.78	2	0.31	0	0
other causes	3	1.13	6	4.13	0	0	13	4.91	1	0.26	0	0
puerperal sepsis & other causes	3	1.13	1	0.30	0	0	22	8.31	8	1.23	5	1.50

Total maternal mortality rates for total births for:
BMB 0
EEMH 1.37
Hampstead 3.78
England & Wales (1925–9) 1.73

Sources: EEMH and BMB, *A/Rs* (1926–30); Hampstead MOH, *A/R* (1930), 71–3; Registrar General, *Annual Reports of Births, Deaths and Marriages for England and Wales* (London: 1926–30).

While the small sample here makes the evidence from Hampstead inconclusive, such a high rate of maternal mortality, particularly in connection with puerperal sepsis, suggests that the maternity care in Hampstead was less adequate than in some poor areas.[108] The contrast is particularly striking when we consider the very low maternal mortality recorded not only for the whole of Stepney, but also in relation to one of its major hospitals, the East End Maternity Home. In the wider community the East End Maternity Home was often praised as exemplary in its maternity care, and was commended for its success in lowering maternal mortality despite the high number of abnormal cases received. Of the 33,116 mothers delivered as in-patients by the East End Maternity Home in the years 1905–39 there were 58 deaths, which was a rate of 1.8 per 1,000 births. The maternal mortality rate for in-patients was much higher than for out-patients, partly because of the high proportion of abnormalities admitted into hospital. Out of a total 27,310 out-patient deliveries there were 13 fatalities, or a rate of 0.50 per 1,000 births.[109] Overall the maternal rate for all categories of patient was 1.17. Its rate of puerperal sepsis was also very low. The total number of in-patients dying from puerperal sepsis for these years was six, the equivalent rate of 0.18 per 1,000 births.

While it is difficult to compare these rates with other hospitals in Stepney, Kensington or Hampstead, they were slightly below those of the British Hospital for Mothers and Babies in Woolwich. This hospital also had a low rate of maternal mortality. Between 1905 and 1929 there were 29 deaths out of the 14,577 in-patients, a rate of 2 per 1,000 births. Among the 6,372 out-patients five deaths occurred, an equivalent rate of 0.8 per 1,000 births. The hospital's overall maternal mortality rate was 1.6.[110] Mothers who were confined in the British Hospital for Mothers and Babies appear to have had an advantage over the local population. Out of a total of 40,396 births in the years 1916–30 146 mothers died in the borough, a rate of 3.61 per 1,000 births, while of the 9,959 births cared for by the hospital 11 mothers died, a rate of 1.1 per 1,000 births.[111] Puerperal sepsis was also rare. None of the births were septic at the British Hospital for Mothers and Babies between 1922 and 1935.[112]

One of the reasons for the good record at the East End Maternity Home and British Hospital for Mothers and Babies was their clinical practice, which ensured not only strict antisepsis, but also minimal medical intervention. This policy partly stemmed from the fact that these institutions were primarily staffed by midwives, but it was also due to the tight precautions they took in antenatal screening to select abnormal cases for hospital confinements. Their approach in this regard can be seen from the comments of one medical officer, who stated 'The essence of the East End Hospital practice is not wait and see, but see and wait. That that is the basis of sound midwifery, results abundantly testify.'[113] This conclusion is proved by the very low rate with which instruments were applied to births at the hospital. Although the rate at which it used forceps for its deliveries varied over the years, its overall rate of forceps delivery was 2.9 per cent of all births, much lower than the rate of 6.4 found among the Queen Victoria Jubilee Nurses who only worked with district cases. Indeed, it was less than half the 7 per cent, the standard rate considered reasonable for forceps.

Table 6.23: Percentage of in-patient and out-patient deliveries at the EEMH, BMB and CLMH in which forceps were used

Date	CLMH	EEMH	BMB Forceps
1913	5.9	–	5.68
1914	9.9	–	5.59
1919	11	–	–
1923	7.37	–	–
1925	–	2.5	6.58
1931	–	4.8	6.79
1934•	–	4.1	6.08
1936	–	4.2	6.58
1938	–	5	3.16

•In 1933–4 the forceps rate at Queen Charlotte's Hospital was 9.64% and 5.89% at the Salvation Army's Mothers Hospital. In 1934 the forceps rate in LCC hospitals was 3.54%.

Sources: EEMH, BMB and CLMH A/Rs (1905–1938; LCC, *Maternity Services of London, Report of the County MOH to the Hospital and Medical Services Committee* (London: 1934), 20 (GLRO Library LP 26.8 LCC); 'Booked Cases after 28 weeks', in L. Fairfield's Papers (GLRO file: PH/Gen/3/6).

The East End Maternity Home also had a low induction rate of 1.21 per cent which favourably matched that registered in London County Council hospitals in 1934 of 1.72. At London County Council hospitals only 0.1 per cent caesarian sections were performed for every 1,000 births, which again was below the average practice for this period.[114] No figures remain for the rate of inductions and caesarians at the British Hospital for Mothers and Babies, but it too had a good record in forceps deliveries. As Table 6.23 shows the British Hospital for Mothers and Babies was not as good as the East End Maternity Home in this respect, but it was comparable to other maternity hospitals such as the City of London Maternity Home.

The treatment provided by the East End Maternity Home and the British Hospital for Mothers and Babies was not only reflected in their good records in maternal mortality, particularly septic deaths, but also in their rates of neonatal mortality, the incidence of which can partially be linked to the quality of midwifery care during birth. Table 6.24

shows that the overall neonatal death rates per 1,000 births was much lower for the East End Maternity Home and the British Hospital for Mothers and Babies than for England and Wales nationally, and compared favourably with rates also found at the City of London Maternity Home. When broken down by in-patients and out-patients, however, it would seem that there was a slightly higher number of neonatal deaths among the in-patients of the two hospitals, but this probably reflected the fact that a high proportion of the in-patients were abnormalities (Table 6.25). Whatever the reason for the difference between in-patients and out-patients, these hospitals' overall low rates of neonatal mortality suggests that they provided for safe deliveries.

Table 6.24: Neonatal mortality rate for England and Wales, and for total infants born at the CLMH, EEMH and BMB, 1929–39

Year	England & Wales	CLMH	EEMH	BMB
1926–30	46.8	14.9	15.1	10
1931–5*	50.5	16.4	14.4•	12•
1936–40	52.8	18.3	13.1•	12•

Neonatal mortality rate = deaths per 1,000 births.
• The rates for the EEMH and BMB are for 1925–30 and 1936–8.
* The neonatal mortality rates for Queen Charlotte's Hospital in 1933–4 was 20.8, while at the Salvation Army Mothers' Hospital it was 17.6.

Sources: CLMH, EEMH, BMB *A/Rs* (1926–1939), and A. MacFarlane and M. Mugford, *Birth Counts: Statistics of Pregnancy and Childbirth, Tables* (London: 1984), Table A3.4, 10–11; 'Booked cases after 28 weeks', in L. Fairfield's Papers (GLRO file: Ph/Gen/3/6).

Table 6.25: Number and rate of neonatal deaths at the EEMH and BMB, 1925–39

Type of patient	Hospital	Year	Neonatal deaths	Neonatal mortality rate
Out-patient	BMB	1926–30	9	9
		1931–5	8	8
		1936–8	2	3
	EEMH	1925–6	29	15
		1929–30	10	8
		1931–6	21	9
		1938–9	3	6
In-patient	BMB	1925–30	35	11
		1931–5	48	13
		1936–8	35	14
	EEMH	1925–6	30	13
		1929–30	43	15
		1931–6	48	16

Sources: BMB and EEMH, *A/Rs* (1925–39).

234

Table 6.26: Stillbirth rate for England and Wales, CLMH, EEMH and BMB, 1929–39

Year	England & Wales	LCC hospitals	CLMH	EEMH	BMB
1929	40	–	–	25	–
1930	41	–	–	22	28
1931	41	51	–	26	28
1932	41	41	–	22	23
1933	41	44	–	20	–
1934	40	40	44	23	25
1935	41	–	40	22	30
1936	40	–	63	–	28
1937	39	–	63	–	–
1938	38	–	–	25	26
1939	38	–	–	29	–

Stillbirth rate = stillbirths per 1,000 births.

Sources: CLMH, EEMH and BMB *A/Rs* (1929–39), and A. MacFarlane and M. Mugford, *Birth Counts: Statistics of Pregnancy and Childbirth* (London: 1984), Table A3.4, 10–11; *Report to Hospitals and Medical Services (Hospital Management Sub-Committee)* in Fairfield's Papers (GLRO file: Ph/Gen/3/6).

Table 6.27: Number and rate of stillbirths at the EEMH and BMB, 1911–39

Type of patient	Hospital	Year	Total births	Stillbirths	Stillbirth rate
Out-patient	BMB	1911–15	920	23	25
		1916–18	552	17	31
		1925–8	803	17	21
		1930–5	1,148	30	26
		1936–8	637	9	14
	EEMH	1911–14	3,961	85	21
		1925–6	1,989	38	19
		1929–30	1,237	26	21
		1931–6	2,382	37	16
		1938–9	550	8	15
In-patient	BMB	1926–30	3,925	109	28
		1931–5	3,764	116	31
	EEMH	1911–14	2,131	49	23
		1925–6	2,337	31	13
		1929–30	2,781	69	25
		1931–6	9,032	230	5
		1938–9	2,805	83	30

Sources: BMB and EEMH, *A/Rs* (1911–39).

Although less directly linked to the quality of midwifery care, both hospitals had low rates of stillbirths. Table 6.26 also demonstrates that the rate was much lower for these hospitals than for the whole country and compared favourably with the City of London Maternity Home. This rate might have been the result of the scrupulous attention the hospitals paid to the mothers during their pregnancies. There was no perceptible difference in stillbirth rates found among the different categories of patient, indicating no difference in the antenatal provision made to each type of patient (Table 6.27).

Unfortunately no statistics remain for measuring the effectiveness of the type of care that was available to mothers through the institutions in Kensington. None the less, the standard of care offered to mothers in North Kensington by pupil midwives from Queen Charlotte's Hospital was probably good given the strict supervision they received from the hospital.[115] The medical officer's policy of keeping institutional births to a minimum within Kensington, also probably protected many of its mothers. Yet its rate of maternal mortality was continually higher than that found in East London, and for the country nationally.

Impact of Antenatal Care on Maternal Health

The care of the mother was not only dependent on good supervision during delivery, but also in the antenatal phase. As we have seen above antenatal coverage was very high in Stepney and coordination was extremely good, which could again be another explanation for its low rate of maternal mortality. Such provision, however, was not enough on its own to counter maternal mortality, as is testified by the case of Kensington, where antenatal provision was also good, but high rates of maternal mortality persisted. As the case of Stepney illustrates, a mother's chance of survival in childbirth depended on a high degree of antenatal supervision followed by a delivery which ensured antisepsis and minimized unnecessary interference. While the multiplicity of bodies involved in providing such a service made this an ideal which was hard to attain in reality in all the boroughs, Stepney probably came closest to achieving the goal.

Conclusion

Following its tradition of a highly centralized and strong hospital-based medicine, maternity provision in London appears to have been dominated by a large number of hospital-based deliveries from early on. Within London such provision was unevenly spread, and tended to be most prominent in working-class boroughs such as Stepney.

Part of this reflected the high number of voluntary teaching hospitals in the area, as well as its great poverty and overcrowding which made hospital births a more attractive option. London also tended to have a greater number of mothers who were attended by doctors than by midwives, reflecting both the dominance of the medical profession within the capital as well as the prosperity of many of its residents. As in the case of hospital births, the number of doctors attending women in childbirth varied between boroughs and was greatest in richer areas such as Hampstead.

London was not only unique in respect to its dominance of hospital and doctor births, but also in its overall good provision of antenatal care. Within London, however, this varied greatly not only between boroughs but also between institutions. Those women who were living in Stepney and Woolwich tended to be assured of better antenatal coverage than those in the two other boroughs. Overall women were more likely to receive a better standard of antenatal care and one which ran throughout the pregnancy from a hospital than if she was cared for by a general practitioner.

Such variations in the provision of maternity care had important consequences for the safety of births in each borough and their levels of maternal mortality. As we have seen, in contrast to health visiting and infant welfare centres which could do little to improve health standards among those they cared for in the face of acute social and economic deprivation, good maternity provision appears to have been a crucial force in the preservation of a mother's life and seems to have outweighed other factors such as poverty and over-crowding. The determinants of maternal mortality were less suscep-tible to external social and economic circumstances than infant mortality, and more closely associated with the quality of medical care received during pregnancy and childbirth. Stepney's remarkably low rates were achieved despite very high levels of poverty and deprivation, as a result of the very good charitable maternity services in the area. By contrast, residents in Hampstead although richer than those in Stepney, appear to have had access to an inferior type of care, which is revealed by very high rates of maternal mortality.

Much of this chapter and the previous one has been based on an assessment of aggregate attendances numbers and mortality statistics with little reference to individual experience. Yet the success of the services in reaching those they most wanted to target was highly dependent on meeting the expectations and perceptions of those they served. What these demands were and how they were met by the different facilities described in this chapter are crucial if we are to understand what the overall impact of the services were on health standards among mothers and infants. The degree of success a service enjoyed was influenced not only by the cooperation between different agencies involved in maternal and child welfare, but also by the willingness of mothers to follow proffered advice. As the following chapters will show, mothers' attitudes depended on the attitude of the professionals towards them, as well as on the perceptions and expectations that the mothers themselves held of the services provided.

Notes

1. MH, *Final Report of Departmental Committee on Maternal Mortality and Morbidity* (London: 1932), 144.
2. See, for instance, MH, *Memorandum in Regard to Maternity Hospitals and Homes* (London: 1920); and J. Campbell, *Maternal Mortality: Report on Public Health and Medical Subjects,* 25 (London: 1924). See also N. Pfeffer, *The Stork and the Syringe: A Political History of Reproductive Medicine* (Cambridge: 1993), 95.
3. For a good summary on the high degree of welfare provision in London see R. Lee, 'Uneven Zenith: Towards a Geography of the High Period of Municipal Medicine in England and Wales', *J. Hist. Geog.,* 14/3 (1988), 260–80.
4. L. Marks, 'Medical Care for Pauper Mothers and Their Infants: Poor Law Provision and Local Demand in East London, 1870–1929', *Econ. Hist. Rev.,* 43/3 (1993), 518–42.
5. EEMH, *A/Rs* (1913), 19–20; and (1934), 12.
6. BMB, *A/R* (1913), 12–13. See also *Pioneer,* 16 July 1913.
7. BMB, *A/Rs* (1905), 11; and (1912), 14.
8. 'The Beveridge Committee Report', Material from C. J. Holloway, March 1942, 2 in Nuffield College Social Reconstruction Survey, Box 161.
9. For more information on hospital provision in London see F. K. Prochaska, *Philanthropy and the Hospitals of London: The King's Fund 1897–1900* (Oxford: 1992).
10. A. Crowther, *The Workhouse System, 1834–1929,* 162; F. Driver, 'The Historical Geography of the Workhouse System in England and Wales, 1834–1883', *J. Hist. Geog.,* 15 (1989), 267–86.
11. Lee, *op. cit.* (note 3), 268.
12. In 1928 there were 885 voluntary hospitals in England, Wales and Scotland providing 60,153 beds. Institutions under the Board of Guardians for this year provided 200,000 beds, and municipal and district council hospitals 130,000 beds. 'Maternity Hospitals and the Public', in *Onward,* 6, 1925, and 'In the Melting Pot', *Onward,* 17, 1928 (GLRO files: H10/CLM/Y3/1 and H10/CLM/Y3/2); *Onward* was the newspaper of the City of London Maternity Hospital.
13. *Onward,* 25, 1930, 712 (GLRO file: H10/CLM/Y3/3).

14. St Pancras had a high rate of hospital births because of the large number of teaching hospitals and lying-in institutions in the area. J. Lewis, *The Politics of Motherhood: Child and Maternal Welfare in England, 1900-1939* (London: 1980), 120–1.

15. The Jewish Maternity Home specifically provided domiciliary and in-patient midwifery care to the Jewish population in the neighbourhood but was open to non-Jewish women. L. Marks, "'Dear Old Mother Levy's": The Jewish Maternity Home and Sick Room Helps Society 1895–1939', *Soc. Hist. Med,* 3/1 (1990), 61–88.

16. Stepney Borough, 'MCW Full Report' (1932), 5 (PRO file: MH 66/392).

17. For more detailed information on these hospitals see L. Marks, *Model Mothers: Jewish Mothers and Maternity Provision in East London, 1870–1939* (Oxford: 1994), Ch. 4.

18. The Princess Beatrice Hospital, formerly known as Kensington, Fulham and Chelsea General Hospital was rebuilt during 1930 and reopened in 1932. The hospital included an antenatal clinic and a maternity ward and in 1934 the hospital accommodated 276 maternity patients. Kensington MOH, *A/Rs* (1923), 13 and (1934); 'Kensington Public Health Survey', 1932, 15–16 (PRO file: MH 66/359 and MH 66/360).

19. Insured patients made up about two-thirds of the patients covered by these midwives, and they were expected to pay 5s. to the hospital. The average contribution of non-insured mothers was 6d. 'Acting MOH Report for Kensington', 5 July 1916 (PRO file: MH48/164).

20. Kensington MOH, *A/R* (1922), 31; Kensington Council Minutes, 25 June 1935, 321.

21. Kensington Council Minutes, 25 June 1935, 321.

22. Each case booked was submitted to the MCW (Applications) Sub-Committee. The maximum fee charged was two guineas, and charges were made according to a family's income. Kensington MOH, *A/R* (1934), 12.

23. R. S. Salaman, 'The Helmsman Takes Charge', unpub. memoirs, n.d., 27-8 (Cambridge University: Salaman papers). Miss M. B., interviewed by L. Marks, 7 July 1987, transcript, 4. See also London Hospital, *A/Rs* (1921), 187; (1922), 181; and (1924), 187.

24. 'A Wireless Appeal' by Rt. Hon. Lord Balfour of Burleigh for Princess Louise Kensington Hospital for Children, December 1925 (KLHL file: KP 797); Kensington MOH, *A/R* (1923), 13; Archer Street Infant Welfare Clinic, *A/R* (1928–9).

25. Woolwich MOH, *A/R* (1914), 135; BMB, *A/R* (1915), 5; see also D. Weinbren, "'The Peace Arsenal" Scheme: The Campaign for Non-munitions Work at the Royal Ordnance Factories, Woolwich after the First World War', unpub. Ph.D., Thames Polytechnic, 1990, 229 and D. Thom, 'Women Munitions Workers at Woolwich Arsenal in the 1914–18 War', unpub. M.A., Warwick, 1976.

26. London Hospital, *A/R* (1925), 197.
27. Woolwich MOH, *A/Rs* (1925), 67–9; (1926), 74, (1930), 65–6; 'Woolwich Public Health Survey', 1934, 5 (PRO file: MH 66/404).
28. BMB, *A/R* (1925), 4–5.
29. BMB, *A/R* (1931), 5.
30. EEMH, *A/Rs* (1913), 12; and (1925), 13.
31. EEMH, *A/R* (1931). See also London Hospital, *A/R* (1930), 210 and Stepney, MOH, *A/R* (1930), 12.
32. E. W. Morris, 'Report of a Visit to the District Maternity Charity with Miss Nicholls, District Midwife', 19 December 1922, 3–4 in London Hospital papers; BMB, *A/R* (1932), 4–5; MH, *Memorandum* (note 2), 1.
33. Hampstead MOH, *A/R* (1919), 65.
34. MH, *Memorandum* (note 2), 1.
35. London Hospital, *A/Rs* (1924), 187; and (1927), 201. See also 'Maternity Mortality', in *Onward*, 3, 1925, 58 (GLRO file: H10/CLM/Y3/1), which attributes the growing demand for in-patient care with the contact women had with hospitals as a result of the First World War.
36. BMB, *A/R* (1932), 4–5. Hospital patients not only increased in these years of depression, but also the number of mothers attending infant welfare centres. See Ch. 5.
37. BMB, *A/R* (1924), 9.
38. BMB, *A/R* (1932), 4–5.
39. London Hospital, *A/R* (1921), 186.
40. M. Llewellyn Davies, *Maternity: Letters from Working Women* (London: 1915; repr. 1984), 5.
41. *Onward*, 49, January 1936, 36.
42. 'Maternity Hospital and the Public', *Onward*, 6, 1925, 132 (GLRO file: H10/CLM/Y3/1).
43. Woolwich MOH, *A/R* (1927), 18.
44. BMB, *A/R* (1930), 5; (1934), 4.
45. Kensington Council Minutes, 25 June 1935, 321.
46. Lewis, *op. cit.* (note 14), 121. Home confinements were also cheaper for the hospital than hospital births. In 1914 the total cost of each in-patient per week amounted to 17s. 7d., whereas the average cost of each out-patient cost 6s. 10d., less than half of the sum to keep an in-patient in for a week. EEMH, *A/R* (1914).
47. I am grateful to Irvine Loudon for pointing this out to me. See also E. P. Peretz, 'A Maternity Service for England and Wales: Local Authority Maternity Care in the Inter-War Period in Oxfordshire and Tottenham', in J. Garcia, R. Kilpatrick and M. Richards (eds), *The Politics of Maternity Care: Services for Childbearing Women in Twentieth Century Britain* (Oxford: 1990), 33; and Lewis, *op. cit.* (note 14), 121.
48. Kensington Council Minutes, 25 June 1935, 321.

49. Miss M. B. interview, transcript, 6.

50. Stepney Public Health Memo. to the MH, 8 May 1920 (PRO file: MH 52/202).

51. London Hospital, *A/R* (1929), 209.

52. I. Loudon, *Deaths in Childbirth: An International Study of Maternal Care and Maternal Mortality 1880–1950,* (Oxford: 1992), 90–1.

53. G. F. McCleary, *The Maternity and Child Welfare Movement* (London: 1935), 56–7.

54. LCC, *Maternity Services of London: Report by the County MOH to the Hospitals and Medical Services Committee* (London: 1934), 20 (GLRO Library: [LP] 26.8 LCC).

55. MH, *Final Report,* (note 1), 145.

56. L. Fairfield, 'Maternal Deaths in the Council's Hospitals – Report for the Year ending December 31 1933', 1 (GLRO file: Ph/Gen/3/6).

57. *Maternal Mortality and Childbirth – Ante-Natal Clinics. Their Conduct and Scope,* Memo. 145, MCW 1929.

58. L. Fairfield, 'Ante-natal Care and Hospitals', in *Nosokomeion* 5/3 (1934), 203-4 (GLRO file: Ph/Gen/3/6), and 'Report to Hospital and Medical Services (Hospital Management Sub-Committee): Maternal Mortality', *c.*1934, 3 (GLRO file: Ph/Gen/3/6).

59. Kensington MOH, *A/R* (1935), 10; 'Stepney Public Health Survey', 1932, 42–3 (PRO file: MH 66/391); LCC, *op. cit.* (note 54), 7; Fairfield, *op. cit.* (note 58), 203–4, and 'Report to Hospital' *op. cit.* (note 58), 3, 4.

60. Part of this stemmed from the pressure on these hospitals for taking in patients, which resulted in the hospitals positively discriminating towards those who booked early.

61. LCC, *op. cit.* (note 54), 7–9.

62. Association of Infant and Maternal Centres, *Report on Enquiry of Existing Ante-natal Centres,* (London: 1925), 8 (Fawcett Library).

63. LCC, *op. cit.* (note 54), 15.

64. St George's Hospital was one of the providers. 'Report of the Work of Infant Welfare in the Borough of Kensington', 24 July 1914. (PRO file: MH 48/164). See also MOH Report submitted to the Medical Sub-Committee, 30 January 1917 (PRO file: MH 48/164).

65. In 1915 221 women were seen under this scheme. Report of Acting MOH for Kensington, 5 July 1916 (PRO file: MH 48/164). See also Kensington MOH, *A/R* (1923), 13.

66. Stepney MCW Committee Minutes, 10 July 1928, letter from W. McClelland dated 9 July 1928; and 2 October 1928.

67. McCleary, *op. cit.* (note 53), 56–7.

68. Fairfield, *op. cit.* (note 58), 202.

69. Stepney MOH, *A/R* (1935), 48. The EEMH which was based near the London Hospital, was often cited as having one of the lowest rates of maternal mortality as a result of its good antenatal department. See *Br. Med. J.,* 1 February 1930, 294–5 and also *Med.*

Offr., 25 August 1928, 79–80; 31 January 1931, 45. See also Stepney MCW Committee Minutes, 10 March 1931.

70. Hampstead MOH, *A/R* (1930), 62.

71. Hampstead MOH, *A/R* (1924), 45.

72. No reason was given by the MOH for the increase. (Hampstead MOH *A/R* (1933), 33). Such a boost in attendance might have stemmed partly from the economic recession in the late 1920s and early 1930s which prevented many women from purchasing the private antenatal care they had easier access to in earlier more prosperous years.

73. Hampstead MOH, *A/R* (1932), 39. In 1934 an agreement was also reached for the coordination of antenatal care for maternity cases confined at New End Hospital. Hampstead MOH, *A/R* (1934), 49.

74. This high percentage can be gauged from Birmingham where there are comparable figures. In Birmingham the percentage of mothers considered eligible for welfare provision receiving such antenatal attention was much lower, estimated to be 25 per cent in 1924. By 1932 it had reached 50 per cent. V. Cox, 'Team Work and Post-Natal Care', *Mother and Child,* 5/9 (1934), 348–9, 349.

75. Kensington Council Minutes, 25 February 1930, 172–3.

76. LCC, *op. cit.* (note 54), 20; Fairfield, *op. cit.* (note 58), 203–4 and 'Report to Hospital', *op. cit.* (note 58), 3.

77. Kensington MOH, *A/R* (1934), 10.

78. Kensington Council Minutes, 18 December 1934, 65.

79. Kensington MOH, *A/R* (1935), 26. In 1934 antenatal sessions were also held at Princes Beatrice Hospital.

80. Kensington MOH, *A/R* (1934), 10. In 1930 it had been reported that there had been a problem of getting midwives to send in their cases to antenatal clinics. Kensington Council Minutes, 25 February 1930, 172–3.

81. Kensington MOH, *A/R* (1937), 30.

82. Kensington MOH, *A/R* (1936), 11.

83. 'Stepney Public Health Survey', 1932, 42–3 (PRO file: MH 66/391).

84. London Hospital, *A/Rs* (1925), 197 and (1927), 201.

85. London Hospital, *A/R* (1922), 181. 'Stepney Public Health Survey', 1932, 42–3 (PRO file: MH 66/391).

86. Woolwich MOH, *A/R* (1927), 201; and 'Woolwich Public Health Survey', 1934, (MH 66/405).

87. 'Report to Hospital', *op cit.* (note 58), 4; and LCC, *Maternal Mortality: Hospital and Medical Services' (Hospital Management Sub-Committee) Report by MOH,* 10 May 1935, 2 (GLRO file: Ph/Gen/3/7/7).

88. LCC, *op. cit.* (note 54), 20; Fairfield, *op. cit.* (note 58), 203–4; and 'Report to Hospital', *op. cit.* (note 58), 3.

89. BMB, *A/Rs* (1931–5). The average attendance recorded for these years in another voluntary hospital, the CLMH was slightly lower

than the BMB, at 4.12. See CLMH, *A/Rs* (1931–5) and Marks, *op. cit.* (note 17), Ch. 4.

90. LCC, *op. cit.* (note 54), 15.
91. 'Report to Hospital', *op. cit.* (note 58), 3.
92. Lewis, *op. cit.* (note 14), 124.
93. I. Loudon, 'Some Historical Aspects of Toxaemia Pregnancy. A Review,' *Br. J. Obstet. & Gynaecol.*, 98 (1991), 1–6.
94. For more information on the way in which midwifery and obstetrics was treated as an inferior specialty in medicine see O. Moscucci, *The Science of Woman: Gynaecology and Gender in England, 1880–1929* (Cambridge: 1990).
95. For the recollections of obstetric training offered at the London Hospital at the turn of the century see Salaman, *op. cit.* (note 23), 27–8. See also Dr E. Holland, 'Report on the External Maternity District and on the Urgent Need of Reforming the Work of Students thereon', April 1919, 5 (London Hospital Archive file: LH/A/17/35).
96. Lewis, *op. cit.* (note 14), 146–7.
97. *Ibid.,* 120.
98. *Maternal Mortality: Report of the Meeting held at Friends House, Euston Road November 15 1932* (London: 1932), 27. See also Alice Gregory's comments in *Report of the Proceedings of the English-Speaking Conference on Infant Mortality* (London: 1913), 284–5. Both sources at the Fawcett Library.
99. In 1937 the Kensington MOH reported that there was a higher rate of maternal mortality among the wealthier mothers in the borough. Of the four deaths belonging to this group, three had died from toxaemia. Kensington MOH, *A/R* (1937), 10.
100. 'Report of the CMB from its formation to 31 March 1908', PP 1909, Cd. 4822, p.xxxiii.
101. See Table 5.1 in Lewis, *op. cit.* (note 14), 142.
102. *Nursing Notes,* December 1915, 279, cited in I. Dove, 'Powerful and Peripheral: A History of Alice Gregory, Lelia Parnell and Maud Cashmore, Founders of the British Hospital for Mothers and Babies and the National Training School for Midwives', unpub. M.A., Thames Polytechnic, 1985, 37.
103. *Hampstead and Highgate Advertiser,* 9 February 1918, 5.
104. In 1917 it was estimated that about 50 per cent of all the births in Kensington were being attended by midwives. Letter from Kensington Acting MOH to MCW Committee, 5 July 1917 (PRO file: MH 48/164).
105. In 1923 Dr Janet Campbell reported that the rate of maternal mortality in Stepney in the years 1919–22 was 2.42, which was not only lowest of any district in London, but also of any county borough or administrative county in England and Wales. Stepney MOH, *A/Rs* (1923), 4; and (1931), 5.
106. Kensington MOH, *A/R* (1937), 10. This data needs to be treated with

caution because it is based on a small sample and is therefore more likely to be inaccurate. Accurate statistics have to be based on 10,000 births.

107. Hampstead MOH, *A/R* (1930), 71.

108. The high rate of maternal mortality in Hampstead did not necessarily stem from a negligence on the part of the council to try to provide a good service. In 1924 Hampstead was one of the first boroughs to establish a special committee for investigating all the maternal deaths each year. Hampstead was also one of the pioneering councils to provide the services of specialist obstetrician for difficult or abnormal labours in 1926. Hampstead MOH, *A/R* (1930), 73.

109. The low rate of maternal mortality at the EEMH was discussed in the *Br. Med. J.* (5 February 1930), 294–5, 294; *ELO*, 17 May 1930, 5, and 23 May 1931, 6; and *Med. Offr.*, 25 August 1928, 79–81 and 31 January 1931, 45.

110. BMB and EEMH, *A/Rs* (1905–38). The rates of maternal mortality at the EEMH and the BMB compared very favourably with other hospitals. In the years 1870–1939 out of a total of 62,143 in-patients there were 374 deaths at the CLMH or a rate of 6.01 per 1,000. Its record for out-patients was 123 deaths out of 74,049 deliveries, the equivalent of 1.66 per 1,000 births. CLMH, *A/Rs* (1870–1939).

111. Figures based on those provided in Dove, *op. cit.* (note 102), 36. These figures do not separate out the number of deaths in the hospital from those in the borough, and the hospital deaths might include women who were not from Woolwich.

112. *Ibid.*, 37.

113. 'The East End Maternity Hospital', *Med. Offr.*, 31 January 1931, 45.

114. The standard rate considered reasonable for forceps was 7% of all deliveries. See W. H. F. Oxley, 'Prophylaxis in Midwifery', *Med. Offr.*, 25 August 1928, 80; and 'The East End Maternity Hospital', *Med. Offr.*, 31 January 1931, 45; and LCC, *op. cit.* (note 54), 20.

115. In 1930 of the 2,526 births notified, 1,076 or 43% were notified by midwives, and of these 696 (28%) were attended by midwives from Queen Charlotte's Hospital, 380 (15%) of the births being attended by other midwives, 335 (13%) of the births were attended by doctors, 481 (19%) of the mothers were confined in St Mary Abbot's Hospital, 564 (22%) were notified by institutions outside the borough, and 14 were notified by other sources. 'Kensington Public Health Survey', 1932, 14–15 (PRO file: MH 66/359).

7

Listening To and Involving Mothers in the Provision of Services

All the activities of a Maternity Centre depend on the district and the needs of the women who live in it ... the important point to emphasise is that the women should feel that the Centre is for them, and it is largely for them to decide what functions it can usefully undertake.... It is essential not only to provide favourable conditions for the expectant mother, but to make use of them. For this reason there must be provision for different needs and different tastes, and there must be not a trace of patronage, officialdom or charity. Coercion in any form is useless; the best maternity scheme will fail unless it has the co-operation and approval of the mothers. For this reason, it is essential that working women should be fully represented on all committees controlling pre-natal work, and no effort must be spared in finding out their views. The best paper scheme will have no results if women feel that it interferes with their freedom, and the most beautifully equipped Maternity Centre or Maternity Home will be avoided and empty if the staff are unsympathetic and the rules irksome.[1]

These words, written by Edith Eckhard (a lecturer at the London School of Economics)[2] in 1921, highlight the numerous factors that were involved in making maternal and infant welfare services successful. As this and the next chapter will show, the success of a service was not only contingent on the supply of certain facilities and treatments, but also on the degree to which those running such services ascertained and listened to their client group, and fulfilled their expectations and needs. This not only varied between the boroughs, but also between institutions within each borough.

Much depended on the attitude of the individual personnel caring for the mothers as well as the aims of the institution. Central to this issue was the degree to which the independence and autonomy of mothers was upheld. Much of the approach taken by the personnel was contingent on the nature of the institution and the clients it intended to serve. Poor Law provision, for instance, which was aimed at relieving the most needy, and often the most inarticulate, often differed from the care offered by voluntary and municipal agencies which catered to a clientele who were usually seen as more respectable and independent. Equally important was the wider political mobilization within the area particular services were situated. Political participation not only shaped the type of services provided, but also the degree to which they were accepted and utilized by the local population.

One of the most striking features of Eckhard's above statement is her emphasis on the need for the participation of mothers if maternity centres were to achieve any success. Such an appeal is especially interesting in the light of the current political discussions taking place over the degree to which individuals should have a say in the planning and running of health and social services. One of the catch-phrases that has emerged in this debate is that of active citizenship. Yet what is meant by this term and how it is to be realized is continually being contested.[3]

Controversies over the meaning of citizenship and how it is to be achieved were no less apparent in Eckhard's day. For Eckhard, and for many other women, particularly those involved in the Women's Labour League and the Women's Co-operative Guild, the new services that were developing around maternal and infant welfare offered a vital opportunity for encouraging women to escape from their role as passive clients and to start taking an active role in the facilities being run for them. Part of this goal was to be achieved by encouraging mothers to become representatives on the committees that were planning and running such services. Indeed, welfare centres were thought to provide an ideal setting for educating mothers on the meaning of active citizenship.[4] Yet it would be a mistake to think that this attitude was universal during these years. Many medical and social welfare experts continued to see maternal and infant welfare as a matter of drilling mothers in the rigours of motherhood and infant care without paying any attention to their needs or in any way allowing for their voices to be heard.[5]

To what extent such conservative attitudes dominated the provision available in the four boroughs, or were beginning to move more towards those of Eckhard, is the subject of this chapter. A key question addressed is the degree to which the attitudes and policies of different agencies and their personnel were influenced by the

246

increasing state intervention in maternal and infant welfare in the early twentieth century, as well as the shifts that were occurring to the vision of citizenship as a result of the expansion in suffrage, particularly for women.[6]

At the heart of the chapter is the extent to which the changing nature of women's political and social power within society as a whole altered the vision of mothers and their infants as objects of charity to one which envisioned them as equal citizens with special needs and requirements and who had a voice of their own. This shift not only shaped the attitudes of the givers and receivers and their perception of what should be provided, but what direction the services should take. The chapter explores the degree to which institutions were willing to take mothers' perceptions of their own needs into account and involve them and their husbands in the services provided. Throughout the chapter I draw heavily on material from Kensington, which is unusually rich for exploring these questions.

Involving and Listening to Mothers in the Provision of Services

When setting principles for her model maternity centre, Eckhard was quick to stress the need to involve all its mothers in the day-to-day running of the enterprise. As she stated,

> The argument is often used that mothers are too busy and too unused to united action to be capable of taking part in the control of the Centre. This may be true in some places, but much can be done to stimulate, encourage and help the mothers to take the reins into their own hands.[7]

Mothers were going to feel that a maternity centre was for them and that it existed for their benefit if they had something to say in running the place. According to her the only way this could be achieved was if mothers were allowed to 'share with the workers the responsibility of making it as useful and pleasant a place as possible'. She stressed not only that mothers had many organizational and financial talents that were all too often ignored, but that their presence might help draw in mothers at the bottom of the social ladder whose social alienation with those running the centres often prevented their attendance.[8]

Eckhard's advice, based on the success of some centres, was for centres to establish a Committee of Mothers. She warned against the mothers being chosen by the Superintendent or Secretary of the centre. Instead, she advocated, mothers should be 'elected by members of the

Centre', and that those voting should be required to be members of the centre for a certain period. She recommended that all the routine arrangements should be left to this committee, and that it should be encouraged to make suggestions as to useful developments for the work. Similarly she urged for a box to be placed in a prominent place in every centre so that members could make written suggestions, the use of which she argued could act as a valuable measure for gauging the degree of influence the centre had on its members.[9]

Yet the extent to which Eckhard's ideas were put into practice varied greatly. In the following sections I will be examining how such ideals were applied to three specific services: infant welfare centres, Fathers' Councils and the North Kensington Women's Welfare Centre. These services were chosen not because they were necessarily representative of all the services in these years, but because they provided some innovative and surprising examples of the way in which certain institutions and personnel could and did reach out to the people they intended to serve.

Infant Welfare Centres 1902–36

In Hampstead, Kensington, Stepney and Woolwich many infant welfare centres provided a host of social activities for their mothers as well as providing medical advice. In offering such services these centres were carrying on a tradition which had long been established through mothers' meetings in the nineteenth century. By the inter-war years most centres were holding teas for their mothers and offered Christmas entertainment along with day outings. For many mothers such social activities provided a valuable opportunity to meet others facing similar problems to their own and to exchange ideas, as well as a much needed break away from the isolation of their home. None the less, few of these centres provided activities and a structure which encouraged the participation of mothers in the planning and running of services in the way advocated by Eckhard.

One infant welfare centre in Woolwich, however, which drew heavily on the help and support of women as early as the First World War was the one based on the Well Hall Estate. Much of the women's participation in the running of this centre can be linked to the high degree of political mobilization on this estate particularly in connection with the cooperative movement and the trade unions of the Arsenal, as well as the powerful influence of the Labour Party in Woolwich as a whole. Indeed, the estate was a hive of social activity, with fortnightly discussion groups and a very active Tenants' Association. In all these areas women were given a prominent role.

On the Tenants' Association, for instance, women were given an equal voice and held an equal number of places on the executive committee. Many of the women active in these spheres were the wives of Arsenal workers or had some job connected to the Arsenal.[10] Much of these women's active involvement in the running of the welfare centre was, therefore, an extension of their political action in other spheres.[11]

A high degree of political mobilization on the part of the Labour movement, however, was not the only factor which spurred the participation of women in the running of a maternal and infant welfare centre. This is illustrated in the case of the Raymede School for Mothers established in the 1930s. Based on the newly built housing estate established by the Sutton Housing Trust in Dalgrano Gardens in the St Charles ward of North Kensington, this centre had no direct ties with the Labour movement,[12] but it was situated in an area where there was high commitment to social and communal action. This took the form of lectures and talks on the importance of citizenship to young girls and boys. The spirit of the estate was later reinforced by the establishment of a community centre by the London County Council in 1936.[13]

Prior to the opening of the community centre, however, those running the infant welfare centre had already actively begun to encourage the direct involvement of mothers in the centre through the establishment of a Mothers' Council. Mothers standing on this council were elected annually, and played a crucial part in fund-raising for the centre and other charitable bodies. Their power is testified by the fact that they were able to persuade the centre to provide a nursery four afternoons a week so that mothers could leave their children while attending a class or consultation at the centre. Mothers attending the centre could also participate in other social activities, one of which was a choir, which provided social contact alongside a means of fund-raising through its concerts.[14]

Fathers' Councils 1921–36

Mothers were not the only ones who were being encouraged to participate in the running of the welfare services in these years. Fathers' Councils established in Kensington fostered a remarkable degree of participation, and highlight the degree to which some health professionals and social workers were willing to support this goal. The first Council was set up in 1921 encouraged by Dr James Fenton, who early on had observed that many fathers in his borough resented their wives' attendance at welfare centres. On some occasions, Fenton had noted, fathers prevented mothers carrying out the advice they had been given, and forbade certain treatments and operations for their children. This problem was reinforced by the fact that many fathers were at work all day and did not have any contact with workers in these centres.[15] Fathers were often 'inclined to regard an Infant Welfare Centre as a kind of club for mothers and, although they see no objection to visiting their own clubs they think the mother's place is in the home, especially if she has young children'.[16] He thought that fathers tended to be ignored by maternal and infant welfare workers, and warned that such neglect had a detrimental effect on the overall success of infant welfare centres.

In order to resolve the problem Dr Fenton began lecturing to a small group of fathers at the maternal and infant welfare centres in the evenings on issues relating to maternal and infant welfare. These meetings became increasingly popular, which can partly be attributed to Dr Fenton's realization that their success was largely dependent on them fitting in with the daily demands of the fathers he was trying to reach. The place of the meeting was, therefore, always held near the homes of the fathers and meetings were held 'not earlier than 8.30 p.m., thus allowing the men to get home, have a meal, wash and change'.[17] An added incentive to attend came from the free coffee and cigarettes provided during these meetings by ladies on the infant welfare centre committees.[18]

While Fenton's prime purpose was to educate the fathers in matters concerning infant welfare, his action prompted an enterprise which embodied the idea of active citizenship to a remarkable degree. Soon after he started his lectures, a number of fathers at the Lancaster Road infant welfare centre in North Kensington banded together to raise funds for the centre. This initiative led to the establishment of the first Fathers' Council in 1921. What is most striking about this Council was that although originally inspired by Dr Fenton's lectures, it was initiated by the fathers themselves.[19] The three main objectives of the Council were:

1. to bring to the father the responsibility which rests upon them in giving the child a proper start in life;
2. to advance the interest of the new centres;
3. to raise funds for the centres by means of entertainments etc.[20]

Within a few years such councils had spread to other centres within Kensington as a whole and there was widespread interest in the enterprise not only nationally, but all over the world, including Japan.[21]

Overall the structure of the council was democratic. While Dr

Fenton acted as the President of Council, all the officers and members of the Executive Committee were appointed by members of the Council. Those belonging to the Council were required to pay an annual subscription of 1s. which entitled them to vote for the Executive Committee, and to attend a monthly Council meeting in the evening at the centre. These meetings usually consisted of a lecture by Dr Fenton or another trained health worker on subjects concerning hygiene. Fathers also prepared lectures for the meetings. In this way the Council was not only providing education, but actively encouraged fathers to participate in the meetings and the running of the Council. Council members were also encouraged to do their own publicity, which was usually allotted to one particular father who wrote articles for the local press. Members of the Fathers' Council were also called on to act as representatives for the Council, and to address various meetings in the neighbourhood.[22] Fathers themselves, and not other health workers, were thus the active promoters of their own work. Similarly, fund-raising, an activity frequently left to middle-class volunteers running a maternal and infant welfare centre, was also actively taken up by the Fathers' Council. The fathers often organized concerts to collect money, some of which was used to send a 'limited number of mothers and children to convalescent homes at the seaside during the summer months'.[23]

The work of the Fathers' Council was not only confined to maternal and child welfare work, but played an important role in involving its fathers and other residents in public health work as a whole. One of the most important items on the agenda of the Fathers' Council in Kensington was the consideration of health conditions within their districts. Fathers were encouraged to 'report to the meetings if yards were not kept clean, dustbins without lids or with lids not kept in position, manure heaps in mewsways not regularly removed, and matters of this kind'. Sometimes members were deputed to speak to offenders, or the matter was reported to the medical officer of health. In highlighting this work Dr Fenton was quick to point out that in the context of the meetings held by the Fathers' Council,

> Public health knowledge grows rapidly. Moreover the men are learning to be good citizens and to take an interest in local public life, which is for the benefit of themselves and their neighbours, and finally, they are better occupied in smoking, chatting and meeting in this way than by spending their time in public houses.

Moreover, as he went on to say,

> One difficulty of infant welfare in the past has been to get at the fathers. Experience shows that this is easy once tackled. They not only become keen, but they want to act as disciplines of hygiene and influence other men and women.[24]

Such attempts to raise people's consciousness about the need to take an active role in health matters was not unique to the Fathers' Councils, but were also apparent in the policies of other institutions such as the Hampstead Health Institute.[25]

While the Fathers' Councils clearly stimulated wide participation on the part of the fathers and can be seen as one health professional's attempt to listen to their demands, the underlying aim of their creation can be seen to bear some hallmarks of a more conservative attitude. One of Dr Fenton's original aims in his talks to fathers, which had partly inspired the establishment of the Fathers' Councils, had been to eradicate their 'prejudice' against maternal and child welfare. In this respect he was not far from the founding ethics of health visiting and maternal and child welfare work as a whole, the aim of which was to educate the 'ignorant' and 'feckless' poor and to induce the notion of self-help.[26] Yet rather than looking to health professionals to undertake such work, in educating the fathers, Dr Fenton enabled the fathers to take matters into their own hands, a key element in the ethic of self-help and active citizenship. In this sense Dr Fenton could be seen as achieving the aim of helping the poor to help themselves. The fathers, rather than health workers, were now seen to be the ambassadors of maternal and infant welfare among the poor. While Fenton's approach might hint of the 'self-help' attitude often adopted by other more patronizing middle-class workers, the spirit in which he worked implies a much more democratic approach.

Where perceptions of women's participation and citizenship were concerned, however, Fenton's initiative might be thought to be double-edged. In recognizing that many women could not act in their own, and their children's, best interests without the support of husbands, he acknowledged and endorsed the weakness of women's position and reinforced the gender differences that continued to frame the notion of citizenship.

North Kensington Women's Welfare Centre, 1924–36

One institution in Kensington which was more directed towards empowering women was the North Kensington Women's Welfare Centre. Founded in 1924 by Margery Spring Rice[27] and other women campaigners to provide birth control, this centre encouraged women to participate in the development and running of services.

Such representation was partly achieved by the establishment of a mothers' club, which had a committee controlled and elected by the mothers themselves. Membership of the club was to be by subscription, but this, it was specified, should not be too high so as not to deter the poorest. As in the case of the Fathers' Councils, the North Kensington Women's Welfare Centre also encouraged its mothers to act as representatives for the centre. Mothers were approached by the organizers of the centre to speak at publicity meetings within the neighbourhood.[28] Former patients were seen as 'the best propagandists'.[29] Within the centre mothers were also given a room where they could rest during the day, which it was hoped would not only provide them with a chance to temporarily escape their often monotonous and solitary routine, but also to meet other mothers with whom they could share their concerns.[30] Partly reflecting the close ties that the centre had with Dr Fenton and the contact that it had with Eckhard, such schemes paralleled some of those established by the Fathers' Councils and some maternal and infant welfare centres.

Such involvement of mothers within its organizational structure enabled women to have a more direct and powerful role within the centre than they were allowed in many institutions. The degree to which the North Kensington Women's Welfare Centre attempted to empower women was apparent in a much wider sense. Originally established to provide birth control, the subject of great taboo and controversy in the outside world, those running the centre not only had to have a high degree of tact and sympathy for those they served, but were also spurred into taking a very different approach from those involved in the provision of other maternal and infant welfare services. One of the underlying principles in providing birth control was also to enable women to take more control over their fertility, and thus provide them with the means to lead healthier lives which would afford them greater opportunities of independence. Within a few years of its foundation Margery Spring Rice and her co-workers, through their very direct contact with women and the very intimate problems they confronted, realized that birth control was not the total solution to women's problems and that more comprehensive facilities were required if birth control services were to be of any use.

One of the most important services they set up was a gynaecological clinic. Established in 1931, the clinic was the first of its kind in the country. Providing not only advice, but also treatment, the clinic was particularly important given that most working-class mothers had no national insurance to cover the expense of a doctor, and only received medical treatment during pregnancy and child-birth. With no recourse to medical care, many women were, there-fore, forced to suffer many discomforts such as prolapsed wombs which could lead to infections and incontinence.[31] Alongside this clinic by the 1930s the North Kensington Women's Welfare Centre also began to offer emotional counselling, which was later formalized into the first Marriage Guidance Clinic in the country.

In providing emotional and gynaecological help together with birth control, staff at the North Kensington Women's Welfare Centre were acknowledging the complex dynamics at work in deter-mining women's health. Their attitudes can be seen most clearly by a statement made by the Executive Committee in 1938:

> It is ... clear that health education and ample medical facilities for every sort of ailment are not all that the working woman needs to lead a healthy and happy life. Some of the remedies needed are outside the scope of such a clinic as this viz: the provision of suf-ficient and well-paid work for the father of every family, the provision of a labour-saving, adequately equipped home, and pos-sibly the rationalisation of a great part of the housewife's domestic work. It is arguable that if all these 3 reforms were achieved, the individual woman might safely be left to herself with the certainty that her salvation would lie in her own hands. But as things are at present, her life is in general one of such unceasing toil and anxiety that she has neither the money nor the time to seek or pursue those social, educational and recreational activities which are as essential to health, (in fact *more* essential to the *maintenance of health*,) as the doctor's advice and treatment. It must never be forgotten that for the woman her home is her workplace, and her family however devoted she may be to them, create her work. The result of this is that she cannot *rest* in her home as her husband, returning from work outside can; and her children, although they can give her much happiness cannot in themselves provide recreation for her in the sense in which she, of all human beings, needs it most.[32]

Central to those working in the centre, was that their work should enable women to take health matters into their own hands, of which the provision of birth control was seen as the first step. As Dr Helena Wright argued, most of the patients she saw at the centre lived in perpetual anxiety of having another child, and every month lived through 'nightmares of terror'. By educating women on methods of birth control it was hoped women would no longer suffer in this way and generally raise their conditions of health. As Helena Wright outlined,

What can be hoped for from the dissemination of adequate Birth Control instruction? We can free mothers entirely from the fear of unwanted pregnancies. We can free them from the danger of the fact of repeated pregnancies and so conserve their health to a very large extent. We can free the sex life of these people from the unnatural and bad psychological restrictions that are at present happening. We can produce that state of happiness, stability and normality which we have observed very often in the cases of our patients who have been our patients for 2 or 3 years, and have had a chance to see what a difference it makes to their lives.[33]

In addition to extending women's knowledge about contraception, the centre aimed to raise women's consciousness about their overall health. Margery Spring Rice, in carrying out an investigation of the health of 1,250 women nationally, indicated that much of the ill health women suffered was the result of the apathy they felt towards their own bodies. As she argued,

A difficulty about treatment is woman's heroic, often indeed very foolish indifference to her own health, and the absence of any teaching or empirical knowledge which might have enabled her to form a high standard of good health. Knowing as she does that upon her ability to keep going depends the well-being of her family, she will only ask advice in the very last resort, ie when her condition gets to the point of crippling her work.[34]

Many medical experts and social reformers argued that it was this factor which was one of the major causes of the high rate of maternal mortality.[35] By providing gynaecological treatment the North Kensington Women's Welfare Centre hoped to strike at 'the roots of maternal ill-health'. Such treatment was not only aimed at married women, but also young unmarried women who it was hoped, would come to 'the gynaecological session in order to learn the care of their own health before they embarked on childbearing.'[36] As they stated,

12 years of welfare work among married women have confirmed the opinion of the committee and medical staff of this centre that many of the failures to achieve or maintain health in mind and body are the direct results of insufficient or injurious instruction during adolescence or early womanhood.

They went on to argue,

Through the nature of the work at this centre a relationship of intimacy and sympathy is established between patient and doctor. There is no personal difficulty of domestic life – whether of health, emotion or understanding, that patients will not discuss with the doctor whom they consult here. The clinic therefore possesses unique qualifications to help to dispel the widespread ignorance and inhibitions which contribute to the unhappiness and ill-health of hundreds of patients which, with continuance of the present activity in these matters, will be passed [on] to their children.[37]

Much of the instruction provided concerned 'physiology and sex hygiene', as well as the rudiments of women's bodies and their health. This policy could be considered radical for this period, particularly when we consider that from the mid 1930s the centre began to direct some of this education towards unmarried adolescent women.[38] It was also very different from the lessons on mothercraft and child rearing offered in maternal and child welfare centres which was largely based on the premise of women's passivity and made very little attempt to enlighten women on reproduction and the means of preserving good health.

Yet while the centre was pioneering in this respect, many of the motivations behind the work were rooted in the more traditional aims of eugenics and nationalism.[39] It is clear that one of the prime purposes of the centre was to teach birth control to the working class so as to improve the quality of the race. Organizers of the centre, for instance, discouraged childless married women from having contraception until they had at least one baby, unless they had good reasons such as bad health, a hereditary disease, or straitened economic conditions.[40] By helping women to space out their births and to improve their health the North Kensington Women's Welfare Centre hoped to raise the standard of health not only of the mothers and their infants but of the whole nation.[41] Margery Spring Rice's letter to Dr Fenton highlights this attitude:

> I am an unrepentant believer in *voluntary* rather than enforced parenthood, I believe that the best service a married couple can do to themselves and to the community of which they are members is to rear as large a family as their health and resources allow. I also firmly believe that the power of deciding the number of children and the times of their birth is a direct and powerful stimulus to parenthood amongst healthy and public-spirited people.[42]

Nevertheless, while these attitudes underlay the facilities provided, within the clinics themselves it would seem that a more pragmatic approach was taken even when it contradicted the policies laid down by eugenic supporters.[43] The gratitude and high attendance of the women who attended the centre examined in the next chapter indicates that this approach was successful. Indeed, it would seem that the centre provided a service which answered a real need not answered elsewhere.

Overall Attitudes of Health Workers in Listening to Mothers

While it would seem both from the Fathers' Councils and from the North Kensington Women's Welfare Centre that a number of health professionals and social reformers were willing to listen to and involve those they catered to in the early twentieth century, it is difficult to judge how far these attitudes extended to other workers. Dr M. P., who worked widely in maternal and infant welfare centres as well as birth control clinics in the 1930s and 1940s, including the North Kensington Women's Welfare Centre, recalled that among her peers there was the feeling, 'that one didn't want to have the idea that we, the people who know, are trying to teach the poor ignorant mothers how to bring up their children. This was an idea that was very much frowned upon....' She stressed that the feeling was, 'that one is only helping mothers to do it themselves, that they are the right people to bring up their children, and all they need is a little support and backing to do it themselves'. She and her colleagues were adamant that they must 'get away from the idea that people in the know were doing [the] teaching'.[44]

These ideals were not always easy to achieve. As Dr M. P. admitted, there was a mixture of attitudes among maternal and infant welfare workers even in the 1930s. She recalled that the voluntary lady workers with whom she collaborated with 'were very good', but that 'they always knew better, they were always self-appointed "do-gooders". Some of them were rather a menace.' According to her some of these ladies had difficulties in listening to the health professionals as well as the mothers. Some of them gave 'advice that was quite contrary to what the health visitors were saying, but they, because they were voluntary, because they were on the Committee of this Centre would over-rule the health visitors'. Much of the tension surfaced in arguments 'about what sort of food the children ought to have, whether it should be dried milk, whether it should be condensed milk, or whether it should have sugar added.' Such conflicts were reinforced by the differing levels of knowledge, which was constantly altering. The battles not only emerged between voluntary workers and the professionals, but also between the long-experienced professionals and those who were more recently trained. Similarly some health visitors were more old-fashioned than some voluntary workers.[45]

Listening to and involving mothers within maternal and infant welfare work was therefore not only determined by the attitudes towards the mothers of the personnel running the facilities, but also by the continual fights among the professionals over what mothers should be taught and how they should be included. Clearly the question as to who had the ultimate authority to dictate these terms was closely tied to the power dynamics of each institution. In this situation the voice of the mother and her priorities could be lost in the midst of the hierarchical struggles between staff.

Conclusion

As we have seen in Chapter 1 women had varying perceptions of their roles as wives and mothers. While motherhood was prized, for many mothers it brought as much toil as it brought pleasure. Much of their experience of motherhood was greatly dependent on their social and economic conditions. While many working-class mothers were keen to have children, they were constantly hampered by the scarcity of resources as well as the lack of decent accommodation. The threat of an appearance of another child was therefore a perpetual anxiety. Adding to these pressures was also often the poor facilities women had for controlling their fertility and the difficulties they frequently experienced in negotiating the sexual relations with their husbands. From the testimony of many women from these years it would seem that a number of husbands were reluctant to use any contraception and that the responsibility of motherhood rested solely on the shoulders of the mother.

While a mother's lot was largely shaped by her marital relationship, it was also influenced by the degree of support she could also expect in the outside world. To what degree her perceptions and needs were heeded, however, was largely dependent on the attitudes of the professionals running services for their aid and the space that they were willing to allow for mothers' voices to be heard. Some of the clearest examples we have of the degree to which health professionals and their staff were willing to listen and involve those they were trying to reach were the Fathers' Council and the North Kensington Women's Welfare Centre.

Such institutions were quite unusual, but should be viewed within the wider context of the growing crusade in the 1920s and 1930s for citizen participation in civic life[46] together with the winning of the vote for women. This campaign was particularly forceful in Kensington. As already outlined in Chapter 2, Kensington from early on had a strong suffragette movement with large support at the grassroots level, and was among the first areas in the country to have women elected to the council. Kensington was also an area where there was a long tradition of philanthropy which promoted the ethics of self-help, as well as a growing solidarity for the Labour Party. Combined, all these factors were probably a potent force in challenging professionals to listen to and include those they were trying to serve.

Kensington was not unique in having such institutions. Similar moves were also undertaken in Woolwich, most clearly seen in the Mothers' Committee at the infant welfare centre on Well Hall Estate. Arising partly as a result of the strong tradition of trade unionism and in an area of large Labour Party support such a committee seems to have emerged from a different political and social context than that of Kensington. While such differences are important to bear in mind when considering the extent to which different schemes allowed for the participation of mothers, as the following chapter will show, the real test of whether those running the schemes listened to the mothers and how far they met their demands is to examine the extent to which women used the services.

Notes

1. E. V. Eckhard, *The Mother and the Infant* (London: 1921), 61.
2. Born in 1885, Edith Eckhard originally came from Manchester and was the daughter of Gustav and Mary Eckhard, and a cousin of Lord and Lady Simon Wythenshawe. Starting as an assistant lecturer in the Ratan Tata Department (later known as the department of Social Science and Administration) at the LSE in 1919, Eckhard rose in 1928 to become senior lecturer in social administration and deputy-head of the department, where she remained for over 30 years. Very little material remains on her life but various obituaries state that she was a quiet, unobtrusive, and creative person who was not only widely admired by those she taught, but was also powerful in moulding and shaping the ideas and policies of the department of social administration. For more information on Eckhard's life see the obituaries in *Manchester Guardian,* 11 August 1952 and 10 December 1952; *The Times,* 19 August 1952; and *London School of Economics Magazine,* No.5, January 1953, 25–6. For more information on the influence of the Department of the Social Administration at the London School of Economics and its influence on the training of social workers and the formulation of social policy see J. Harris, 'The Webbs, The Charity Organisation Society and the Ratan Tata Foundation: Social policy from the perspective of 1912', in M. Bulmer, J. Lewis, and D. Piachaud (eds), *The Goals of Social Policy* (London: 1989), 27–63.
3. In many of the current debates the term citizenship is frequently

confused with that of consumer rights, which has very different implications from citizen rights. For more information on the present controversy over these issues see A. J. Kearns, 'Active Citizenship and Urban Governance', *Trans. Inst. Br. Geog.*, 17 (1992), 20–34; S. J. Smith, 'Society, Space and Citizenship: A Human Geography for the "New Times"', *Trans. Inst. Br. Geog.*, 14 (1989), 144–56; R. Lister, 'Tracing the Contours of Women's Citizenship', *Policy and Politics,* 21/1 (1993), 3–16; N. Black, 'Private Health Care: Patients' Beliefs and Practice', *Br. Med. J.,* 307 (10 July 1993), 81; N. Pfeffer and A. Pollock, 'Public Opinion and the NHS', *Br. Med. J.,* 307 (27 September 1993), 750–1; N. Pfeffer and A. Coote, *Is Quality Good for You: a Critical Review of Quality Assurance in Welfare Services,* Institute for Public Policy Research, Social Policy Paper No. 5, 1994; M. Hodge, *Quality, Equality, Democracy: Improving Public Services,* Fabian Pamphlet 549, (1991); D. Edgar, 'Are You being Served?', *Marxism Today,* (May 1991), 28; G. Mather, 'Serving You Rights', *Marxism Today,* (May 1991), 29; and J. Stewart, N. Lewis and D. Longley, 'Accountability to the Public', paper presented to the European Policy Forum for British and European Market Studies Conference, December 1992.

4. Eckhard, *op. cit.* (note 1), 63–4.
5. See, for instance, the advice given in a parallel service, the child guidance clinics described in C. Urwin and E. Harland, 'From Bodies to Minds in Childcare Literature: Advice to Parents in Inter-War Britain', in R. Cooter (ed.), *In the Name of the Child: Health and Welfare, 1880–1940* (London: 1992).
6. One of the most concrete signs of this was the Maternal and Child Welfare Act of 1918 which insisted on women being represented on Maternal and Child Welfare Committees. Woolwich Council Minutes, 8 May 1918, 333.
7. Eckhard, *op. cit.* (note 1), 63–4.
8. *Ibid.*
9. *Ibid.,* 63.
10. D. Thom, 'Women Munition Workers at the Woolwich Arsenal in the 1914–18 War', unpub. M.A., Warwick, 1976, 110. Thom does not specify whether constitutionally the Association was bound into giving women an equal number of places on the committee.
11. Such participation is particularly interesting within the context of women's participation in politics as a whole, which is often explained in terms of their work patterns. For an example of this see J. Mark-Lawson, M. Savage and A. Warde, 'Gender and Local Politics: Struggles over Welfare Policies, 1918–39', in Lancaster Regionalism Group, *Localities, Class and Gender* (London: 1985).
12. Until 1934 St Charles ward continually returned Municipal Reform candidates in the borough council elections. See *Kensington News and the West London Times* and *Kensington Citizen.*

13. Raymede School for Mothers, *A/R* (1930–1), 3 (PRO file: MH66/659); The Community Centre, Dalgrano Gardens, leaflet for the session 1936–7 (CMAC file: SA/FPA, Box 649 NK158).

14. Raymede School for Mothers, *A/R* (1930–1).

15. Dr Fenton, speech in 'Fourth English-Speaking Conference on Infant Welfare' (London: 1926), 62–3; 'Kensington Public Health Survey', 1932, 14 (PRO file: MH66/359).

16. For more information on Dr Fenton see Ch. 2. Fenton, *op. cit.* (note 15), 63. Fenton's talks to fathers was not totally new. In the 1880s fathers' classes were established alongside mother's meetings by religious organizations. The classes included hymn singing and secular instruction. Much of the activity of their classes was to 'promote male respect for Christian family life and motherhood'. F. Prochaska, 'A Mother's Country: Mothers Meetings and Family Welfare in Britain, 1880–1950', *Hist.,* 74 (1989), 379–99, 388.

17. Such stipulations indicate that the meetings were biased towards those fathers who were considered to be the more respectable poor.

18. Fenton, *op. cit.* (note 15), 63.

19. *Ibid.,* 64.

20. *Ibid.;* 'Kensington Public Health Survey', (note 15), 14.

21. Such widespread interest had even inspired one film company to make a talkie picture of the Fathers' Council at work. Fenton, *op. cit.* (note 15), 64–5, and also see the discussion emerging from his paper, 69–70. See also 'Kensington Public Health Survey', (note 15), 14. One similar scheme was set up at the East Street Welfare Centre in East Street in Lambeth known as the Working-Men's Propaganda Committee. See C. Kenner, 'The Politics of Married Working Class Women's Health Care in Britain, 1918–39', unpub. M.Phil, Sussex, 1979, 184–5.

22. The fathers were limited financially in how they could travel, and were dependent on financial assistance from the Ladies Committee to attend meetings taking place far from Kensington. In order to get around this problem fathers were encouraged to come from other districts to the meetings in Kensington. Fenton, *op. cit.* (note 15), 66, 69.

23. *Ibid.,* 65.

24. *Ibid.,* 66.

25. HCSW, *Biannual Report of the Executive,* (1921–2), 38.

26. Fenton, *op. cit.* (note 15), 65.

27. For more information on Margery Spring Rice see Ch. 2.

28. NKWWC Executive Committee Minutes, 14 December 1934, 9.

29. NKWWC, *A/R* (1925–6), 2. The justification for this belief is discussed in the next chapter.

30. 'The NKWWC – Suggested Lines of Development' (July 1938), (CMAC file: SR15/19, Box 665).

31. 'The NKWWC – Suggested Lines of Development' (note 30); Dr M. P., interviewed by L. Marks, London, 23 November 1992, transcript,

15–16.

32. 'The NKWWC – Suggested Lines of Development' (note 30).

33. *Report of the Conference on the Giving of Information on Birth Control by Public Health Authorities* (4 April 1930), 15–16 (CMAC file: SA/FPA/SR 24A/7). See also Dr M. P., interviewed by L. Marks, transcript, 17.

34. M. Spring Rice, 'The Health of Working Women', *The Eugenics Review,* 32/2 (1940), 50–44, 52–3.

35. 'Protect the Nation's Mothers', Report by the Standing Joint Committee of Industrial Women's Organizations – Labour Party's Advisory Committee on Women's Questions, to the National Conference of Labour Women, Sheffield, May 1935 (CMAC Box 340, SA/FPA/ A.13/38–42), 9–10.

36. NKWWC, *A/R* (1933–4), 2.

37. NKWWC, Executive Committee Minutes, discussion on 'The Need for Education in Physiology and Sex among Girls and Women', 1938 (CMAC file: SA/FPA/NK 215).

38. NKWWC, *A/R* (1936–7), 3.

39. For the links between birth control, eugenics and nationalism see Ch. 4.

40. NKWWC, *A/R* (1927–8), 3. See also NKWWC, Medical Committee Minutes, 16 April 1940, 57 (CMAC file: NK226, Box 657).

41. NKWWC, *A/R* (1935–5).

42. M. Spring Rice's letter to Dr J. Fenton, 12 December 1938. (CMAC file: SR/NK 87, Box 640).

43. Such a contradiction also prevailed among the clinics provided by Marie Stopes. See D. Cohen, 'Private Lives in Public Spaces: Marie Stopes, The Mothers' Clinics and the Practice of Contraception', *Hist. Workshop J.,* 35 (1993), 95–116.

44. Mrs M. P., interviewed by L. Marks, transcript, 18.

45. *Ibid.,* 9.

46. S. and E. Yeo, 'On the Uses of "Community": from Owenism to the Present,' in S. Yeo (ed.), *New Views of Co-operation* (London: 1988), 235–43.

8

The Approval of Mothers: Popularity
and Uptake of Services

Today one of the most important debates around the future of the National Health Service is the degree to which it is providing for the needs and demands of its consumers. Much of this discussion is framed around the concept that people have a choice in the services provided, and can influence the direction the provision takes. The recent Citizen's Charter, under which patients are assured of their rights to a high quality and easily accessible provision of medical care, has provided an important focus for this discussion. According to the Charter citizens are seen as being given powers of assertion to demand certain services. Yet, as Kearns has pointed out the Charter 'has more to do with consumerism than with citizenship, for the rights it seeks to realize are those arising out of contractual relations rather than out of the citizen's membership of a political economy'. Indeed, this new emphasis on citizenship and rights in fact hides the increasing erosion of both democratic participation and the ability to demand welfare services.[1]

This chapter takes the discussion further, exploring within the historical context the degree to which the growing awareness of the need to involve and listen to mothers in the inter-war years, as outlined in the previous chapter, was reflected in the popularity and uptake of provision.

Chapters 5 and 6 indicate that the attendance numbers at various maternal and child services were rising in these years. Yet while these figures indicate that the services were reaching a high proportion of those that they intended to serve, they are drawn from aggregate statistics which reveal little about the experience of individuals. Indeed, these figures disguise the very complex processes involved in the choices mothers made in using the services. In this chapter I will show that the popularity and uptake of services was dependent on a host of issues and not solely confined to the attitudes of the staff running the services.

Some idea of the range of factors that were involved can be gauged from one survey carried out by the Women's Sections of the Labour Party in 1935 which explored women's views of maternity services. From this survey it was clear that women's attendance at antenatal clinics, for instance, was greatly dependent on the degree of promotion the services were given by health visitors which in turn was dependent on the number of health visitors in particular areas. The support local midwives and doctors gave to certain clinics was also influential on women's attendance. None the less, even when well informed, many women admitted they were reluctant to attend a clinic if it was situated in a depressing building, and they faced sitting many hours in uncomfortable waiting rooms followed by the demand that they fill in complicated forms. Many women reported having to wait over two hours before being seen. Women also complained that they often had no privacy with the doctor and on many occasions felt patronized by the doctor attending them. They were more likely to attend a session if the doctor was a woman and if the workers within the institution refrained from making them feel like objects of charity. Among the other factors listed for women's reluctance to use facilities was if they were not provided with an opportunity to rest after a painful medical examination. Women were also less likely to attend a clinic if it was too far from their homes and involved expensive bus or tram fares.[2] Clearly from these answers, the degree to which a maternal and child welfare centre heeded women's demands and served their needs had an impact on the degree to which women used specific services.

While most of the women questioned in the Labour Party survey were active members of the Labour Party, who were more highly politically motivated to improve new facilities, the positive and negative reasons they listed as influencing their uptake of provision were not unique. To what extent were these also reflected in the attitudes of those mothers using the services in Hampstead, Kensington, Stepney and Woolwich? This question is difficult to answer, partly because, as we have already seen in previous chapters, facilities varied greatly between boroughs and attitudes differed sharply between institutions. It would be difficult to provide a comprehensive examination of all the services in each borough and to describe the perceptions of all the women who used the services. What follows, therefore, is only a sample of the mothers in the boroughs and their reaction to a handful of the services available. Like the previous chapter much of this focus is on the services in Kensington, where the sources are particularly good for analysing these questions. While a sample from Kensington cannot be taken as representative of all the women in each borough or indicate the true extent of the popularity or distaste of certain institutions, such a sample gives us some understanding of the factors which influenced women's perceptions of the services. This will be examined firstly in relation to the services provided for infants, such as health visiting, infant welfare centres and the Kensington Baby Clinic, and then in relation to the care available to mothers, particularly the North Kensington Women's Welfare Centre.

Popularity of Services for Infants
Health Visiting, 1902–36

One of the first reasons listed in the Labour Party's survey for the lack of use of clinics was the inadequate promotion of the services by health visitors. As already stated in Chapter 5, the health visitor was the key liaison officer for maternal and child welfare services. It was she who visited all the notified births in the district and encouraged mothers to attend infant welfare centres, and chased up the mothers if they failed to make follow-up visits to the clinic. She was also the one who checked to see if mothers were carrying out the instructions and treatment advised by the infant welfare centre. But, as Peretz has pointed out, health visitors were often in an ambiguous and difficult position. In many instances they were the buffer between the medical officer or the clinic doctor, and the mothers and infants themselves. Thus health visitors were 'poised between speaking for families and policing them'.[3] This ambiguous position of the health visitor had an important impact throughout the early twentieth century not only on the relationship between health visitors and the mothers, but also on the degree to which their advice was accepted.

It is clear that for some poor mothers the appearance of a health visitor felt like an infringement of their personal liberties, and saw their visit as a sign that something was wrong and that a complaint had been made against them.[4] Such views, although misinterpreting the purpose of the health visitor's call, are not surprising given that on some occasions health visitors did report their cases to policing agencies such as the National Society for the Prevention of Cruelty to Children.[5] In Kensington health visitors also sent their needy cases for assistance to the Charity Organization Society, an agency not known for its sympathy.[6] Given the strong stigmas attached to receiving charity and the hostility many of the poor felt towards the

Charity Organization Society and the National Society for the Prevention of Cruelty to Children, any associations the health visitor had with such organizations could provoke antagonism among those they visited, and make mothers feel stigmatized.

It is interesting to note that the greatest resistance to health visitors appears to have occurred at the time of their original appointment in the years before the First World War. This hostility partly reflected the nature of maternal and child welfare services in this period, which were not so much about listening to mothers as inducing them to change their ways. In all the boroughs health visitors continually cited difficulties in persuading mothers to improve their feeding habits, cooking, household skills, and general infant care.[7] Many of these mothers could not see why the advice given by the health visitor should take precedence over their own knowledge, or that learned from their mothers.[8] In order to placate the health visitor some mothers would give accounts of the baby that the health visitor wished to hear when not necessarily following the advice given.[9]

Some of the greatest resistance health visitors faced came from those mothers who were older and had more children and therefore had much more experience. Not surprisingly the health visitors tended to concentrate their efforts on younger mothers who had just had their first child.[10] By catching mothers at a young and impressionable age it was hoped that the advice a health visitor gave would not only be followed in the case of the first child but also for subsequent ones, and that their advice would later be passed on to the next generation. This attitude was expressed by a health visitor in Woolwich, who hoped 'that from this beginning – this acquiescence in being instructed – many develop the general convictions, that child-rearing is a difficult art, requiring special knowledge and definite preparation.'[11] Within this context childrearing and care was seen as a skill which did not come naturally and had to be taught. Rather than boosting the role of mothers and the work they performed, this policy in fact disenfranchised mothers of their status. By pressurizing mothers to ignore their own common sense in childcare matters and to follow the advice of the expert instead, health visitors and other maternal and child welfare workers were often robbing mothers of their own skills.

Much of the conflict between health visitors and the mothers was rooted in general perceptions over what constituted good health. This tension is illustrated by the comments made by a health visitor in Woolwich, who stated,

It is difficult to distinguish between apathy and ignorance. What appears to be apathy on the mother's part is often at bottom a profound ignorance of meaning of the symptoms, which tell their tale plainly enough to the experienced observer. Imminent danger of death, and illness acute enough to require the doctor, they understand. All conditions short of this they would class as healthy, or to use the favourite term, 'wiry'. Many hundreds of pallid, rickety children have been pointed out to me by proudly complacent mothers as 'wiry'.[12]

Indeed, for this health visitor, as for most health visitors, the prime aim of her work was to change these attitudes. As she said, 'One of the first things to be aimed at in practical work is the implanting in the mother's mind of some standard of what constitutes a healthy vigorous mind.'[13]

Much of the tension not only emerged as a result of the differences in perceptions, but also because in many instances mothers were inhibited from carrying out the advice given to them because of the conditions they were living in. As a health visitor in Woolwich pointed out in 1906, 'in several instances extreme poverty renders the carrying out of proper precautions and treatment impossible or very difficult'.[14] Similarly, in Stepney many mothers were reported as having been forced to neglect their infants in order to earn the family income. As a health visitor indicated, 'work had to be finished and returned to the employer's premises before the next meal could be provided'.[15] In some cases mothers were forced to leave the care of their infants to unsuitable carers.[16]

While much of the attitude of health visitors in these years appears to have been patronizing and not necessarily heeding the voice of the mothers, reports from the health visitors in the four boroughs suggest that despite initial resistance, most mothers welcomed them with open arms. As the health visitor in Woolwich claimed in 1906, 'My visits are almost invariably well received; the exceptions are so few as to be really a negligible quantity.' She went on to note, 'As soon as visiting after the notification of the birth of a child becomes the rule in any district, it seems to be taken as a matter of course and to be looked for.' By 1907 she further reported, 'As a matter of fact, it is not the paying of a visit, but the omission of a visit which is more often regarded as a grievance.'[17] Health visitors claimed that any objections a mother might have to the visit soon disappeared when they revealed 'that it is not criticism but help and sympathy which is offered'.[18]

While the lowering of mothers' resistance to health visitors might have been exaggerated on the part of the health visitors wanting to emphasize the value of their work, it would be a mistake to dismiss their evidence as false. For many mothers the health visitor was not necessarily a draconian figure, but rather someone who could provide useful information and support. The help that health visitors provided was highlighted not only in the case of the survey carried out by the Women's Section of the Labour Party in the 1930s, but also from the letters written by mothers to the Women's Co-operative Guild in 1913. Much depended on the personality of a health visitor and her ability to combine advice and education with tact and sympathy for the situation of the mother she was visiting. From the evidence available it would seem that while critical of the habits of some mothers, health visitors did have some appreciation of the circumstances mothers faced. Indeed, if the health visitor was to succeed and not be ignored she had to take these factors into account and listen to the demands of the mother.

Infant Welfare Centres, 1902–36

The health visitor was often addressing a captive audience. Mothers who were approached by a health visitor in their own homes could do little to escape her attention. Those who visited welfare centres, however, had slightly greater autonomy. It was up to each mother to choose whether or not to attend. A woman's attendance at an infant welfare centre was, therefore, more representative of her views of the facilities, than her response to a health visitor. Even so, the decision to attend an infant welfare centre was not entirely free of pressure, which began as soon as the health visitor, often an agent for the infant welfare centre, visited the mother. The tactics of the persuasion on the part of the health visitor could often be hard to resist.

   If we look at the rise in the number of attendances as outlined in Chapter 5, it would seem that the new centres increasingly enticed mothers to their doors. These figures, however, hide the very personal and individual nature of the choices that women made in attending such centres. A mother's decision over whether to attend a welfare centre was governed by many of the same questions as those which confronted her in accepting advice from a health visitor knocking on her front door. For some the decision to attend had to be made in the face of opposition from relatives and friends, and, of course, husbands.[19]

   Their determination to attend was also influenced by the ease with which they could reach a clinic. Appendices 1 to 4 show where the various infant welfare centres and other maternal and child welfare services were sited within each borough. From these appendices we can see that services were the least spread out and most easily accessible within Stepney, partly reflecting its greater poverty and larger population than the other boroughs. In all the boroughs infant welfare centres were primarily sited in the poorest areas where infant mortality was perceived to be highest.[20] The targeting of poor areas can most clearly be seen from the map for Kensington in Appendix 2, which shows a much stronger clustering of infant welfare centres in the North of the borough where infant mortality and poverty were higher. By placing centres in these locations it was hoped that they would be accessible to those who most needed to attend them. Despite this aspiration, however, there were some variations in the kind of neighbourhoods that the centres were based in, with some poorer than others and some more politically organized and galvanized to make use of the services. These factors had an impact on the degree to which individual centres could attract those that they most wanted to reach.

Table 8.1: Numbers and percentages of infants and mothers attending different IWCs in Kensington, 1921–38

MCW Centre	Date	Infants attending IWC			Expectant mothers attending IWC		
		Total number	As % of births designated suitable for welfare relief	Average number of visits per infant	Total number	As % of births designated suitable for welfare relief	Average number of visits per mother
Earl's Court	1921–5	837	50	–	266	16	2.6
	1926–30	881	68	–	451	35	2.5
	1931–5•	1,154	94	11.5	499	41	3.6
	1936–8	868	125	–	335	48	4.9
Golborne	1921–5	1,296	72	–	168	9	2.1
	1926–30	1,523	117	–	226	15	2.2
	1931–5•	1,278	117	10.5	253	23	2.8
	1936–8	689	133	10.3	334	65	3.5
Lancaster	1921–5	1,496	88	–	298	17	3.5
	1926–30	1,647	97	–	384	23	3.8
	1931–5•	1,701	147	11.2	537	30	3.7
	1936–8	2,297	128	9.4	638	55	4.7

• Up to 1930 all figures for infants are taken from those listed as new patients, while those from 1931 are from infants 0–1 year.

Source: Kensington MOH, *A/R* (1921–38).

The importance of geographical location was highlighted in Woolwich where the medical officer of health found that the number of mothers attending infant consultations was limited by the long distances they had to travel to visit a centre.[21] Similarly in Woolwich poor mothers often refused to attend the nearest and more modern centre for fear of embarrassment because of their poor clothes in front of the 'better class of mothers'. Sympathetic to these mothers' feelings the medical officer kept open another centre, known as the Ferry centre, which, although situated in an older building with duller accommodation, was nevertheless more attractive to such women. It was located in the poorest quarter of Woolwich, resulting in a clientele who had more in common with each other than if they travelled to another centre in an area with a greater mixture of social classes.[22] Such reluctance to attend on account of the class of other clients was not only apparent among working-class mothers. Middle-class mothers also sometimes showed reluctance to attend centres in poor areas.

The location of an infant welfare centre was important, therefore, in determining both the type and number of mothers it targeted. Kensington provides particularly rich material for examining this issue, because detailed records were kept both for the number of births each individual centre aimed to cater for, as well as the numbers of infants they saw. From this evidence it would seem that in Kensington the location of an infant welfare centre had a slight impact on the level of attendance. Table 8.1 shows that the infant welfare centre in Earl's Court initially attracted fewer mothers and infants than the Golborne infant welfare centre or that in Lancaster Road. Only in the late 1930s did the infant welfare centre in Earl's Court begin to cover as large a percentage of the total births seen as suitable for welfare attention as the other two centres.

Such differences in attendance at the Kensington infant welfare centres are particularly interesting when studied in relation to their geographical setting. Figure 8.1 shows that the three centres were based in very different parts of the borough. The 'Earl's Court' centre was sited on the edge of Earl's Court and Redcliffe. These wards were much richer, less overcrowded and experienced lower infant mortality rates than those served by the other two centres, and overall were strongholds for the Conservative Municipal Reform Party.[23]

Figure 8.1: Map showing the selection of maternal and child welfare services in Kensington with political composition of borough councillors elected in each ward, and their rates of infant mortality, 1906–37

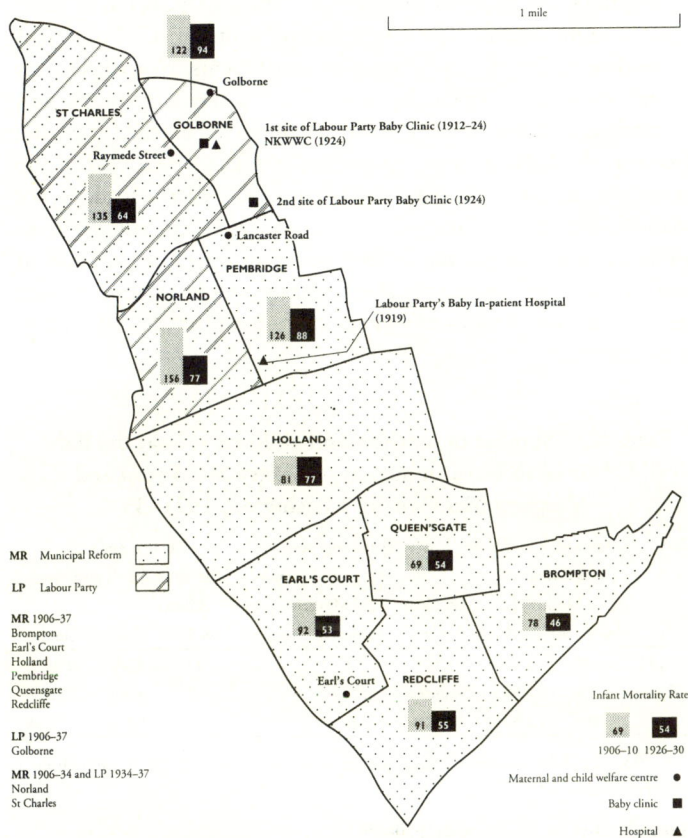

Sources: 'Kensington Public Health Survey', 1932, (PRO File: MH 66/359); Kensington MOH, A/Rs (1906–37); *Kensington News and West London Times*, 1906–37.

By contrast the centre in Golborne was located in the poorest and most overcrowded part of Kensington with very high rates of infant mortality, and where the Labour Party had a stronghold from early on.[24] It might be inferred that the high attendance of infants at the Golborne centre partly stemmed from the high degree of political mobilization in the area which might have raised mothers' consciousness about their entitlement and where to get help. Poorer mothers are usually assumed to have a poorer record of attendance than other mothers on account of their generally lower literacy levels and greater difficulties in dealing with bureaucracy. Health visitors often commented that irregular attendance was more common among the wives of casual labourers than those of husbands in more regular employment.[25] The infant welfare centre in Golborne had more than its fair share of such poor constituents. Nevertheless, its attendance figures suggest that it did reach a very large proportion of mothers and infants. The centre might have benefited from the fact that the Labour Party was particularly active here, and in the early years established its own baby clinic in Telford Road. As we shall discuss below, this clinic, set up in 1911, had cultivated an audience very ready to use facilities when provided. In addition to this factor, there was also the sheer poverty and desperation for free medical support in Golborne which might have enhanced the attendance figures.

Table 8.2: Number of mothers and children seen at the Baby Clinic established in memory of Mary Middleton and Margaret MacDonald, Kensington, 1921–35

Date	Number seen by doctor at consultations		Average number seen by doctor at consultation		Total attendance at clinic for all purposes			
	Mothers		Children	Mothers		Children		
	Antenatal	Postnatal	0–5 yrs	Antenatal	Postnatal	0–5 yrs	Mothers	Children
1921–5	1,331	1,704	33,926	5	7	45	3,040	29,993
1926–30	1,271	2,652	30,627	5	11	41	4,691	72,928
1931–5*	868	2,371	26,734	4	14	44	5,163	71,884

* In 1935 the Baby Clinic no longer served as an infant welfare centre, remaining a treatment centre only.

Source: Kensington MOH, *A/R* (1920–38).

In contrast to the other two centres, the infant welfare centre in Lancaster Road was based in a district which was much more socially mixed. Sited on the edge of the wards of Golborne and Pembridge, the centre catered for residents who were not as devastatingly poor as those living in the northern part of Golborne, but who still had their fair share of social and economic deprivation. Located in Pembridge ward, the centre, like Earl's Court, was in an area where the Municipal Reform Party was strong. Such political affiliations of the overall district, however, disguise the political and communal ties that existed within the neighbourhood immediately surrounding the centre. The establishment of the Fathers' Council at the centre[26] suggests that it was located in an area where there was a high degree of awareness and mobilization around welfare activities. Such high participation partly resulted from the centre being on the edge of the Labour ward of Golborne, and the presence of the baby clinic of the Labour Party which in later years transferred to a road near to the centre. It could also be linked to the ideals of independence and self-help promulgated by the Municipal Reform party in Pembridge. Whatever the root of the awareness, its very presence might explain the high proportion of infants attending the centre at Lancaster Road.

While the type of staff running a centre and its geographical setting were critical to the success of a maternal and child welfare centre, an even more important factor was the kind of support it offered. If a centre did not provide the service a mother wanted she often went elsewhere. As we have seen in Chapter 5 most infant welfare centres aimed to provide advice and not medical treatment. None the less, while maternal and child welfare centres strove to be educational institutions, many mothers viewed them as medical institutions. Some went so they could get their children immunized or get some minor treatment for their child, and also because they could get milk or other forms of nourishment which was sold at cost price, rather than because of the educational advice they provided.[27] Mothers were thus not merely passive recipients of health and welfare provision, but were active choosers of the types of services most suiting their needs and those of their children.

Kensington Baby Clinic, 1912–36

One of the clearest examples of the ways in which the type of service attracted mothers was the Kensington Baby Clinic in North Kensington. As already discussed in greater detail in Chapter 4, this clinic, established in 1912 by the Women's Labour League, differed from most maternal and child welfare services in these years in that it provided medical treatment alongside advice. Soon after its foundation, in 1913, the clinic was already recording a high attendance indicating that the services it provided met a real need not being met elsewhere. In that year 1,210 children aged up to five years were attending the clinic, with 5,382 attendances in all. Of these many were coming in for medical treatment, with 33 out of every 100 requiring some kind of surgical attention: 'the opening of an abscess, the setting of a bone, stitching a split lip, to the removal of tonsils or adenoids'. Medical cases included those suffering from rickets, skin diseases, blepharitis (sore eyes), otorrhea (earache), diarrhoea, bronchitis and many other complaints.[28] In the years to come the numbers attending increased as did the types of patients. Tables 8.2 and 8.3 show the increasing number of mothers and children attending the clinic and the hospital in the years 1920 to 1938.

**Table 8.3: Number of admissions and
average stay of each patient at the Baby Hospital,
Ladbroke Grove, Kensington, 1920–38**

Date	Number of admissions	Average number of days spent in hospital
1920–5	559	56
1926–30	771	52
1931–5	1,284	34
1936–8	750	32

The Baby Hospital was seen as the in-patient extension of the Baby Clinic established in memory of Mary Middleton and Margaret MacDonald.

Source: Kensington MOH, *A/R* (1920–38).

The degree of popularity of the baby clinic is not so much measured by the numbers of attendances as much as the threat infant welfare centres felt from the clinic. In 1922 complaints were heard by Kensington borough council that Raymede, Golborne and Lancaster Road infant welfare centres were losing their clients to the baby clinic which was near by (see Figure 8.1). As members of the Council reported,

> Specific cases were cited in which mothers and children had ceased to attend their respective Centres because of certain attractive features, such as the issue of free drugs etc., offered by the Clinic Authorities, which the Welfare Centres could not, in conformity with the Council's Scheme, offer to mothers attending the respective centres. The evidence offered, it is only right to state, was qualified by the remark that the facts were based on what the mothers had said.
>
> Some of the Welfare Centres referred to the Telford Road Clinic certain children requiring special treatment or surgical operations, but it was found that, not only did these children fail to return after convalescence, but that other children from the same family, and in good health, who might reasonably have been expected to visit the Centres, were taken by their mothers to the Clinic instead, as were any subsequent additions to the family. In consequence of experiences of this kind the Centres practically ceased to refer cases to the clinic, and now recommend St Mary's or some other conveniently situated hospital for any surgical operations or special treatment which may be required.[29]

While the Council was most concerned that the services of the baby clinic should not overlap with those of other infant welfare centres, clearly what was at stake was the fact that the mothers preferred the services offered by the baby clinic. The tension was also heightened by the fact that the clinic refused to cooperate with the other infant welfare centres. Part of this stemmed from the opposition imposed by its founder Dr Ethel Bentham, who objected to such cooperation on the grounds that these centres were voluntarily run.[30] While the clinic itself had been founded by the voluntary funds of the Labour Party, those running it saw it as a model on which to build municipally funded maternal and child welfare services. Any collaboration with voluntary infant welfare centres was seen, therefore, as undermining this goal. To try and overcome the problem the council suggested that the baby clinic should become solely a treatment centre and not undertake the same functions as an infant welfare centre. Such a proposal, however, was resisted by those running the baby clinic, who felt it important to integrate treatment with other maternal and child welfare services on the same premises. Nevertheless, finally in 1935 the clinic was changed to a treatment centre.[31]

Whatever the tensions between the council and the baby clinic, it is clear from the evidence that mothers themselves favoured the clinic over other centres. The popularity of the clinic was probably not only due to the medical treatment it offered and its hospital provision, but also to the overall attitude of the place. From the beginning the clinic was open to all Kensington residents, and any child under five years of age was admitted 'without any charge being made of any kind'. All the attention a child received from the doctor, dentist and nurse was free as were the medicines provided and the operations performed. Those who desired to contribute to the funds of the clinic were encouraged to do so, but it was underlined by the clinic policy that there should be no 'enquiry into the character of the parents – except in so far as the doctor may require information in order to do the best for the little one'.[32]

These views were quite unusual for this time. While most infant welfare centres made no charge for their services, mothers were expected to pay for any supplements or food they obtained and to cover any costs incurred when referred on to another institution for medical treatment. Those who could not afford to pay were assessed according to their income. Mothers were often asked detailed personal questions, which could result in embarrassment. Such questioning was not only common in infant welfare centres, but also in hospitals and Poor Law institutions. Indeed, a number of women interviewed remembered the resentment they felt when asked questions in such institutions.[33] It was this discomfort which the organizers of the clinic were so keen not to repeat. However, rising costs meant that in later years patients visiting the hospital attached to the clinic were expected to pay for treatment, which was assessed according to the parents' income. The average fee charged in 1931 was 3s. 6d. per week.[34]

The organizers of the clinic showed themselves sympathetic towards those they cared for not only in the context of fees, but also in their overall attitude towards mothers. While, like many health visitors, they listed ignorance among the causes of infant mortality, the annual reports indicate that they were less likely to blame the mothers for the neglect of their children. As writers of one report outlined, 'It is recognised that the more careless a mother may be, the greater the need for the best treatment for the child and the most enduring patience with the mother. Not that the careless mothers are often to be found.' They went on to state that when living conditions were taken into consideration, 'the want of knowledge, the careless-ness and neglect of parents ... sink almost to insignificance'. Indeed, they argued that even where ignorance was present it was clear that parents struggled 'to do their best'. As they concluded,

> all mothers know that breast or cow's milk is the best for infants. When the one fails and another cannot be obtained they do not know the best substitutes and make many harmful mistakes. They know that daily washing is good for children – but the provision of the necessary hot water and appliances is beyond either their finan-cial or physical capacity and they compromise by a daily bath for the infant and a Saturday night bath for bigger children. They all know that a child sleeps better in a bed to itself with clean bed-clothes, but with a mixed family in two rooms, they must resign themselves to the inevitable three children in a bed and the two youngest with their parents, with the scanty supply of bedclothes, which often have to be washed and used again the same night... It is most striking, especially in view of the opinions often expressed that mothers need so much training in cleanliness, to see how well kept most of the children are.[35]

Such sympathy for mothers was not unique to the baby clinic. None the less, the popularity of the clinic, together with the comments by its organizers, suggest that the atmosphere and the services it pro-vided went a long way to understanding the needs of the mothers and supporting them. Part of the sympathy offered by the clinic to its mothers might have stemmed from its attachment to the local Labour Party which saw the clinic as an important means of winning votes. As I have argued in Chapter 4, on a national level the clinic also embodied the model for how women within the Labour Party wanted maternal and child welfare services to be developed, putting emphasis as much on medical treatment as preventive measures. It was important, therefore, for the clinic to listen to the demands of those it strove to represent. Whatever the politics behind the baby clinic its services clearly provided a service that mothers wanted for their infants. For many mothers, however, it was not only the services on offer that attracted them, but also whether they saw them to be effective and convenient.[36]

Popularity of Services for Mothers: North Kensington Women's Welfare Centre, 1924–36

The North Kensington Women's Welfare Centre was another institution which showed the degree to which the popularity of a service was dependent on the sympathy and tact of the personnel as well as the help it provided. Records from this centre provide remarkably rich material for studying this question because of the detailed surveys the centre undertook to judge the effectiveness of their work and was in line with the institution's commitment of empowering women noted in Chapter 7. Such evidence provides a unique opportunity for understanding women's response to certain health services in these years. In addition, the North Kensington Women's Welfare Centre is an especially interesting case because of the considerable taboos and controversies it had to overcome to reach those for whom it catered.

Reports from the North Kensington Women's Welfare Centre indicate that it was often very difficult for women to even take the first step to visit the clinic. When the clinic first opened very few women initially came, because many were too shy to attend. As one woman admitted to an abortion survey carried out on the clinic premises in 1937, 'I was shy at asking about birth control – I didn't think it was quite nice.'[37] Similarly another woman confessed, 'I had heard of the birth control clinic, but didn't like to talk about things like that.'[38] Some were able to get over their embarrassment by attending the clinic in the evenings when they could slip in and out unnoticed.[39] For a number of women the possibility of a medical examination was frightening. One Catholic woman, for instance, who had been brought up in a convent, could not bear to think of her inside, or to be touched.[40] Similarly another Catholic woman was horrified by the idea that she would have to undress.[41]

Sensitive to these issues, those running the centre were eager not to increase the discomfort of their clients by pressing on them too many questions. As they emphasized, 'Anyone who has worked at a Hospital or Welfare Centre realises that there is a certain proportion of women who are particularly sensitive, and the same applies of course to the patients at a birth-control clinic. Our experience is that in the majority of cases the information required is readily given...'[42] The centre also made a point of ensuring that all women were examined by a woman doctor both for issuing contraceptive devices and gynaecological treatment. All consultations were conducted in strict privacy and confidentiality was maintained.[43] According to the sociologist Norman Himes and his wife Vera, who undertook a detailed survey of the workings of the centre in 1929, all women examined by the doctor for contraception received 'as much time and skill and patience as if they were private patients'.[44] In this way the centre fulfilled many of the demands listed above of the women surveyed by the Women's Section of the Labour Party in 1934.

Every care was also taken by the North Kensington Women's Welfare Centre to help the women to find a contraceptive device that was most appropriate for them and easy to use. Each woman was given instruction by a nurse in how to use the device and presented with a printed card of instructions. They were expected to make a return visit for a check-up one week later and then to return again in six months. Those who did not return were traced by the centre. Such follow-ups were aimed at seeing whether the woman was still following the instructions correctly as well as to see whether they were satisfied with the help they had received.[45]

From the evidence available it would seem that the efforts the clinic made to win the approval of women met with a high degree of success. As one 32-year-old woman who had three children and was married to a builder's labourer wrote to the centre,

> My hubby is so pleased that he is helping me (to pay), and it has made such a lot of difference to us. I have proved it is all right, and I have told several friends about it. I don't know if any have been; I expect they are like I was at first – rather shy.[46]

The initial visit of this woman had been spurred on by the delicate health of her youngest child as well as her own poor health which her doctor had warned would make further pregnancies dangerous. The satisfaction with the clinic was also apparent in the letter of another woman, who had been married to an operative in a tobacco factory for nine years and had three children. She stated,

> I and my husband are delighted with the appliance I purchased from you and we have the greatest confidence in it. We think it is such a boon to poor mothers who cannot really afford large families... I

cannot say enough of the courtesy and kindness shown to me at your Clinics I am sure I shall never be afraid to visit you again.[47] The approval of mothers was not confined to letters of gratitude, but can also be seen in the attendance figures. Within the first nine months of opening, the clinic received 250 women and 196 had returned for a second visit. Such attendance was much higher than other comparable clinics.[48] By the second year the attendance numbers had doubled (Table 8.4). The popularity of the clinic was not only measured by the number of patients attending, but also by the high number of women who came as a result of the recommendation of old patients. Table 8.5 shows that by 1929 over 51 per cent of the patients who had come to the clinic came as a result of their contact with old patients. This was much higher than those referred by doctors from an infant welfare centre or those who had heard about the clinic through a meeting.

Table 8.4: Number of patients and their attendance at the NKWWC, 1924–39

Date	Birth-control Patients			Gynaecological Patients		
	Number	Attendance	Average visit per patient	Number	Attendance	Average visit per patient
Nov. 1924	255	–	–	–	–	–
July 1925–6	403	–	–	–	–	–
1926–7	432	–	–	–	–	–
1927–8	351	–	–	–	–	–
1928–9	372	–	–	–	–	–
1929–30	546	–	–	–	–	–
1930–1	653	–	–	–	–	–
1931–2	722	–	–	–	–	–
1932–3	915	–	–	–	98•	–
1933–4	1,082	–	–	–	–	–
1934–5	1,184	4,102	3.5	–	659	–
1935–6	1,134	4,532	3.9	388	880	2.3
1937	1,235	5,510	4.5	496	1,274	2.6
1938	1,383	6,154	4.4	587	1,750	3.0
1939	1,352	6,727	4.9	638	1,925	3.0

• Figures refer only to a six month period.
All the numbers refer to women listed as new patients.

Sources: NKWWC, *A/R* (1924–39), (CMAC, Box NK 206).

Table 8.5: Means by which new birth-control patients heard of the NKWWC, 1926–34

		1926–7	1927–8	1928–9	1929–30	1934*
	Total Patients	432	351	372	546	1,000
	Contacts through:					
Lay Sources:	Old patients and friends	151	173	185	277	535
	% of total patients	40	49	50	51	54
	Meetings/Canvassing	92	44	12	38	–
	% of total patients	21	13	3	7	–
	Books & other publicity	–	–	–	–	108
	% of total patients	–	–	–	–	11
	Total by Lay Sources	243	217	197	315	643
	% of total patients	56	62	53	58	64
Medical/	MCW Centres	74	79	85	139	129
Professional	% of total patients	17	23	23	25	–
Sources:	Private doctors	–	–	–	–	182
	% of total patients	–	–	–	–	–
	Hospitals	–	–	–	–	28
	% of total patients	–	–	–	–	–
	Health Visitors & Nurses	–	–	–	–	18
	% of total patients	–	–	–	–	–
	NKWWC Committee Member/Social Worker	–	–	–	57	–
	% of total patients	–	–	–	10	–
	Total of Medical & Professional sources	74	79	85	196	387
	% of total patients	17	23	23	36	39

* All figures for 1934 relate to a survey of 1,000 cases visiting the clinic.

Sources: NKWWC, *A/Rs* (1926–30); 'Survey of Cases Attending the Centre during 1934, 1,000 cases', 3 (CMAC file: NK 93, Box 641).

Such evidence not only confirms that the centre was popular, but that it was successfully fulfilling an acknowledged need. Many women were desperate both to learn how to limit their families and to have access to cheap and effective gynaecological care.[49] An overwhelming proportion of women who came to the centre for birth control were doing so for economic reasons as well as medical ones. In a survey carried out of 1,000 cases in 1934, 43 per cent were coming to the centre for economic reasons, while 24 per cent were coming for medical help.[50] Many of the women who came to the centre already had a small family, the average number of pregnancies each woman having had before attending being 3.9 in 1929 and 2.4

in 1934. On average these women had been married at least six years before seeking contraceptive measures.[51] Most of these women sought advice from the clinic either because they wanted a rest between births or because they wanted to limit the size of their families so they could give their children a better chance than they had had themselves.[52]

Table 8.6: Social grade of 1,000 birth-control patients attending NKWWC, 1934

| | Attending | | Lapsed |
	No.	%	% of total
Grade I (professional)	47	4.7	•
Grade II (clerks, travellers, etc.)	120	12	•
Grade III (policemen, busmen, postmen, shop assistants)	326	32.6	27
Grade IV (carmen, lorry drivers, porters)	299	29.9	31
Grade V (general labourers, odd jobbers & unemployable)	208	20.8	27

• Percentages not given, but Grade I and II were the least represented among the lapsed patients.

Sources: 'Survey of Cases Attending the Centre during 1934, 1,000 cases', 2–3, (CMAC file: NK 93, Box 641).

Table 8.7: Income per week of birth-control patients attending NKWWC, 1934

Income	Number
Between 17s. 7d. and £1 17s. 6d.	65
Between £1 17s. 7d. and £2 17s. 6d.	313
Between £2 17s. 7d. and £3 17s. 6d.	269
Between £3 17s. 7d. and £4 17s. 6d.	117
Between £4 17s. 6d. and over £5 2s. 7d.	42
Unemployed	76
No income given (including some unemployed)	40
Total	922

Sources: 'Survey of Cases Attending the Centre during 1934, 1,000 cases', 2–3 (CMAC file: NK 93, Box 641).

The importance of economic reasons was confirmed by the fact that the clinic tended to be visited most by those who were in social grade III or below (see Table 8.6). Table 8.7 also shows that the majority of women attending had an income of between £1 17s. 7d. and £2 17s. 6d. The high number of these patients partly reflects the priority of the clinic to help provide contraception for patients who could not otherwise afford to pay for such devices. Organizers of the clinic were very clear that they should not be catering for women who could purchase the help of a private clinic or doctor.[53] However, while it seems that the centre was able to reach a very high proportion of the women it targeted, it continually struggled to attract women on the lowest incomes. As was highlighted in an *Annual Report* for 1927–8, 'the very poorest type of woman' was 'slow in attending this clinic, just as she is in taking her children to the Welfare Centre. She is still liable to rely on muddling through in the belief that she may not become pregnant, or on attempts at abortion when pregnancy is an established fact.'[54]

The success of the centre cannot be measured only by the numbers it attracted, but by the degree to which women returned for their second visit and had absorbed the advice they had been given. Vera and Norman Himes found in 1929 that of the 855 patients who were fitted with a contraceptive appliance, 76.5 per cent returned for a second visit and of these 513 or 78.5 per cent showed that they successfully learned how to use the device they had been given. While it was difficult to determine the outcome in 3.2 per cent of the cases, those who needed to be retaught the method constituted 18.3 per cent. From this they concluded that the patients 'for the most part' were 'co-operative, quick to learn and easy to teach'. Nor was the success of the instruction short-lived. From a follow-up survey carried out of 365 cases, 72 per cent were found to still be carrying out the advice they had been given six months to two months earlier. Only 28 per cent were found to have problems.[55]

Much depended on the original motivation that pushed the women to attend the centre in the first place. As one survey of lapsed patients in 1934 pointed out,

> It would seem that patients brought or recommended by their friends would have more inclinations to pursue the method, but that those who have been sent by doctors and welfare centres very probably come after considerable persuasion and are therefore less likely to *wish* to use the method prescribed.[56]

The decision to attend the North Kensington Women's Welfare Centre was not a matter which solely concerned the woman. Clearly the motivation women had to attend the Centre was dependent on the relationship they had with their husbands. This was highlighted by Dr Violet Russell when she emphasized the need for tact on the part of her staff. As she said, providing contraception was very different from other forms of care, such as dental treatment,

> since husband and wife are equally involved and yet one seldom has

the opportunity of speaking to more than one of them. Once the husband has refused his consent it seldom serves to discuss the matter further with the wife – quite often I have asked her permission to write to him and ask him to come for an interview with regard to his wife's health, but for married happiness I think better to take the line that the husband's decision be accepted. Many women have told me that the husbands prefer to deal with contraception themselves rather than leave it to their wives...[57]

In addition to the importance of the husband, there were the wider kinship and family influences.

The success of the North Kensington Women's Welfare Centre was not only based on the fact that the centre provided a service mothers could not find elsewhere, but also the welcoming attitude of the staff. From material available it would seem that on occasion the personnel at the centre were judgemental about those they cared for, labelling those women who failed to return for visits as of 'low mentality' and irresponsible.[58] Despite this, the staff tended to understand the difficulties their patients experienced. Of those patients who failed to return for follow-ups virtually none listed the personnel as the reason for their reluctance to attend.[59] Similarly, the assistant medical officer of health in Kensington, Dr Violet Russell, reported that the only criticisms she had had of the centre had come from patients she had seen at the antenatal sessions who, while admitting 'their dislike of the birth control methods', had never let this prevent them 'from expressing their appreciation of the kindness of all the personnel attached to the centre'.[60]

Two of the most important factors listed by lapsed patients for their reluctance to reappear at the North Kensington Women's Welfare Centre was firstly their inability to learn the method they had been taught, and secondly the amount of money they owed the clinic. In both cases, the organizers of the clinic tried their utmost to get over these problems. In reviewing the difficulties some women experienced with certain contraceptive methods, such as the cap, organizers of the centre realized,

> that women, often flustered, very nervous, shy, entirely new to the idea of Birth Control and with no physiological knowledge, have to take in and *remember* a number of important instructions. Frequently they forget which way the cap should be inserted; what they should syringe with, and how, and other points.

For this reason the centre began to provide their clients with a simple card of instructions with diagrams.[61]

In attempting to alleviate the anxiety patients felt when they owed money to the centre, the organizers put up a notice in the waiting room 'to urge the point that patients must not worry if they owed money', and entreated dispensers to lay particular emphasis on this point.[62] Dr M. P. who worked occasionally at the centre in the 1930s remembered that where a poor mother could not afford to pay, the money was 'forked out for her'. She recalled that she had absolute powers of discretion, as she said, 'One could issue things free or you could reduce it, you could say pay a shilling now and pay another shilling in six months time, something like that.'[63]

Clearly the North Kensington Women's Welfare Centre went a long way in trying to understand the women's needs and to fulfil them. Their success is shown by the fact that many of the women who were investigated for follow-up work by Norman and Vera Himes in 1929 proved 'very friendly and gave whatever information they could'. As they stated, 'several people were particularly co-operative, invited the investigator into their homes and spoke of their experiences at length'.[64] The respect that women had for the centre was also shown in their implicit trust in the centre. As Dr M. P. highlighted, even when the contraceptive device failed, the women 'didn't come complaining that they had become pregnant in spite of it'. As she went on to say,

> Now this is rather interesting, people who become pregnant in spite of coming to the clinic would always admit that it was their fault they had forgotten to do what they ought to and they were always very contrite about it... I think they got a very strong sense of allegiance to the clinics that the method was alright and the Clinic can go on, the method was alright it was just I who failed. Yes, I think ... it was a real ... a sense of gratitude that they had been given this wonderful way of controlling birth and were grateful for it... Not that there was anyone to blame.[65]

In this respect, it would seem that many of the women who came to the North Kensington Women's Welfare Centre were so happy to have a means of limiting their families which previously had been denied to them that they were also more ready to accept failures. Indeed, for many women another pregnancy was almost accepted as a matter of course. Such attitudes, however, might also have been a reflection of the fact that many of these women were scared of being told off by the professionals, and also found it difficult to criticize those in authority.

Conclusion

As outlined in this chapter, the success of maternal and child welfare facilities in winning the approval of mothers was dependent on a wide variety of factors. A woman's enthusiasm to take up such services not only reflected the type of help provided, but also the distance she had to travel to reach the centre and the time she had to wait before being seen. In addition, she had to consider the expenses she had to cover in attending the centre and in purchasing the treatment they advised. Much also depended on the atmosphere of the institution she was expected to visit. This was determined by the physical environment in which the facility was housed as well as its social and emotional conditions. As illustrated above in the case of Woolwich, even in the most modern and accessible infant welfare centre a poor woman could be put off from attending because of the embarrassment she experienced in facing mothers who were better dressed and more obviously wealthy than she. It was important that a mother felt that the service was part of her world.

The degree to which women felt welcomed by an institution was greatly influenced by the attitude of those running the service. As we have seen this changed greatly in the period 1902 to 1936. While the prime focus of maternal and child welfare during these years remained on educating the mother, by the 1920s a new approach emerged which started to take women's opinions and interests much more seriously. This is not to argue that the patronizing attitude found among health visitors and other health experts at the beginning of the century had been totally eradicated, but some steps had been taken to understand and involve mothers in a way that had been previously denied. Such a shift in attitudes was not smooth, and was greatly dependent on the political complexion of an area, the attitudes of the professionals and volunteers running an institution and the nature of the services they provided, as well as the perceptions of the mothers themselves.

Clearly a woman's choice to attend a centre was based on a range of decisions which is difficult to understand in aggregate terms. The growing attendance figures for different services, however, indicate a growing acceptance and use of the provision made as well as a change in the attitudes of the staff and the treatment available. Part of this also reflected the overall changes that had occurred in the attitude towards the provision of services. Indeed, health and welfare services, so often seen as an individual responsibility in the nineteenth century had become a collective responsibility by the 1920s and one which was seen as having to take the needs and demands of mothers into account. Mothers and their infants were no longer seen as the passive receivers of health and welfare services.

Notes

1. A. J. Kearns, 'Active Citizenship and Urban Governance', *Instit. Br. Geog. Trans.*, New Ser. 17 (1992), 20–34, 22. See also G. B. Doern, 'The UK Citizen's Charter: Origins and Implementation in Three Agencies', *Policy and Politics*, 21/1 (1993), 17–29.

2. 'Protect the Nation's Mothers', Report by the Standing Joint Committee of Industrial Women's Organizations – Labour Party's Advisory Committee on Women's Questions, to the National Conference of Labour Women, Sheffield, May 1935 (CMAC Box 340, SA/FPA/ A.13/38–42). Such attitudes were not confined to the inter-war years, as can be seen from a survey of birth control services in the 1970s. See A. Cartwright, *Parents and Family Planning Services* (London: 1970), 114–18.

3. E. P. Peretz, 'Maternal and Child Welfare in England and Wales between the Wars: A Comparative Regional Study', unpub. Ph.D., Middlesex University, 1992, 107 and 110.

4. Woolwich MOH, *A/R* (1907), 89–90. Today mothers continue to resent the appearance of health visitors. See E. J. Allen, 'Child Health Care in the Inner City: Perceived Roles and Responsibilities', unpub. Ph.D. Queen Mary and Westfield College, London 1994.

5. Stepney MOH, *A/Rs* (1910), 42 and (1912), 54. See also Peretz, *op. cit.* (note 3), 140.

6. 'Kensington Public Health Survey', 1932.

7. Kensington MOH, *A/R* (1906), 65; Stepney MOH, *A/Rs* (1910), 42; (1912), 54; and (1914), 57.

8. *Ibid., A/Rs* (1910), 42 and (1912), 54.

9. *Ibid., A/R* (1914), 57.

10. Kensington MOH, *A/R* (1909), 9; Stepney MOH, *A/Rs* (1910), 41 and (1911), 52; and Woolwich MOH, *A/R* (1922), 67.

11. Woolwich MOH, *A/R* (1906), 92.

12. *Ibid.*, 89.

13. *Ibid.*

14. *Ibid.*, 102, and Kensington MOH, *A/R* (1909), 9.

15. Stepney MOH, *A/R* (1910), 41 and (1914), 60.

16. Kensington MOH, *A/Rs* (1909), 9, and (1906), 65. Similar remarks were made by a health visitor in Stepney, see Stepney MOH, *A/R* (1912), 57.

17. Woolwich MOH, *A/Rs* (1906), 92 and (1907), 89–90. See also (1925), 149.

18. *Ibid., A/R* (1921), 89.

19. Stepney MOH, *A/R* (1914), 59.

20. Compare the maps in the appendices with the maps in Figures 2.12 to 2.15.

21. Woolwich MOH, *A/R* (1910), 116–17, and (1928), 165–6.
22. 'Woolwich Public Health Survey: Maternal and Child Welfare Report', 1934, 4–5 (PRO file: MH66/404).
23. For more detailed information on the degree of overcrowding in each area see Ch. 2.
24. See Ch. 2.
25. Stepney MOH, *A/R* (1914), 59.
26. Discussed in Ch. 7.
27. J. Lewis, *The Politics of Motherhood: Infant and Maternal Welfare Services* (London: 1980), 105.
28. *The Labour Woman,* 1/8, December 1913, 139.
29. Kensington Council Minutes, 7 February 1922, 135. See also 'Kensington Public Health Survey', 1935, (PRO file: MH 52/177).
30. *The Labour Woman,* 1/8, December 1913, 139. See also Ch. 2.
31. Kensington MOH, *A/R* (1935), 26. Part of the change in the attitude and policy of those running the baby clinic probably stemmed from the council's increasing responsibility for maternal and child welfare services. By 1935 the council had taken over the organization and running of a couple of maternal and child welfare centres and had appointed two full-time medical officers to conduct infant consultation sessions in the place of the 14 part-time doctors. Such changes were more in line with Bentham's thinking.
32. *The Labour Woman,* 1/8, December 1913, 139.
33. Miss T. G. interviewed by L. Marks, 22 January 1988, transcript, 8; Mrs A., interviewed by L. Marks, 8 June 1992, transcript, 9–10. See also 'Protect the Nation's Mothers' (note 2).
34. 'Notes on Visit to the Baby Hospital', 18 November 1931, 2 in 'Kensington Public Health Survey', 1935.
35. *The Labour Woman,* 1/8, December 1913, 139.
36. Woolwich MOH, *A/R* (1928), 165–6.
37. Dr Fenton's forms, Box 171, case no. 365. These forms are kept with the questionnaires from the abortion survey noted in Ch. 1 filed under SA/NBTF/S.93. See also NKWWC leaflet asking for money 1935 (KLHL file 362 Nor K62/717). Similar reticence was observed among the women attending the Marie Stopes clinic. See D. A. Cohen, 'Private Lives in Public Places: Marie Stopes, The Mothers' Clinics and the Practice of Contraception', *Hist. Workshop J.,* 35 (1993), 95–116, 103–4.
38. Dr Fenton's forms, Box 171, case no. 382.
39. NKWWC, *A/R* (1924–5), 2.
40. Dr Fenton's forms, Box 171, case no. 185.
41. *Ibid.,* case no. 426.
42. NKWWC, A/R (1927–8), 4–5; N. and V. Himes, 'A Study of the First Thousand Cases to Visit an English Birth Control Clinic', unpub. MSS. *c.*1929, 9, (Francis A. Countway Library, N. Himes Collection BMS C77 [Box 83 fo. 883]).

43. NKWWC leaflet asking for money, (KLHL file 362. Nor K62/717); NKWWC, Executive Committee Minutes, 2 July 1936, 51.

44. Himes, *op. cit.* (note 42), 8.

45. *Ibid.*, 'Notes on Method at the North Kensington Clinic', 2 (CMAC file: NK 93, Box 641).

46. NKWWC, *A/R* (1929–30), 3–4.

47. NKWWC, *A/R* (1929–30), 4.

48. Himes, *op. cit.* (note 42), 8.

49. See Ch. 1.

50. 12% of the women coming to the centre were doing so to space their families, and 11% because they already had enough children, while 7% were wanting to wait before having children. The remaining percentage came for miscellaneous reasons, including disease in the family, being too old for children and disliking children. 'Survey of Cases Attending the Centre during 1934, 1,000 cases', 3 (CMAC file: NK 93, Box 641).

51. *Ibid.*

52. NKWWC, *A/R* (1927–8), 2–3.

53. Letter from M. Spring Rice to Dr A. Wright, 13 June 1935 (CMAC file: NK 160); NKWWC, A/R (1928–9), 2; and Letter from M. Spring Rice to Dr J. Fenton 12 December 1938 (CMAC file: SR/NK 87, Box 640).

54. NKWWC, A/R (1927–8), 2–3; 'Survey of Cases Attending the Centre during 1934' (note 34). The difficulty of attracting women on the lowest income is a problem which continues to plague women's welfare clinics today. See M. Pearson, S. Spencer and M. McKenna, 'Patterns of Uptake and Problems Presented at Well Woman Clinics in Liverpool', *J. Public Health Med.* 13/1 (1991), 42–7.

55. N. E. Himes and V. C. Himes, 'An Analysis of the First Thousand Cases at the North Kensington Working Women's Clinic and A Special Study of the Effectiveness of the Clinic's Work by Means of Patients' Follow-Up Visits and an Investigator's Home Visits', 5–6 in NK 91 (Box 640). The success of the teaching of the techniques appears to have been higher in the NKWWC than for other birth control clinics. For a discussion of this see Cohen, *op. cit.* (note 37), 108–9.

56. 'Survey of Cases Attending the Centres during 1934' (note 50), 4.

57. It was for this reason that Dr Russell argued that the centre should provide a male doctor, whom she claimed would convince husbands of the utility of contraception. Such a measure could be seen as comparable to Dr Fenton's talks to fathers in infant welfare centres. (Letter from Dr Violet Russell to Margery Spring Rice, 15 March 1939, in CMAC NK 87, Box 640).

58. 'Notes on Method at the North Kensington Clinic', 2 (CMAC file: NK 93, Box 641); 'Survey of Cases Attending the Centre during 1934' (note 50), 4.

59. 'Survey of Cases Attending the Centre during 1934' (note 50), 4.

60. Letter from Dr Violet Russell to M. Spring Rice, 29 November 1938 (CMAC file: SR/NK 87, Box 640).
61. 'Notes on Method at the North Kensington Clinic' (note 58), 2.
62. Clinic Sub-Committee Minutes, 28 January 1935, 22 (CMAC file: SA/FPA/NK 213, Box 656). Cohen has noted that at the Marie Stopes clinics the midwives were often keen to enforce payment from their mothers which they saw as a form of a contract in which patients were demonstrating that they appreciated the help they were being given and that the services they provided were given in a 'respectable' manner. Marie Stopes objected to this attitude but nonetheless in a number of instances women were turned away when found they could not pay. Cohen, *op. cit.* (note 37), 108. Such a conflict between the organizers and the staff was not apparent at the NKWWC.
63. Dr M. P., interviewed by L. Marks, 23 November 1992, transcript, 12.
64. Letter from M. Spring Rice to Dr A. Wright, 13 June 1935 (CMAC file NK 160), NKWWC, A/R (1928–9), 2; and Letter from M. Spring Rice to Dr J. Fenton, 12 December 1938 (CMAC file: SR/NK 87, Box 640).
65. Dr M. P., interviewed by L. Marks, transcript, 19; see also Dr Fenton's forms Box 171, case no. 192.

Epilogue

From the preceding chapters we can see that the early twentieth century was a time of expansion in maternal and child welfare services. These years not only witnessed an increase in the types of facilities available to mothers and their children, but also in their accessibility. As *Metropolitan Maternity* has shown, however, the provision of services was far from comprehensive. Much depended on the geographical area in which a mother and her child lived as to the service they would receive. London mothers and children tended to be better served than those in provincial cities or rural areas. Yet even in London some areas were better served than others. From this survey of four boroughs, it is clear that the quantity and quality of maternal and child services was dependent on a range of factors besides central government policy: including the social and political character of a locality and the resources available for funding such provision. Of the four boroughs examined, municipal maternal and child welfare provision tended to be most extensive in the poorer boroughs of Woolwich and Stepney which had strong Labour borough councils, in contrast to the richer boroughs of Hampstead and Kensington, where provision was more limited and viewed as an individual rather than a municipal responsibility, reflecting these boroughs' more conservative political and social character.

The boroughs not only differed in the degree to which they utilized municipal or voluntary resources for funding and organizing services, but also in the types of services they offered. Stepney and Woolwich provided many more health visitors and infant welfare centres and provided for a much larger proportion of their population aged under five years than Kensington or Hampstead. Such differences in provision had an important impact on the health standards of infants in each of the boroughs. Although the overall rate of infant mortality declined in all four boroughs in the years between 1900 and the late 1930s, the most drastic reduction occurred in Stepney, where the fall in infant mortality is especially noticeable given the very poor socio-economic conditions in the area, and when compared to Kensington where infant mortality remained static until the Second World War. Stepney also compares favourably with Hampstead in this respect.

Stepney's reduction in infant mortality might indicate an improvement in living and economic conditions within the borough during the early twentieth century, but it also reflected the local borough council's strong commitment to infant welfare services. The importance of such services in helping to reduce infant mortality is borne out by the evidence from Woolwich and Hampstead, which at the turn of the century had equally low rates of infant mortality within London. By the 1930s Woolwich had a greater number of municipal infant health services and greater coverage for its population, and had experienced a much greater reduction in its mortality rates than Hampstead. None the less, while infant health standards seem to have improved most in the poorer boroughs which gave greater priority to maternal and child welfare services, the presence of these services was not necessarily a guarantee of better health. In North Kensington, for instance, infant mortality remained very high despite numerous measures to curb the problem. Desperate social and economic deprivation in the area diminished any value children gained from such services.

While the success of medical and welfare services depended greatly on the social and economic circumstances in which an infant was born and reared, the success of maternity services was much less dependent on these factors. Part of the difference lay in the different determinants of maternal and infant mortality. As we have seen, while an infant's survival depended on good social and economic conditions, a mother's was determined more by the quality of her obstetric care. The remarkably low rates of maternal mortality in the poverty-stricken area of Stepney testify to this fact. Stepney not only had the lowest rate of mortality within London, and nationally, but was the only London borough to experience any significant reduction in maternal mortality between 1900 and 1936.

The low rate of maternal mortality in Stepney can partly be explained by the very good charitable midwifery and obstetric care available within the borough. Various voluntary teaching and municipal hospitals offered mothers a high quality of domestic and institutional obstetric care. The low maternal mortality is particularly interesting given that by the late 1920s Stepney had an unusually high number of hospital births. Strict adherence to antisepsis and minimal medical intervention was the key to the successful hospital births within Stepney. Overall the risk of infection was much greater in hospital than at home. Medical students and midwife pupils attached to the hospitals were also under strict supervision whether attending deliveries at home or in the hospital.

Contrary to received wisdom, richer mothers in Hampstead faced a much greater risk of dying than the poor mothers in Stepney. Mothers in Hampstead were much more likely to hire a general practitioner to attend their delivery than in many other parts of London. Yet, the general practitioner faced far less regulation and supervision than midwives or hospital-based doctors, and was often less rigorous in practising antisepsis and more likely to intervene unnecessarily. Unlike Stepney, Hampstead did not experience any significant reduction in maternal mortality during the early twentieth century.

This study has not only exposed the complex relationship between socio-economic conditions, medical provision, and health standards among mothers and children, but also the complexities which underlay the success of services in terms of access. As we have seen the numbers of mothers and children attending maternal and child welfare clinics increased greatly in the early twentieth century. Part of this growth in attendance stemmed from the real need among mothers and children for medical advice and care prior to the National Health Service, and their exclusion from national insurance. It also, however, reflected a shift in attitude in health and the entitlement to good health care. Growing concern for the nation's future economic and military capacity made the health of mothers and their children a national preoccupation in the early twentieth century. Increasingly, politicians, social reformers and medical practitioners realised that the health of its future soldiers and workers relied on state sponsorship of health services and could no longer be seen as merely an individual's responsibility. Good state health care services for all citizens was increasingly linked to the survival of the nation as a whole: raising health standards among the population, and enabling individuals to realize their full potential as citizens, particularly as soldiers and workers.

Such a vision contrasts with that espoused by the Conservative government today, which although inspired by similar concerns about Britain's international economic and military reputation, regards too much state involvement in health services as economically unsound and liable to encourage a 'culture of dependency'. Part of this shift in vision might be attributed to the different political economy now in existence. The emergence of a highly technical society and the growing use of computers both in the work-place and for warfare have increasingly reduced the need for healthy workers and soldiers, which is evidenced by the mass casting off of workers from industry and the defence force in recent years.

The current economic recession and the growing numbers becoming reliant on state aid in the last decade has also intensified the questions concerning state welfare provision and its efficiency and the ability of the nation to shoulder such expenditure.[1] In 1992–3 the British Government's direct funding of the main welfare services (education, health, housing, personal social services and social security) came to £160 billion, amounting to almost two-thirds of all government funding and over a quarter of national income (GNP).[2] Soaring costs in medical technology and the growing proportion of elderly people within the population has made the question of state financed health care and welfare particularly acute. The government's dilemma appears to focus upon whether state health services should be provided on a comprehensive basis for all citizens or whether such services should serve merely as a safety net for those who cannot afford to purchase private forms of care. Clearly the degree to which the state should take responsibility for the health of its citizens and how this responsibility is viewed in terms of its economic and military stability and future differs over time, and must be understood within particular historical contexts. Calls for greater state involvement in the provision of health care at the turn of the century were made at a time when there was no real state provision of health and welfare services and standards of public health were much lower than today.

The early twentieth century saw not only a significant expansion in maternal and child welfare services, but also an increasing willingness to heed the voice of those they were intended to serve. The Kensington Baby Clinic, the Fathers' Council and the North Kensington Women's Welfare Centre, for instance, who encouraged the active participation of mothers and fathers in the running of services during the 1920s and 1930s, reflected a very different approach from the more patronising one apparent among health visitors and other infant welfare staff earlier in the century. This shift in attitude reflected an increasing realization that the success of maternal and infant welfare rested not only on education, but on the cooperation and response of mothers and fathers, which could be achieved only by listening more to parents and providing what they needed.

Not all institutions were so democratic and open in the 1920s. Nevertheless, the approach taken by the three institutions mentioned above is particularly interesting in the light of debates over the accountability and openness of health services today. While completing this book I became keen to examine what had happened to the boroughs I had studied for the early twentieth century. Much to my surprise I discovered that this was a much more difficult task than I had anticipated. I soon realized that it was far easier to do research on maternal and infant health services in the 1920s and 1930s than it is today.

Some of the institutions I studied in the book have remained, notably the North Kensington Women's Welfare Centre (now called the Raymede Clinic). Indeed, this centre has continued to have an interesting history, having helped initiate the Birth Control Investigation Committee in 1926 and coordinated trials of various contraceptives, the Centre became a major part of the Family Planning Association in 1939, and by the 1960s was carrying out some of the early trials on the oral contraceptive pill. The Lancaster Road infant welfare clinic in Kensington continued well into the 1960s to provide infant welfare services. Today, however, it is an institution catering for the mentally ill. The East End Maternity Home in Stepney, once a leader in obstetric care, has become Steel's Lane Clinic, renowned for its links with radical general practice, particularly when David Widgery was alive. Other institutions, however, such as the British Hospital for Mothers and Babies have been closed and totally disappeared.

Such changes in institutions are not that surprising, but what I found worrying was the difficulty of assessing the types of maternal and child welfare services presently being provided in each borough. In all cases the health reforms of recent years and the many changes in the boundaries of health authorities make research on this subject almost impossible.[3] The health authorities governing Kensington and Woolwich, for example, have changed their boundaries more than twice in the last three years and are presently facing upheaval again. The confusion this has caused is reflected in the difficulty of obtaining a directory of the maternal and child welfare services provided in each area. Some of the material I received had extremely glossy photographs with smiling nurses and patients, arguing that the health authorities and trusts were promoting better health care within their particular areas, but this publicity included no factual information on what services were actually being provided, or their impact on health.[4] Uniform data which can be used as a basis for comparing services in particular areas and across time are also difficult to find. When viewed in relation to the documents from the early twentieth century, such a dearth of information is particularly disturbing. Annual reports from medical officers of health in the 1920s and 1930s, for instance, often provided a directory of all the maternal and child-health services in the borough, and a detailed summary of what was occurring to standards of health among their population. Kensington Medical Officer of Health reports were particularly good in this respect.

In carrying out the work for today's services, I soon realised the lack of accountability of health authorities to the local community they served. The contrast with the past is palpable: while supported by central government finance, most maternal and child welfare services in the 1930s were under the auspices of the local borough council which was responsible to a local electorate. Residents within particular boroughs had some say over how their services were run. In 1948 many of the health services within Britain were centralized under the National Health Service, making them subject to central, rather than local, control. Maternal and child welfare services remained under the jurisdiction of local authorities until the 1974 National Health Service reorganization, when they were handed over to central government. Local residents lost their voice in the planning and development of maternal and infant health services within their own area.

A more drastic erosion of accountability has recently occurred to health services as a result of the introduction of a competitive internal market within the National Health Service, which has blurred boundaries between the state and the private sector in the provision of services. Many of the services which were previously financed and run by the state are now being 'contracted out' to private bodies.[5] The creation of a market system within the National Health Service not only blurs the distinctions between private and public services and the values attached to each, but represents an even more fundamental revolution in the ways in which the public sector is controlled. The shift to a market economy has resulted in the break-up of national pay scales and a radical transformation of administrative relations. What we are witnessing, therefore, is a much more fragmented and mixed structure to the service.[6] One of the most important structural changes is the move towards a National Health Service based on compulsory insurance collected through taxation, with local health authorities acting as the insurance companies who themselves are the direct purchasers of health services from hospitals and general practitioners.[7]

Many of these changes have been introduced by the current Conservative Government on the grounds that they will enable services to be provided on a more competitive and efficient basis. In widening the scope for private enterprise the Government also claims to be extending the range of services available to patients and enhancing their powers of choice.[8] However, while this might have empowered a minority of the population, particularly those in the higher income brackets, it has done little for a large proportion of the population on lower incomes who have had their options limited rather than extended by the 'enterprise culture' now pervading the National Health Service.[9]

My experiences in trying to gather information on current maternal and child welfare provision and health standards in the four boroughs studied in this book, appears to bear out the argument that in farming out services to the private sector, the public sector is now less liable to be accountable for the services provided.[10] Health service workers are also increasingly facing censorship and are unable to reveal the problems they experience in the services they provide.[11] Such a trend away from accountability and from providing free information to the public, is particularly noticeable when we compare the current situation with that in the 1930s, when many institutions were improving and increasing the accessibility of their services so as to involve and help those they were intended to serve. The expansion of municipal maternal and child welfare services in the early twentieth century also stands in marked contrast to the contraction of state-funded health services today.

In comparing the past with the present, the degree to which poverty and deprivation continue to undermine health is evident. While infant mortality has fallen substantially since the 1930s, great disparities still exist between the social classes, with the poor suffering the worst mortality rates. In 1991, for instance, the infant mortality rate for social class I (professional) was 5.1 per 1,000 live births, while among social class V (unskilled) it was 8.2. Similar differences exist for the perinatal, neonatal and post-neonatal rates.[12] Interestingly, North Kensington, which was one of the most underprivileged areas in my study and had some of the highest rates of infant mortality, continues to manifest this trend today.[13] Stepney, which witnessed poverty equal to that in Kensington and had high infant mortality at the beginning of the century, is today seen as a black spot.[14] Sadly, Woolwich, which had very low rates of infant mortality in the early twentieth century now has a very poor record, reflecting the demographic changes in the area since the Second World War. Today unskilled, rather than skilled workers dominate the population and the area suffers high levels of unemployment.[15] While the national infant mortality rate has continued to drop since the Second World War, the rate of decline has begun to slow and Britain is now lagging behind other developed countries in this respect. Why this should be the case is the subject of much dispute, but some attribute it to the increasing deprivation and to a lowering of health care standards.[16]

Maternal mortality rates for England and Wales have fallen almost continuously from a peak of 440 per 100,000 total births in 1934 to a level ranging between 7 and 8 per 100,000 in the late 1980s. Since then they have remained static.[17] An enquiry into confidential maternal deaths in the United Kingdom for the years 1988 to 1990 revealed that nearly half of the deaths had occurred as a result of substandard care. It pointed out that many of these women had been cared for by junior doctors and that their deaths had resulted from difficulties resulting from inadequate staffing levels, inappropriate service provision and poor clinical standards.[18]

Fortunately only a small number of women die in childbirth today, but recent surveys in the Grampian region of Scotland, Reading and Birmingham have indicated that there is extensive morbidity among mothers in the first eight weeks after birth which is not being picked up by professionals. Some of the difficulties these women suffer include breast pain, bleeding problems, bowel irregularities, painful intercourse, backache, stress incontinence, urinary frequency, headaches, haemorrhoids, depression and extreme fatigue.[19] Sadly for those who have read the pages of this book, such complaints will be all too reminiscent of the suffering of many women a century ago. While much has changed in the provision of maternal and child welfare services since that time, motherhood continues to bring as many burdens as it brings joy.

Notes

1. Department of Social Security, *The Growth of Social Security* (London: 1993), 2. See also J. Hills, *The Future of Welfare: A Guide to the Debate* (London: 1993), 8–14; and J. Le Grand, 'Can We afford the Welfare State?', *Br. Med. J.*, 307 (23 October 1993), 1018–19.

2. When looked at over a long period this figure does not show a dramatic rise in expenditure. For more information on how such expenditure compares with earlier periods see Hills, *op. cit.* (note 1), 8–10.

3. The difficulties this is creating in assessing the quality of maternal and infant health services is explored in A. Macfarlane, *et al.*, *Counting the Changes in Childbirth: Trends and Gaps in National Statistics* (Oxford: 1995) and A. J. Macfarlane, 'Review and Assessment of Models of Care Using Research Information and Data: The Role of Routinely Collected Data', in G. Chamberlain and N.

Patel (eds), *The Future of Maternity Services* (London: 1994).

4. See for instance Parkside NHS Health Trust, *A/R* (1994).

5. Expenditure on private residential care for the elderly and the mentally ill, for instance, has risen from £10 million in 1979 to over £2.5 billion in 1993. This contrasts the stagnation of services provided by local authorities in these years. The number of elderly people in residential care provided by local authorities has fallen from 102,000 in 1979 to just over 100,000 in 1987. By comparison those cared for within private residential homes in the same period has increased from just under 23,000 to over 77,000. Thus, while the number cared for by local authorities has dropped by 2 per cent, those cared for by the private sector has increased by 234 per cent. The number of elderly cared for by voluntary charitable institutions has remained stationary at about 25,000. (M. Evandrou, J. Falkingham and H. Glennerster, 'The Personal Social Services: "Everyone's Poor Relation but Nobody's Baby"', in N. Barr *et al.* (eds), *The State of Welfare* (Oxford: 1990), 20–1; Labour Party, *Health 2000: The Health and Wealth of the Nation in the 21st Century* (London: 1994), 24.) The push towards private care is not only apparent in expenditure on community care services, but can be seen from the increase in private health insurance. Between 1973 and 1980 the proportion of health spending accounted for by private medical insurance varied between 2.6 and 3.1 per cent per annum. By 1989 the proportion had grown to 6 per cent. (D. K. Whynes, 'The Growth of UK Health Expenditure', *Social Policy Administration*, 26/4 (December 1992), 285–95, 293.)

6. Such fragmentation, however, has not led to decentralization of state power. Indeed, it could be said that, despite their rhetorical calls for greater decentralization, many of the reforms undertaken by the Government have enhanced the control of the central state and made it more coercive. For one critique of this see M. Hodge, *Quality, Equality, Democracy: Improving Public Services,* Fabian Pamphlet 549 (1991).

7. For an interesting analysis of the structural changes in the relationship between the state and welfare provision see *Marxism Today* (May 1991), especially R. Murray, 'The State After Henry', 22–7; M. Robbins, 'Breaking Up the Blocs', 30–3; and G. Mulgan, 'Power to the Public', 14–19.

8. Department of Health, *Caring for People: Community Care in the Next Decade and Beyond,* Cm. 849 (London: 1989). For a critique of this policy see D. Leat, *The Development of Community Care by the Independent Sector* (London: 1993).

9. A. Walker, 'Dependent Relativities', *Times Higher Education Supplement,* 22 April 1988.

10. The Conservative Government argues the reverse, stating that the private organizations are more accountable than the public sector. For

the controversies over accountability for services and its implications see J. Stewart, N. Lewis and D. Longley, 'Accountability to the Public', Paper presented to the European Policy Forum for British and European Market Studies Conference, December 1992.

11. See N. Craft, 'Secrecy in the NHS'; S. Sheard, 'Gagging Public Health Doctors'; and R. Smith, 'An Unfree NHS and Medical Press in an Unfree Society'. All three articles appeared under the title 'The Rise of Stalinism in the National Health Service', *Br. Med. J.,* 309 (17 December 1994), 1640–5.

12. OPCS, *Mortality Statistics: Perinatal and Infant: Social and Biological Factors. Review of the Registrar General on Deaths in England and Wales, 1991,* Series DH3 No. 25 (London: 1993); B. Botting and J. Cooper, 'Analysing Fertility and Infant Mortality by Mother's Social Class as Defined by Occupation – Part II', *Population Trends,* 74 (1993), 27–33 and Commentary in OPCS, *Mortality Statistics: Perinatal and Infant: Social and Biological Factors.* Series DH3, No. 24 (1992), xiii–xvii.

13. B. Botting and A. J. Macfarlane, 'Geographical Variation in Infant Mortality in Relation to Birth Weight 1983–85', in OPCS, *Mortality and Geography: A Review in the mid-1980s England and Wales,* Series DS9, (London: 1990), 48–56; and Kensington and Chelsea and Westminster Family Health Services Authority, *A/R* (1992).

14. Stepney is now considered part of Tower Hamlets, an area which has been the subject of much recent concern for its deprivation and high mortality. According to the Jarman index for deprivation Tower Hamlets has experienced a substantial rise in poverty over the past decade, which is also reflected in the very poor health standards in the area. The area also houses a large immigrant population, who are known to have poor health. See East London and the City, *Annual Public Health Report* (1994–5) and a series of reports in the *Evening Standard,* 9 January 1995 and 12 January 1995.

15. Information supplied by the Bexley and Greenwich Health Authority, January 1995.

16. House of Commons, Social Services Committee, *First Report, Perinatal, Neonatal and Infant Mortality* (London: 1988) and Department of Health, *Perinatal, Neonatal and Infant Mortality: Government Reply to the First Report from the Social Services Committee Session, 1988–89* (London: 1989).

17. Macfarlane *et al., op. cit.* (note 3), 19.

18. Department of Health, Welsh Office, Scottish Home and Health Department and Social Security, Northern Ireland, *Report of Confidential Enquiries into Maternal Deaths in the United Kingdom, 1988–90* (London: 1994).

19. Macfarlane *et al., op. cit.* (note 3), 21–2.

Appendix

Appendix 1: Map of various maternal and child health and welfare services in Hampstead, 1933

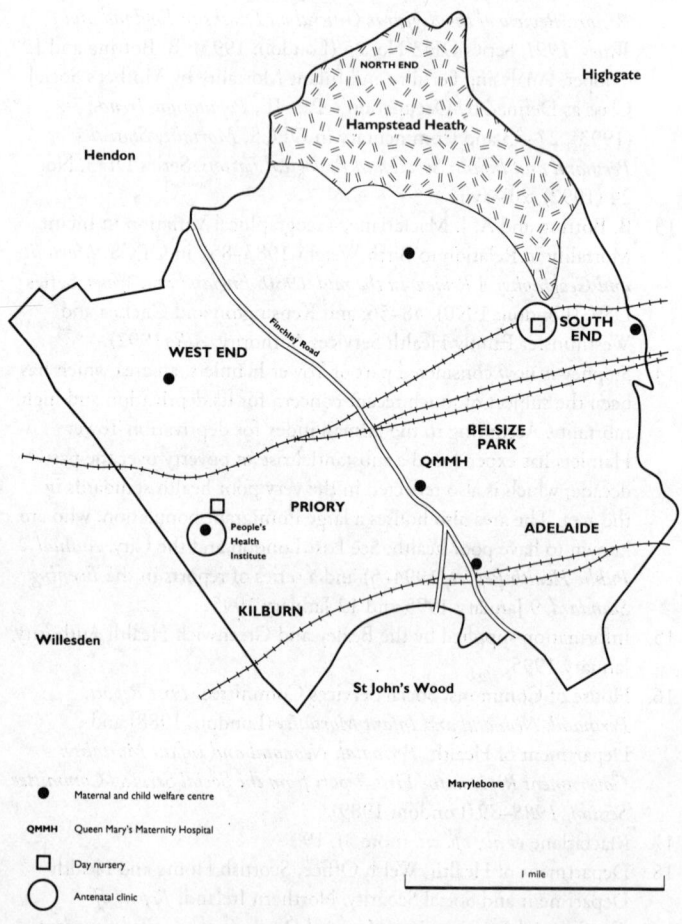

Sources: 'Hampstead Public Health Survey', 1933 (PRO file: MH 66/347); Hampstead MOH, *A/R* (1933).

Appendix 2: Map of various maternal and child health and welfare services in Kensington, 1920s and 1930s

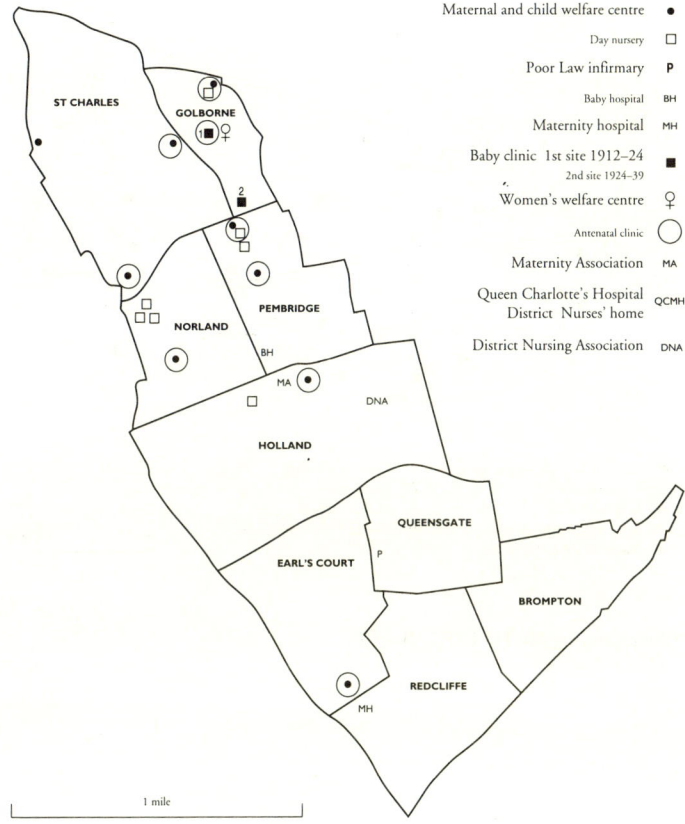

Maternal and child welfare centre	●
Day nursery	□
Poor Law infirmary	P
Baby hospital	BH
Maternity hospital	MH
Baby clinic 1st site 1912–24	■
2nd site 1924–39	
Women's welfare centre	♀
Antenatal clinic	◯
Maternity Association	MA
Queen Charlotte's Hospital District Nurses' home	QCMH
District Nursing Association	DNA

Sources: 'Kensington Public Health Survey', 1932 (PRO file: MH 66/359); Kensington MOH, *A/Rs* (1906–37).

Appendix

Appendix 3: Map of various maternal and child health and welfare services in Stepney, 1901–1930s

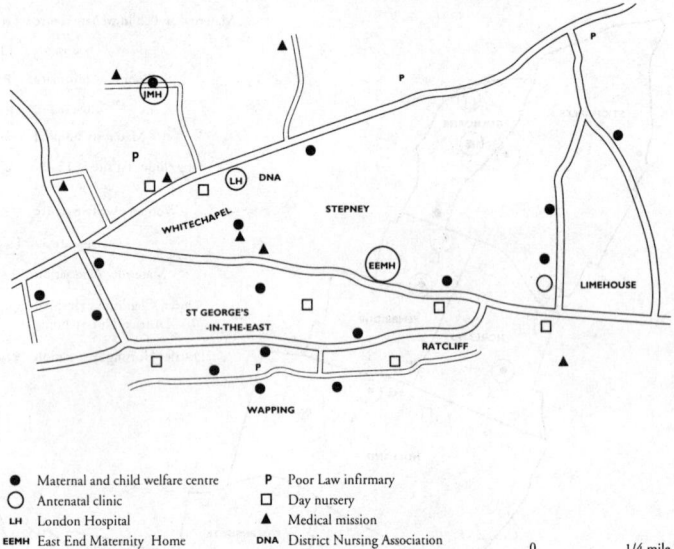

●	Maternal and child welfare centre	P	Poor Law infirmary
○	Antenatal clinic	□	Day nursery
LH	London Hospital	▲	Medical mission
EEMH	East End Maternity Home	DNA	District Nursing Association
JMH	Jewish Maternity Home		

0   1/4 mile

Source: Stepney MOH, *A/Rs* (1920–39).

Appendix 4: Map of various maternal and child health and welfare services in Woolwich, 1920–30s

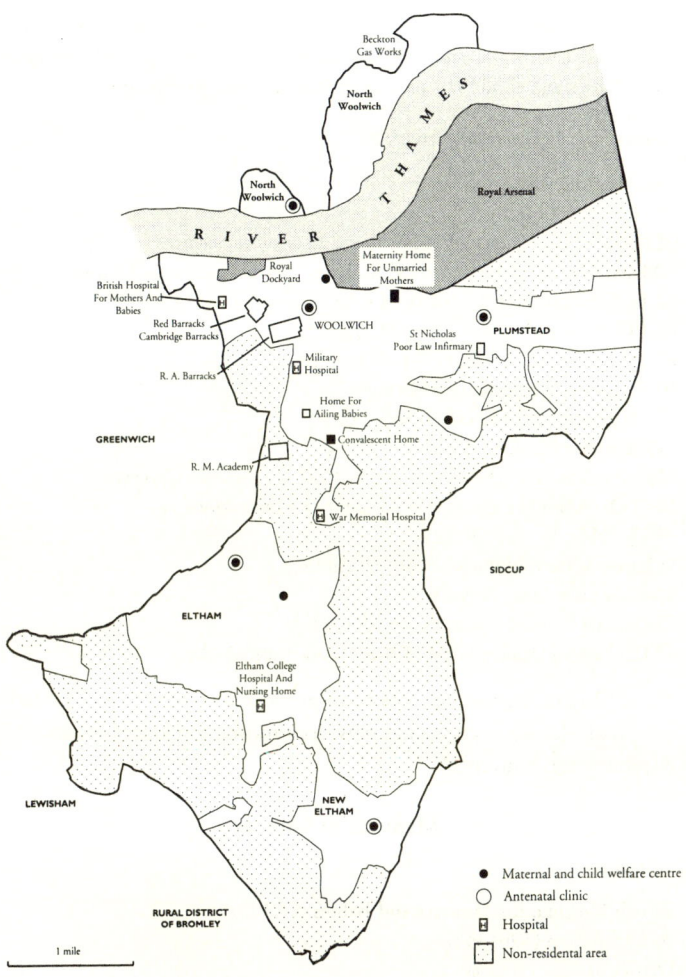

Source: Woolwich MOH, *A/Rs* (1920–30).

Bibliography

The works listed are restricted to those which have been mentioned in the text together with a selection of sources which provide a general history of the welfare state, childbirth and maternal and infant welfare services.

Abbreviations for certain archives:

AJA: Anglo Jewish Archives
BL: British Library
BLPES: British Library of Political and Economic Sciences
CMAC: Contemporary Medical Archives Centre, Wellcome Institute
GLH: Greenwich Local History Library
GLRO: Greater London Record Office
HLHL: Hampstead Local History Library
JWB: Jewish Welfare Board Archive
KLHL: Kensington Local History Library
LH: London Hospital Archive
Mocatta: Mocatta Library, University College, London University
NCVO: National Council for Voluntary Organizations
PRO: Public Record Office
St Barts: St Bartholomew's Hospital Archive
SA: Salvation Army Archive
SS: Sophia Smith Collection, Smith College
THL: Tower Hamlets Local History Library and Archive

Note: Most of the archival collection previously at the Mocatta Library and Anglo-Jewish Archives has now been moved to Parkes Library, Southampton University.

Manuscript Sources

Hospitals

British Hospital for Mothers and Babies (GLRO)
Annual Reports (1905–38)
Diaries of Alice Gregory
Executive Committee Minutes, 1906–10 (H14\BMB\A\1,2)
Miss Gregory's Letterbook (H10\BMB\10\1–10; H14\BMB\A10\1–10;
  H14\BMB\CTM\A1\1)

City of London Maternity Hospital (GLRO)
Annual Reports (1902–40)
Matron's Case Book, 1923–6; 1928–30; 1933–6; 1938–41
Outpatients Admission registers, 1902–35
District Case Books, 1915–35

East End Maternity Hospital (LH)
Annual Reports (1910–39)
Minutes, 1943 (S 591)
Maternity Registers, 1902–35

East London Hospital for Children and Dispensary for Women (LH)
Scrapbook, 1901–14

London Hospital (material at LH, unless otherwise stated)
Annual Reports (1902–39)
House Committee Minutes, 1917
Blue File Committee Minutes (LM/5/22) 1905, Circumcision (LM/5/27) 1906
Maternity Registers of the Medical Students, 1902–35
Marie Celeste Lying–In Wards:
In-patient Registers 1905–35
District Registers: 1905–35
Green and White Charities Registers – numbers 80, 81, 86
Holland, E., 'Report of the External Maternity District and on the Urgent Need of Reforming the Work of Students thereon', April 1919 (LH/A/17/35)
Morris E. W. (House Governor), 'Report of a Visit to the District Maternity Charity with Miss Nicholls, District Midwife', 19 December 1922. Also in *London Hospital Illustrated* (1933), 10–11
Marie Celeste Samaritan Society, *Annual Reports* (1937, 1938) (THL)

Princess Louise Kensington Hospital for Children (KLHL)
Annual Reports (1918–47)
'Brief History, 1840–1935' (KLHL file: K63/902)
Pamphlets and leaflets (KLHL file: KP797)

St Charles Hospital
Pamphlets (KLHL file: 362.11 St Cha/K4626/B)

Salvation Army Mothers Hospital (material at Salvation Army unless otherwise stated)
Admission Registers, 1915, 1925, 1935 (St Barts)
Annual reports (1911–47)
Medical Records, 1902–10
Medical reports, 1924–30 (St Barts)
Midwife case notes, 1929–42
District notes (from 1930s) – City and Hackney, some from Dagenham Management Council Minutes, 1914–23
Salvation Army Mothers' Hospital Minutes, 1914–22
Newspaper Clippings file on Salvation Army Mothers' Hospital

Queen Mary's Maternity Home (LH)
Administrative Records 1919–48 (QM/A/3,4)
Annual Reports (1920–39)
E. H. Benjafield's memories, 1985 (QM/A/7/15)
House Committee Minutes, 1937–9
London Hospital Illustrated 1950
Minute Books, 1919–28

Nursing Associations

East London Nursing Society (THL)
Minutes, 1902–39
Annual Reports (1880–1939)

Kensington District Nursing Association (KLHL)
Annual Reports (1928–39)

Mrs Ranyard's Nurses (GLRO)
Annual Reports (1898–1935)
The Nursing Branch of the Bible Women and Nurses, booklet for future nurses
([n.d.] file no. A/RNY)

St John the Divine Nursing Association (THL)
Annual Reports (1917–18), (1921–2)
St John the Divine's Nurses, 'The Community of Nursing Sisters of St John
the Divine', Centenary Pamphlet (1948)

Shoreditch and Bethnal Green District Nursing Association (THL)
Annual Reports (1927–39)

Other Welfare and Health Organizations

Hampstead (material at HLHL unless otherwise stated)
Hampstead Health Institute *Annual Reports* (1936 and 1939)
Hampstead Hostel for Mothers and Babies:
  Annual meetings and extraordinary meetings, Minutes 1938–9
  Annual Reports (1927, 1929–32, 1937–9)
  House Committee Minutes, 1922–3

Kensington (material at KLHL unless otherwise stated)
Archer Street Infant Welfare Centre, *Annual Reports* (1918–19, 1923–4,
  1924–9)
Bramley Road School for Mothers and Infant Welfare Centre, *Annual
  Reports* (1924–38) (file KP 118–130/class.362.71 bra)
Dalgrano Infant Welfare Centre, *Annual Reports* (1936–8) (file KP
  237–8/class 362.7)
Kenley Street Infant Welfare Centre, *Annual Reports* (1932–9) (file KP

411–18)
Kensington Baby Clinic, papers (National Museum of Labour, Manchester, file: BAB)
Kensington Women (Guardians) Committee Minutes, 1918–28 (GLRO file: K.B.G. 178)
North Kensington Marriage Welfare Centre (files K62/717 andK63/954/class 362.nor)
North Kensington Women's Welfare Centre, *Annual Reports* (1924–39) (CMAC, Fawcett Library and SS)
Clinical Reports and Executive Minutes and other papers among Family Planning Association collection, (CMAC files SA/FPA/NK/84–104, 157–60, 198–214, 224–36)
St Mary Abbots, *Kensington Annual Reports* (1901–39)

Stepney (material at THL unless otherwise stated)
Jewish Day Nursery, *Annual Reports* (1897–1943); Minutes, 1936 (material kept by Mrs C. Rantzen)
Jewish Infant Welfare Centre, *Annual Reports* (1934–5, 1938–9)
Jewish Mothers' Welcome and Infant Welfare Centre, *Annual Report* (1932–3)
Sick Room Helps Society and Jewish Maternity Hospital, *Annual Report* (1931) in Stepney Borough Council, 'Public Health Report', 1925–9 (PRO file: MH55/203–304) *Annual Report* (1936) *Annual Report* (1937) (Mocatta Library)
Newspaper Cutting of Queen Mary's Visit to the East End 1916 (THL file no. O71.1)
Stepney Association for Rescue and Protection Work amongst Children, *Annual Reports* (1933–4)
Stepney Infant Welfare Centre and Babies Nursing Home, *Annual Report* (1926–7)
The Voluntary Maternity and Child Welfare Centres of Bethnal Green, *Annual Report* (1918–19)

Woolwich (GLH)
Health pamphlets (box 614)

Medical Missions:
All Saints Medical Mission, Minutes, Correspondence, Papers and *Annual Reports* (1897–1921) (AJA)
Immanuel's Witness (Barbican Mission to the Jews) 49th *Annual Report* (1937–8), (GLRO file: A/FWA/C/D128/1)

Bibliography

Public Health Committees and Organizations

Hampstead Maternal and Child Welfare Sub-Committee Minutes, 1922–39
  (HLHL)
Kensington Council Minutes, 1900–39 (KLHL)
Kensington Maternity and Child Welfare Committee, 'Report of
  Applications Sub-Committee', 17 October 1933 (held by Jerry White)
Stepney Maternity and Child Welfare Committee Minutes, 1919–39
  (THL)
Woolwich Council Minutes, 1902–39 (GLH)

Medical Officer of Health, *Annual Reports*
  (HLHL, KLHL, THL, GLH and GLRO):
Hampstead (1902–39)
Kensington (1902–39)
Stepney (1902–38)
Woolwich (1902–39)

Charity Organization Society (GLRO)

Annual Reports (1913–39)
Charity files containing correspondence and reports
Council and District Committees, *Annual Reports* (1917–19)
Council Minutes, 1908–13
Correspondence Files
Kensington Philanthropy Society, correspondence and papers, 1902–38
Medical Advisory Committee Minutes, 1915–20
North Kensington COS Committee Minutes, 1922–7

Council for Social Welfare (material at NCVO unless otherwise stated)
Hampstead Council for Social Welfare:
Biannual Report of the Executive, 1921–2
Annual Report of the Executive Committee, 1925–6
Annual Reports included in COS *Annual Reports* (GLRO)
NCVO 1st file: A year's work of the HCSW, October 1932, Box 10
Kensington Council for Social Service:
  Annual Reports
  Finance and pensions sub-committee minutes in COS papers (GLRO)
  Woolwich Council for Social Service, 1938–40 (file 2)
  Draft *Annual Report,* 31 March 1939
  'Thirteen years of Progress: Woolwich Council of Social Service's
  increased Membership: Tributes to Mr C.H. Grinling's Pioneer Work.'

King's Fund Papers (GLRO):
Babies Hospital, Kensington, 1922
British Hospital for Mothers and Babies, 1898–1965

City of London Maternity Home, 1911–65
East End Maternity Home, 1908–67
Hampstead Children's Hospital (formerly Northcourt Hospital) 1910
Hampstead General Hospital, 1905–64
Jewish Maternity Hospital and Bearstead Memorial Hospital, 1925–68
London Hospital, 1897–1967
Princess Beatrice Hospital, 1902–65
Salvation Army Mother's Hospital, 1903–66

London County Council Papers (GLRO)
Files:
  Antenatal clinics in hospitals (LCC/Ph/Hosp)
  Domiciliary Midwifery Service (LCC/Ph/Phs/2)
  Birth Control Clinics (hospitals), 1931–6 (LCC/Ph/Hosp/1/27)
  LCC, Register of Lying-in Homes, 1916–28 (LCC/Ph/Reg/4/1–2)
  Maternity and Obstetrics MOH papers, 1914–66 (LCC/3/6–9)
  Maternity Clinics (LCC/Ph/Phs)
  History of LCC domiciliary midwives service (LCC/Ph/Phs/2/13)
  Midwives training, 1925 (LCC/Ph/Phs/2/8–10)
  Midwives Bill, general papers, 1902–6 (LCC/Ph/Phs/2/14)
  Ministry of Health, Advisory Committee on Nutrition, 1931–9
    (LCC/Ph/hsp/1/42)
  Nursing homes, general papers, 1936–64 (LCC/Ph/Reg/4–7)
  Nursing homes, registers, 1928–65 (LCC/Ph/Reg/4/4–6)
  Nutrition during pregnancy, 1935 (LCC/Ph/Hosp/2/27)
  Pregnancy, general papers, 1937–48 (LCC/Ph/Hosp/2/20–27)
  Puerperal fever, general papers, 1924–63 (LCC/Ph/Hosp/2/34–35, 67–71)
  St Mary Abbots Hospital, general papers, 1935–4 (LCC/Ph/Hosp /3/124–5)
  St Nicholas Hospital, general papers, 1934–48 (LCC/Ph/hosp/3/131–133)
  Abortion, 1931–8 (LCC/Ph/Gen/3/16)
Publications (GLRO library):
  'Report of the Chief Officer of Public Control as to Creches or Day
  Nurseries', No. 884 (file: 22.11 LCC)
  'Joint Survey of Medical and Surgical Services in the Administrative County
    of London: Part II: Municipal Hospital, Clinics and Dispensaries', 1933
    (file: 26.04 LCC)
  'Maternity Services of London: Report by the County MOH to the Hospitals
    and Medical Services Committee', 1934
  Metropolitan Borough Council Election, 'Returns', 1900–62 (file: 15.9 LCC)
  Social Welfare Committee Minutes, 1929–48 (LCC file: 20.58 LCC)
  'Statistics of Metropolitan Boroughs, 1929–30 (expenditure)' (31.6 LCC)
  Hogarth, M., 'A Survey of District Nursing in the Administrative County
    of London', 1931 (file: (P) 26.45 LCC)

Labour Party (GLH)
Labour Representative Association, *Annual Reports* (1903–39)
Minutes, 1903–31
Woolwich Labour Party, Minutes, 1910–20

National Birthday Trust Papers (CMAC)
Papers relating Central Midwives Joint Committee Investigation in Abortion
(file SA/NBT/S.9/3 Boxes 171–5)

Fenton, J. and V. Russell, 'Report of on Contraception an Abortion', a confidential report for the Royal Borough of Kensington, October 1937

Oxley, W. H. F., 'Notes on the Abortion Enquiry', n.d (file:SA/NBT/S2/1)

Society for the Provision of Birth Control Clinics (CMAC and SS)
Annual Reports, (1920–32)

Other Sources

British Library of Political and Social Science Archive
The New Survey of London, papers
Reprint of Speeches made at a public meeting made by Lord Buckmaster, 22
November 1929 in support of the work of the Kensington Housing Trust Ltd

Fawcett Library
Birth Control and Public Health with a preface by Julian S.Huxley (London:
1932)

National Union of Societies for Equal Citizenship, 'Reprint of Speeches
made by Lord Buckmaster in the House of Lords on April 28th 1926'
(File:(P) 363.960941)

*Report of the Conference on the Giving of Information on Birth Control by Public
Health Authorities* (1930) (File: 362.82)

Nuffield College, Oxford
Nuffield College Social Reconstruction Survey

Westminster Diocese Archive
Files:
  Abortion (Hi. 2/2 1935–37)
  Birth Control: Stopes v. Bourne *et al.* (Bo. 1/13 1931–32; Bo. 5/59; Hi. 2/16)
  Catholic Women's League (Bo.1/30 1906–12; Bo. 5/906; Hi.2/34)
  Catholic Nurses Guild (Hi. 2/95)
  Catholic Women's League (Bo. 1/30; Bo. 5/70 (b) 1924–31; Hi. 2/34)
  Hospitals (Bo. 1/63 1905–31; Hi 2/114–15; chaplains: Hi.2/116; statistics:
  Hi 2/190A)
  Marriage, Divorce and Birth Control (Bo. 1/12)

Bibliography

Personal Papers
Booth, Charles (BLPES files A24, A 32, A33, A38, B181, B209)
Fairfield, Leticia (GLRO files: PH/Gen/3/6–7; 11–12; 16)
Himes, Norman (Francis Countway Library of Medicine, Boston, Mass, collection BMS C77)
Salaman, Redcliffe: Scientific papers and personal papers; includes Memoirs 'The Helmsman Takes Charge' (Cambridge University Library)
Spring Rice, Margery (CMAC: Family Planning Association collection FPA/SR)

Government Papers (PRO):
MH48/164 'Report of the Infant Welfare in the Borough of Kensington', and 'Kensington Public Health Survey', 1932
MH48/166 Stepney MOH Report and Public Analyst, 1901–19
MH48/169 Woolwich Metropolitan Borough Council, Sanitary Inspectors, Reports and Correspondence
MH52/31 Local Government Act 1929, Maternity and Child Welfare Scheme for Payments to Voluntary Associations
MH52/55 Maternity Homes Byelaws
MH52/156–7 Bethnal Green Borough Council: Maternity and Child Welfare: Midwifery, 1924–31
MH52/177–179 'Kensington Public Health Survey', 1931
MH52/198a–b Shoreditch Borough Council: Model Welfare Centre, Birth Control Clinic
MH52/202–204 Stepney Borough Council: Maternity and Child Welfare: Home Helps and Maternity Helps, School for Mothers, Jewish Maternity Home, 1920–35
MH66/347–349 'Hampstead Public Health Survey', 1933
MH66/359–361 'Kensington Public Health Survey', 1932
MH66/381–384 'Shoreditch Public Health Survey', Appendices, Correspondence, 1930–3, MOH Report, 1937
MH66/391–393 'Stepney Public Health Survey', Appendices, Correspondence, 1932–4
MH66/404–406 'Woolwich Public Health Survey', 1934
MH66/1081 Public Health Surveys: Chelsea to Hackney, 1932–5
MH66/1083 Public Health Surveys: Lambeth to Shoreditch, 1931–5
MH79/346 Interdepartmental Committee on Milk Consumption, 30 January 1936
HO326/29 W. H. Oxley letter to Secretary of the Interdepartmental Committee on Abortion, 10 October 1937; H. Wright, Memorandum for the Interdepartmental Committee on Abortion (1938)

Bibliography

Oral Materials

Interview tapes and transcripts of L. Marks (deposited at the National Sound Archive)

Mrs A. 8 June 1992 (transcript)

Miss Mary B., 26 March 1992 (tape)

Miss M. B., 7 July 1987 (transcript)

Miss R. C. and Mr W. C., 21 April 1992 (tape)

Mrs E. C., 13 January 1988 (transcript)

Mrs M. H. and Miss B. S., 7 May 1992 (transcript)

Mrs H. and Mrs B., 4 September 1991 (transcript)

Mrs A. L., 15 October 1991 (transcript)

Mrs V. O. and Mr H. O., 14 May 1992 (transcript)

Dr M. P., 23 November 1992 (transcript)

Miss J. W. and Miss D. G, February 1992 (transcript)

Miss T. G., 22 January 1988 (transcript)

Sister P. and Sister T., 14 December 1987 (notes)

North Kensington Community History Group, 25 March 1992 (tape)

Interview transcripts of G. MacFarlane (deposited at the National Sound Archive)

Mrs A. A., 26 May 1992 (transcript)

Mrs P. O., 26 May 1992 (transcript)

Parliamentary Papers

Royal Commission on Alien Immigration, PP 1903, IX (Cd. 1741; Cd. 1742; Cd.1743) Report, Minutes of Evidence, Appendix

Report of the Interdepartmental Committee on Physical Deterioration, PP 1904, XXXII (Cd. 2175 and Cd.2210) Minutes of Evidence, Appendix.

Royal Commission on the Poor Law and Relief of Distress, PP 1909, Reports, Minutes of Evidence and Appendix. SP 1909 XXXVII (Cd.4499); XXXIX (Cd.4625), (Cd.4626), (Cd 4626); XL (Cd.4684); XLI (Cd.4835); XLII (Cd.4850); XLIII (Cd.4653), (Cd.4690); XLIV (Cd.4795), (Cd.4890), (Cd.4632); XLV (Cd.4631)

Bill to Secure Better Training of Midwives and to Regulate their Practice, PP 1900, III, (8) p. 507; (150), p. 517

Midwives Act Committee, PP 1909, XXXIII, (Cd.4822 and Cd.4823), Minutes of Evidence

Reports from Commissioners, Inspectors and Others on the Working of the Midwives Act:

Central Midwives Board, Reports, SP 1909 XXXIII (Cd.4507 and 4725); 1911, XXXV (Cd.5505); 1912–13, XL (Cd.6061); 1913, XXXIV (Cd.6755); 1914, XLI (Cd.7304) ; 1914–16, XXVII (Cd.7784); 1914–16, XXVII (Cd.8142); 1916, XIII (Cd.8408); 1919, XXV (Cd.17)

Bill to Make Further and Better Provision with Respect to Feeble-minded and other Mentally Defective Persons, PP 1912–13 (213) III, Pt II

Maternity and Child Welfare Act, PP 1918 (10) II p. 251

Local Government Board Annual Reports of Commissioners PP 1902–19
  1902, XXXV; 1903, XXIV; 1904, XXV; 1905, XXXI; 1906, XXXV;
  1907, XXVI; 1908, XXX; 1909, Pt. 1 XXVIII, Pt. 2 XXIX; 1910,
  XXXVIII; 1911, XXXI; 1912–13, XXXV; 1913, XXXI; 1914, XXXVIII;
  1915, XII p.511; 1916, XIII; 1917–18, XVI p.131; 1918, XI p.229;
  1919, XXIV p.379

Local Taxation Returns, in Parliamentary Papers (1902–36)

Newspapers and Periodicals

All the World (Salvation Army newspaper)
British Medical Journal.
Charity Organisation Review
Comrade: The Royal Arsenal Co-operative Society's Journal (GLH)
The Deliverer (Salvation Army newspaper)
East End News
East London Advertiser
East London Observer
Evening Standard
Hampstead Advertiser
Hampstead Citizen
Hampstead and Highgate Express
Jewish Chronicle
The Kensington News and West London Times
The Labour Woman
The Lancet
League of London Hospital Nurses Review, (THL and LH)
London Hospital Illustrated, (Newspaper put out by London Hospital),
  (THL and LH)
London School of Economics Magazine
Magazine of the Sacred Heart, (Parish Magazines of Saint Mary and Saint
  Michael Catholic Church, Commercial Road) (THL)
Manchester Guardian
The Medical Officer
North Kensington Citizen
Onward (Newspaper of the CLMH), (GLRO)
The Pioneer (GLH)
Progress
Public Health
Social Service Review (Newspaper of National Council of Social Service)
The Tablet
The Times
The War Cry (Salvation Army journal)
Woolwich Citizen

Occasional Official Papers and Printed Reports

Campbell, J., *Infant Mortality: International Inquiry of the Health Organisation of the League of Nations, English Section Report* (London: 1929)

Census for England and Wales (London: 1901;1911; 1921; 1931)

Department of Health, *Caring for People: Community Care in the Next Decade and Beyond*, Cm. 849 (London: 1989)

Department of Health, *Perinatal, Neonatal and Infant Mortality: Government Reply to the First Report from the Social Services Committee Session, 1988–89* (London: 1989)

Department of Health, Welsh Office, Scottish Home and Health Department and Social Security, Northern Ireland, *Report of Confidential Enquiries into Maternal Deaths in the United Kingdom, 1988–90* (London: 1994)

Department of Social Security, *The Gro.. .h of Social Security* (London: 1993)

House of Commons, Social Services Committee, *First Report, Perinatal, Neonatal and Infant Mortality* (London: 1988)

Interdepartmental Committee on Abortion, 'The Abortion Report', *Br. Med. J.*, (17 June 1939), 1248–51

Report of the Proceedings of the English-Speaking Conference on Infant Mortality (London: 1913)

Report of the Proceedings of a National Conference on Infant Mortality (London: 1919)

Report of the Proceedings of the Second English-Speaking Conference on Infant Welfare (London: 1921)

Report of the Proceedings of the Third English-Speaking Conference on Infant Welfare (London: 1924)

Report of the Proceedings of the Fourth English-Speaking Conference On Infant Welfare (London: 1926)

Maternal Mortality Committee, *Maternal Mortality Report;* (London: 1934)

Ministry of Health *42nd Annual Report on Infant and Child Mortality* (London: 1913)

Memorandum in Regard to Maternity Hospitals and Homes (London: 1920)

Final Report of Departmental Committee on Maternal Mortality and Morbidity (London: 1932)

Memorandum on Milk for Mothers and Children under 5 (July 1937)

Report of an Investigation into Maternal Mortality (1937)

Reports on Public Health and Medical Subjects, No. 25: Maternal Mortality by J. Campbell (London: 1924)

Reports on Public Health and Medical Subjects No. 68: High Maternal Mortality in Certain Areas by J. Campbell (London: 1932)

Bibliography

Report of the Inter-Departmental Committee on Abortion (London: 1939)

Maternal Mortality and Childbirth – Ante-Natal Clinics. Their Conduct and Scope, Memorandum 145, MCW 1929

London County Council, *London Statistics* (London: 1889–1939)

Registrar General, *Annual Reports of Births, Deaths and Marriages for England and Wales* (London: 1870–1939)

Registrar General, *Decennial Supplement of Births, Deaths and Marriages for England and Wales* (London: 1870–1939)

Registrar General, *Quarterly Returns of Births and Deaths for England and Wales* (London: 1880–1910)

OPCS, *Mortality Statistics: Perinatal and Infant: Social and Biological Factors. Review of the Registrar General on Deaths in England and Wales, 1991,* Series DH3, No. 25 (London: 1993)

OPCS, *Mortality Statistics: Perinatal and Infant: Social and Biological Factors, 1990,* Series DH3, No. 24 (1992)

Miscellaneous Reports

East London and the City, *Annual Public Health Report* (1994–5)

Kensington and Chelsea and Westminster Family Health Services Authority, *Annual Report* (1992)

Parkside NHS Health Trust, *Annual Report* (1994)

Unpublished Theses

Allen, E. J., 'Child Health Care in the Inner City: Perceived Roles and Responsibilities', Ph.D. thesis, Queen Mary and Westfield College, London, 1994

Black, G., 'Health and Medical Care of the Jewish Poor in the East End of London, 1880–1939', Ph.D. thesis, Leicester, 1987

Collins, C., 'Women and Labour Politics in Britain, 1893–1932', Ph.D. thesis, London, 1991

Dove, I., 'Powerful and Peripheral: A History of Alice Gregory, Lelia Parnell and Maud Cashmore, Founders of the British Hospital for Mothers and Babies, Woolwich, and the National Training School for Midwives', M.A. thesis, Kent, 1985

Feldman, D. M., 'Immigrants and Workers, Englishmen and Jews: The Immigrant to the East End of London 1880–1906', Ph.D. thesis, Cambridge, 1985

Gillespie, J. A., 'Economic Change in the East End of London during the 1920s', Ph.D. thesis, Cambridge, 1984

Higginbotham, A. R., 'The Unmarried Mother and Her Child in Victorian

London 1834–1914', Ph.D. thesis, Indiana, 1985

Kenner, C., 'The Politics of Married Working Class Women's Health Care in Britain, 1918–39', M.A. thesis, Sussex, 1979

Koven, S., 'Culture and Poverty: The London Settlement House Movement 1870–1914', Ph.D. thesis, Harvard, 1987

Laxton, J., 'The Making of a Labour Victory: Woolwich in the years up to 1903', B.A. thesis, Thames Polytechnic, 1975

Lumley, L. H., 'Obstetric Performance of Women after in Utero Exposure to the Dutch Famine', Ph.D. thesis, Columbia, 1988

Marks, L., 'Irish and Jewish Women's Experience of Childbirth and Infant Care in East London 1870–1939: The Responses of Host Society and Immigrant Communities to Medical Welfare Needs', D.Phil. thesis, Oxford, 1990

Peretz, E. P. 'Local Authority Maternal and Child Welfare Services in England and Wales, 1919–1939: A Comparative Study', Ph.D. thesis, Middlesex University, 1992

Rose, G., 'Locality, Politics and Culture: Poplar in the 1920s', Ph.D. thesis, Queen Mary College, London, 1988

Ross, E. M., 'Women and Poor Law Administration, 1857–1909', M.A. thesis, London, 1956

Smith, E. R., 'East End Jews in Politics, 1918–1939', Ph.D. thesis, Leicester, 1990

Thom, D., 'Women Munition Workers at Woolwich Arsenal in the 1914–18 War', M.A. thesis, Warwick, 1976

Watkins, D. E. 'The English Revolution in Social Medicine, 1889–1911', Ph.D. thesis, London, 1984

Weinbren, D., '"The Peace Arsenal" Scheme: The Campaign for Non-munitions Work at the Royal Ordnance Factory, Woolwich after the First World War', Ph.D. thesis, Thames Polytechnic, 1990

Wilkinson, A. M. 'The Beginnings of Disease Control in London: The Work of the Medical Officers of Health in Three Parishes 1856– 1900', D.Phil. thesis, Oxford, 1981

Williams, N., 'Infant and Child Mortality in Urban Areas of Nineteenth Century England and Wales: A Record Linkage Study', Ph.D. thesis, Liverpool, 1989

Conference Papers and Other Unpublished Works
Lumley, L. H. and Van Poppel, F. W. A., 'Health and Demographic Effects of the Dutch Famine of 1944–45', paper presented to Society for Social History of Medicine Annual Conference on Famine and Disease, 5–7 July 1991, Cambridge

Pitt, S. J., 'Midwifery and Medicine: Gendered Knowledge in the Practice of Delivery', unpublished paper presented to the Conference 'Nursing,

Bibliography

Women's History and the Politics of Welfare', Nottingham University, 21–24 July 1993

Stewart, J., Lewis N. and Longley, D., 'Accountability to the Public', Paper presented to the European Policy Forum for British and European Market Studies Conference, December 1992

White, J., 'Old Worlds for New', unpublished MS

Published Sources

(Place of publication London unless stated otherwise)

Before 1939

Adams, W. G. S., 'Work and Progress in Social Welfare', in *The Archway*, 2/6 (March 1939), 129–39

Ashby, H. J., *Infant Mortality* (Cambridge: 1915)

Association of Infant Welfare and Maternity Centres, *Report on Enquiry on Existing Ante-Natal Centres* (The National League for Health, Maternity and Child Welfare: 1925)

Idem, Talks on Health (The National League for Health, Maternity and Child Welfare: 1929)

Barefoot, W., *Twenty-five Years' History of the Woolwich Labour Party 1903–28* (1928)

Barton, E., *The National Care of Motherhood* (1928)

Battersea, C., *Reminiscences* (1922)

Booth, C., *Life and Labour of the People in London: East London*, 1 (2nd edn, 1889); Ser. 1, *Poverty*, 4 Vols (1902); Ser. 2, *Industry*, 5 Vols (1895–7); Ser. 3, *Religious Influences*, 7 Vols (1895–7); *Notes on Social Influences and Conclusion, Final Vol.* (1902)

Central Bureau for the Employment of Women, *The Fingerpost: Section 1 Public and Social Work* (c.1910)

Cooke, R. G., 'An Analysis of 350 Cases of Abortion', *Br. Med. J.*, 1 (May 1938), 1045–7

Cox, V., 'Team Work and Post-Natal Care', *Mother and Child*, 5/9 (1934), 348–9

Eckhard, E. V., *The Mother and the Infant* (1921)

Fairfield, L. 'Ante-natal Care and Hospitals', *Nosokomeion* 5/3 (1934), 203–4

Idem, 'Maternity Work in LCC Hospitals, 1931–36', *Proceedings of Royal Society of Medicine*, 31 (January 1938), 237–50

Fisher, H. A. L., *The Citizen* (1927)

Franklin, C., *Caroline Franklin 1863–1935 – An Appreciation* (book printed and written by friends for private circulation, 1936 – copy held at BL [1086 cc.15])

Gebbie, N., 'Some Effects of the Local Government Act, 1929, or the Future of Maternity and Child Welfare', *Med. Offr.* (1 November 1930), 193

Heighton, J. H., *The Place of the Voluntary Worker in Civic Life and Social work* (1918)

Himes, N. 'British Birth Control Clinics: Some Results and Eugenic Aspects of their Work', *Eugenics Review* (1928)

Himes, N. and Himes V., 'Birth Control for the British Working-Classes: A Study of the First Thousand Cases to Visit an English Birth Control Clinic', *Hospital Social Service* (1929)

Hope, E. W. 'Observations on Autumnal Diarrhoea in Cities', *Publ. Health* (July 1899), 660– 5

Hope, E. W. and Campbell, J., *Report on the Physical Welfare of Mothers and Children, England and Wales* (1917)

Hurry, J. B., *District Nursing on a Provident Basis* (1898)

Hutchins, B. L., *Working Women and the Poor Law* (1909)

Lane-Claypon, J., *The Child Welfare Movement* (1920)

Llewellyn Davies, M., *Maternity: Letters from Working Women* (1915; repr. with intro. by Gloden Dallas, 1984)

Llewellyn Smith, H., *The New Survey of London,* 9 Vols (1930–5)

Martyn, E. H. and Bird, M., *The Birth Control Movement* (1930)

Maternal Mortality: Report of the Meeting held at Friends House, Euston Road, November 15 1932 (1932) (Fawcett Library 304.64)

McLeary, G. F., *The Early History of the Infant Welfare Movement* (1933)

Idem, The Maternity and Child Welfare Movement (1935)

Mellanby, E., 'Accessory Food Factors (Vitamines) in the Feeding of Infants', *The Lancet* (17 April 1920), 856–64

Morland, E., *Alice and the Stork* (1951)

Munro Kerr, J. M., *Maternal Mortality and Morbidity* (Edinburgh: 1933)

National Birthday Trust Fund, *Maternal Welfare* (1936)

Newman, G., *Infant Welfare. A Social Problem* (1906)

Idem, The Health of the State, edited by P. Alden (1907)

Newsholme, A., *Fifty Years in Public Health* (1935)

Osman Newsland, H., *The Model Citizen* (1907)

Oxley, W. H. F., 'Prophylaxis in Midwifery', *Med. Offr.* (25 August 1928), 79–81

Pember Reeves, M., *Round About a Pound a Week* (1913; repr. with intro. by S. Alexander, 1984)

Pringle, J. C., *British Social Services: The Nation's Appeal to the Housewife and her Response* (1933)

Ramsbotham, E., 'The Eastern District of the Royal Maternity Charity', *London Medical Gazette, New Ser.*, 2 (1843–44), 619–25

'Report of the Infant Committee', *Trans. Obstet. Soc.*, 13 (1870), 132–49

Saleeby, C. W., 'The Human Mother', in *Report of the Proceedings of the Second National Conference on Infantile Mortality* (1908)

Snell, Lord 'Voluntary Assistance in the Modern State', *Charity Organisation Society Quarterly* (January 1939), 1–2

Spring Rice, M. *Working-Class Wives* (1939; repr. with intro. by B. Wootton, 1981)

Idem, 'The Health of Working Women', *The Eugenics Review*, 32/2 (1940), 50–4

Stocks, M. D., *The Meaning of Family Endowment* (1921)

Taussig, F., *Abortion, Spontaneous and Induced: Medical and Social Aspects* (National Committee on Maternal Health: 1936)

Webb, B., *My Apprenticeship* (1926; repr., 1971)

Webb, S., *The Decline in the Birth Rate*, Fabian Tract, No. 131 (1907)

Webb S. and Webb B. (eds), *The Break-Up of the Poor Law: Being Part One of the Minority Report of the Poor Law Commission* (1909)

Whitelegge, B. A. and Newman, G., *Hygiene and Public Health* (1905)

Williams, W., *Deaths in Childbed* (1904)

Young, J., 'Maternal Mortality and Maternal Mortality Rates', *The American Journal of Obstetrics and Gynaecology*, 31/1 (1936), 198–212

After 1939

Abel-Smith, B., *The Hospitals* (1964)

Abrams, P., *Historical Sociology* (Somerset: 1982)

Adelstein A. M. and Marmot, M. G., 'The Health of Migrants in England and Wales: Causes of Death', in J. K. Cruickshank and D. G. Beevers (eds), *Ethnic Factors in Health and Disease* (1989)

Alderman, G., *London Jewry and London Politics 1889–1986* (1989)

Alexander, S., 'Women's Work in Nineteenth Century London: A Study of the Years 1820–50', in E. Whitelegge *et al.* (eds), *The Changing Experience of Women* (Oxford: 1982)

Idem., *Becoming a Woman and Other Essays in 19th and 20th Century Feminist History* (1994)

Alexander, S., Davin, A. and Hostetler, E., 'Labouring Women: A Reply to Eric Hobsbawm', *Hist. Workshop J.* (1979), 174–82

Aronovitch, B., *Give It Time* (1974)

Balarajan R. and Botting, B., 'Perinatal Mortality in England and Wales: Variations by Mother's Country of Birth', *Health Trends*, 21 (1989), 79–84

Bibliography

Baldwin, P., *The Politics of Social Solidarity: Class Bases of the European Welfare State 1875–1975* (Cambridge: 1990, 1992)

Baly, M. E., *A History of the Queen's Nursing Institute 1887–1987* (1987)

Banks, J. A., *Prosperity and Parenthood* (1956)

Barnes, A., *Tough Annie: from Suffragette to Stepney Councillor* (1980)

Bellamy J. M. and Saville J. (eds), *Dictionary of Labour Biography* (1979)

Bermant, C., *Point of Arrival* (1975)

Beveridge, W., *Voluntary Action* (1948)

Black, N., 'Private Health Care: Patients' Beliefs and Practice', *Br. Med. J.,* 307 (10 July 1993), 81

Bock, G. and Thane, P. (eds), *Maternity and Gender Policies: Women and the Rise of European Welfare States 1880–1950* (1991)

Bolster, E., *The Sisters of Mercy in the Crimean War* (Cork: 1964)

Botting B. and Macfarlane, A. J., 'Geographical Variation in Infant Mortality in Relation to Birth Weight 1983–85', in OPCS, *Mortality and Geography: A Review in the mid-1980s England and Wales,* Series DS9, (1990)

Botting B. and Cooper, J., 'Analysing Fertility and Infant Mortality by Mother's Social Class as Defined by Occupation – Part II', *Population Trends,* 74 (1993), 27–33

Brändström, A., 'The Impact of Female Labour Conditions on Infant Mortality: A Case Study of the Parishes of Nedertorneå and Jokkmokk, 1800–1896', *Soc. Hist. Med.,* 1/3 (1988), 329–58

Brasnet, M., *Voluntary Social Action* (1969)

Brenner, M. H., 'Foetal, Infant and Maternal Mortality during periods of Economic Instability', *International Journal of Health Services,* 3 (1973), 145–59

Brookes, B., 'Women and Reproduction', in J. Lewis (ed.), *Labour and Love: Women's Experience of Home and Family 1850–1940* (Oxford: 1986)

Idem, Abortion in England 1900–1967 (Oxford: 1988)

Bryder, L., 'The First World War: Healthy or Hungry?', *Hist. Workshop J.,* 24 (1987), 141–57

Idem, Below the Magic Mountain: A Social History of Tuberculosis in Twentieth Century Britain (Oxford: 1988)

Bulmer, M., *The Social Basis of Community Care* (1987)

Bulmer, M., Bales, K. and Kish Sklar, K. (eds), *The Social Survey in Historical Perspective* (Cambridge: 1991)

Burman, S. (ed.), *Fit Work for Women* (1979)

Caldwell, J. C., 'Cultural and Social Factors Influencing Mortality Levels in Developing Countries', in S. H. Preston (ed.), *Annals of the American Academy of Political and Social Science: World Population: Approaching the*

Year 2000 (Newbury Park, London, New Dehli: 1990)

Idem, 'Major New Evidence on Health Transition and its Interpretation', *Health Transition Review*, 1/2 (1991), 221–9

Campbell, R. and Macfarlane, A., *Where to be Born? The Debate and the Evidence* (Oxford: 1987)

Canon, J., *Princess Louise Kensington: A Hospital's Story 1924–1989* (Kensington and Chelsea Community History Group: 1989)

Carnac Rivett, L., 'The Report of the Abortion Committee of the Joint Council of Midwives', *The Journal of the Royal Institute of Public Health and Hygiene*, 4/11 (November 1941), 263 –70

Cartwright, A., *Parents and Family Planning Services* (1970)

Cartwright, F., *The Story of the Community of the Nursing Sisters of St John the Divine* (1968)

Chamberlain, M., *Old Wives Tales* (1981)

Chamberlain, M. and Richardson, R., 'Life and Death', *Oral Hist.*, 10/1 (1983), 31–43

Cheney, R. A., 'Seasonal Aspects of Infant and Childhood Mortality: Philadelphia, 1865– 1920', *J. Interdisc. Hist.*, 14 (1984), 561–85

Christ, C., 'Victorian Masculinity and the Angel in the House', in M. Vicinus, (ed.), *A Widening Sphere* (Indiana: 1972)

City and Hackney Health Authority, 'The Mother's Hospital', *The City and Hackney Health Authority Newsletter*, Issue 12 (May 1986), 1

Clark Kennedy, A. E., *The London. A Study in the Voluntary Hospital System*, 2 Vols (1962)

Cohen, D., 'Private Lives in Public Spaces: Marie Stopes, the Mothers' Clinics and the Practice of Contraception', *Hist. Workshop J.*, 35 (1993), 95–116

Cohen, S., 'Anti-Semitism, Immigration Controls and the Welfare State', *Critical Social Policy*, 13 (1985), 73–92

Collini, S., *Liberalism and Sociology. L. T. Hobhouse and Political Argument in England, 1880–1945* (Cambridge: 1979)

Cooter, R. (ed.), *In the Name of the Child: Health and Welfare, 1880–1940* (1992)

Craft, N., 'Secrecy in the NHS', *Br. Med. J.*, 309 (17 Dec. 1994), 1640

Crowther, M. A., *The Workhouse System 1834–1929* (1981)

Idem, 'Paupers or Patients? Obstacles to Professionalization in the Poor Law Medical Service Before 1914', *J. Hist. Med.*, 39 (1984), 33–54

Cunningham, A. S.,'Breastfeeding and Morbidity in Industrialized Countries: An Update', in D. B. Jelliffe and E. F. P. Jelliffe, *Advances in International Maternal and Child Health* (Oxford: 1981), 128–68

Davey, C. 'Birth Control in Britain during the Interwar Years: Evidence from the Stopes Correspondence', *Journal of Family History,* 13/3 (1988), 329–45

Davidoff, L. and Hall, C., *Family Fortunes* (1987)

Davies, C. (ed.), *Rewriting Nursing History* (1980)

Idem, 'The Health Visitor as Mother's Friend: A Woman's Place in Public Health, 1900– 1914', *Soc. Hist. Med.,* 1/1 (1988), 39–59

Davis, J., 'Jennings' Buildings and the Royal Borough: The Construction of the Underclass in Mid-Victorian England', in D. Feldman and G. Stedman Jones (eds), *Metropolis London: Histories and Representation Since 1800* (1989)

Davin, A., 'Imperialism and Motherhood', *Hist. Workshop J.,* 5 (1978), 9–66

Dearlove, J., *The Reorganisation of British Local Government* (Cambridge: 1979)

Delamont, S. and Duffin, L. (eds), *The Nineteenth Century Woman: Her Cultural and Physical World* (1978)

Den Otter, S., *Society and Things Social: British Idealists and Social Explanation, 1880–1914* (Oxford: 1995)

Digby, A., *Pauper Palaces* (1978)

Doern, G. B., 'The UK Citizen's Charter: Origins and Implementation in Three Agencies', *Policy and Politics,* 21/1 (1993), 17–29

Donnison, J., *Midwives and Medical Men: A History of the Struggle for the Control of Childbirth* (1977, 1988)

Dougherty, P., *Mother Mary Potter: Foundress of the Little Company of Mary 1847–1913* (1961)

Dove, I., *Yours is the Cause: Suffragettes in Lewisham, Greenwich and Woolwich* (1988)

Idem, 'Women's Suffrage and the Woolwich Labour Party 1908', *South London Record: Southwark and Lambeth History Workshop,* 1 (1985), 24–32

Driver, F., 'The Historical Geography of the Workhouse System in England and Wales, 1834–1883', *J. Hist. Geog.,* 15/3 (1989), 267–86

Ducrocq, F., 'The London Biblewomen and Nurses Mission, 1857–1880: Class Relations/Women's Relations', in B. J. Harris and J. K. McNamara (eds), *Women and the Structure of Society* (Duke, 1984)

Duffin, L., 'The Conspicuous Consumptive – Woman as an Invalid', in S. Delamont and L. Duffin (eds), *The Nineteenth Century Woman: Her Cultural and Physical World* (1978)

Dwork, D., *War is Good for Babies and Other Young Children: A History of the Infant and Child Welfare Movement, 1898–1918* (1987)

Dyhouse, C., 'Working-Class Mothers and Infant Mortality in England, 1895–1914', *J. Soc. Hist.,* 12 (1979), 248–67

Dyos, H. J. and Wolff, M. (eds), *The Victorian City: Images and Reality,* 2 Vols (1973)

Bibliography

Eatwell, R., 'The Woolwich Labour Party, 1903–51', in D. Clark (ed.), *Origins and Development of the Labour Party in Britain at Local Level* (1982)

Edgar, D, 'Are You being Served', *Marxism Today* (May 1991), 28

Edgerton, D.,'Liberal Militarism and the British State', *New Left Review,* 185 (1991), 138–69

Evandrou, M., Falkingham, J. and Glennerster, H.,'The Personal Social Services: "Everyone's Poor Relation but Nobody's Baby"', in N. Barr *et al.* (eds), *The State of Welfare* (Oxford: 1990), 20–1

Ewbank, D. C. and Preston, S. H., 'Personal Behaviour and The Decline in Infant and Child Mortality: The United States 1900–1930', in J. Caldwell *et al.* (eds), *What We Know about Health Transition: The Cultural, Social and Behvioural Determinants of Health,* Vol. 1 (Canberra: 1990)

Eyler, J., 'The Sick Poor and the State: Arthur Newsholme on Poverty, Disease and Responsibility', in D. Porter and R. Porter (eds), *Doctors, Politics and Society: Historical Essays* (Amsterdam: 1993)

Fairbanks, J., *Booth's Boots: Social Service Beginnings in the Salvation Army* (1983)

Feldman D. and Stedman Jones, G. (eds), *Metropolis London: Histories and Representations Since 1800* (1989)

Fildes, V., 'Breastfeeding in London, 1905–1919', *J. Biosoc. Sci.,* 24 (1992), 53–74

Idem, 'Breastfeeding Practices during Industrialization, 1800–1919', in F. T. Falkner (ed.), *Infant and Child Nutrition Worldwide: Issues–Perspectives* (Florida: 1991)

Finlayson, G., 'A Moving Frontier: Voluntarism and the State in British Social Welfare 1911–1949', *Twentieth Cent. Br. Hist.,* 1/1 (1990), 183–206

Idem, Citizen, State, and Social Welfare in Britain 1830–1990 (Oxford: 1994)

Fishman, W. J., *East End Jewish Radicals* (1975)

Idem, East London 1888 (1988)

Fissell, M. E., 'The "Sick and Drooping Poor" in Eighteenth-Century Bristol and its Region', *Soc. Hist. Med.,* 2/1 (1989), 35–58

Flinn, M. W., 'Medical Services Under the New Poor Law', in D. Fraser, (ed.), *The New Poor Law in the Nineteenth Century* (1976)

Fox, D. M., *Health Policies and Health Politics: The British and American Experiences 1911–1965* (Princeton, N. J.: 1986)

Fox, E., 'The Jewish Maternity Home and Sick Room Helps Society 1895–1939: A Reply to Lara Marks', *Soc. Hist. Med.,* 4/1 (1991), 117–22

Idem, 'Powers of Life and Death: Aspects of Maternal Welfare in England and Wales Between the Wars', *Med. Hist.,* 35 (1991), 328–52

Fraser, D., *The New Poor Law in the Nineteenth Century* (1976)

Idem, The Evolution of the British Welfare State (1984)

Freeden, M., *Liberalism Divided* (Oxford: 1986)

Idem, 'The Stranger at the Feast: Ideology and Public Policy in Twentieth Century Britain', *Twentieth Cent. Br. Hist.,* 1/1 (1990), 9–34

Friedman, A., 'Midwifery: Legal or Illegal? A Case Study of an Accused, 1905', in C. Maggs (ed.), *Nursing History: The State of The Art* (1987)

Fuchs, R. G., 'Preserving the Future of France: Aid to the Poor and Pregnant in 19th Century Paris', in P. Mandler (ed.), *The Uses of Charity: The Poor on Relief in the Nineteenth Century Metropolis* (Philadelphia: 1990)

Giddens, A., *The Transformation of Intimacy: Sexuality, Love and Eroticism in Modern Societies* (1992)

Gillespie, J. A., 'Poplarism and Proletarianism: Unemployment and Labour Politics in London, 1918–34', in D. Feldman and G. Stedman Jones (eds), *Metropolis London: Histories and Representation Since 1800* (1989)

Gillis, J. R., 'And the Risks of Illegitimacy in London, 1801–1900', *Fem. Stud.,* 5/1 (1979), 142–73

Gittins, D., 'Women's Work and Family Size Between the Wars', *Oral Hist. J.,* 5 (1977), 84–100

Idem, 'Married Life and Birth Control Between the Wars', *Soc. Hist.,* 3/2 (1975), 53–64

Idem, Fair Sex, Family Size and Structure 1900–1939 (1982)

Glennerster, H., Power, A. and Travers, T., 'A New Era for Social Policy: A New Enlightenment or a New Leviathan?', *J. Soc. Pol.,* 20/3 (1993), 389–414

Graham, N., 'The Epidemiology of Acute Respiratory Infections in Children and Adults: A Global Perspective', *Epidemiol. Rev.,* 12 (1990), 149–78

Idem, Great Britain Committee on Medical Aspects of Food Policy, Present Day Practice in Infant Feeding: Third Report (1988)

Hadfield E. C. R. and MacColl, J. E., *Pilot Guide to Political London* (1945)

Hale, R. 'The History of Health Visiting', in R. Hale, M. Loveland and G. M. Owen (eds), *The Principles and Practice of Health Visiting* (Oxford: 1968)

Hall, R., *Marie Stopes* (1978)

Hall R. (ed.), *'Dear Dr Stopes': Sex in the 1920s* (1978, 1981)

Hardy, A., 'Rickets and the Rest: Diet, Infectious Disease and the Late Victorian Child', *Soc. Hist. Med.,* 5/3 (1992)

Idem, The Epidemic Streets: Infectious Disease and the Rise of Preventive Medicine, 1856–1900 (Oxford: 1993)

Harris, J.,'The Webbs, The Charity Organisation Society and the Ratan Tata Foundation: Social Policy from the Perspective of 1912', in M. Bulmer, J. Lewis, and D. Piachaud (eds), *The Goals of Social Policy* (1989)

Idem, Private Lives, Public Spirit: A Social History of Britain 1870–1914 (Oxford: 1993)

Hennock, E. P., 'Poverty and Social Theory in England: The Experience of the Eighteen-Eighties.', *Soc. Hist.*, 1 (1976), 67–91

Idem, 'Concepts of Poverty in the British Social Surveys from Charles Booth to Arthur Bowley', in M. Bulmer, K. Bales, and K. Kish Sklar (eds), *The Social Survey in Historical Perspective* (Cambridge: 1991)

Higginbotham, A. R., 'Respectable Sinners: Salvation Army Rescue Work with Unmarried Mothers 1884–1914', in G. Malmgreen (ed.), *Religion in the Lives of English Women 1730–1930* (1987)

Idem, '"Sin of the Age": Infanticide and Illegitimacy in Victorian London', *Vict. Stud.*, 32/3 (1989), 319–38

Hills, J., *The Future of Welfare: A Guide to the Debate* (1993)

Hirst, P. Q., *The Pluralist Theory of the State: Selected Writings of G.D.H Cole, J.N. Figgis and H.J. Laski* (1989)

Hodge, M. *Quality, Equality, Democracy: Improving Public Services,* Fabian Pamphlet 549, (1991)

Hodgkinson, R. G., *The Origins of the National Health Service* (1966)

Hollis, P., *Ladies Elect: Women in English Local Government 1865–1914* (Oxford: 1987)

Holloway, S. W. F., 'The All Saints' Sisterhood at University College Hospital 1862–1899', *Med. Hist.*, 3/1 (1959), 146–56

Honigsbaum, F., *The Struggle for the Ministry of Health* (Social Administration Research Trust: 1970)

Idem, The Division in British Medicine (1979)

Idem, Health, Happiness and Security: The Creation of the National Health Service (1989)

Hunter, D. and Webster, C., 'Here We go Again', *Health Services Journal,* 102 (1992), 26– 7

Huss, M. M., 'Pronatalism and the Popular Ideology of the Child in Wartime France: The Evidence of the Picture Postcard', in R. Wall and J. Winter (eds), *The Upheaval of War: Family, Work and Welfare in Europe, 1914–1918* (Cambridge: 1988)

Illingworth J., *et al.,* 'Diminution in Energy, Expenditure During Lactation', *Br. Med. J.,* 292 (15 February 1986), 437–41

Jalland, P., *Women, Marriage and Politics* (Oxford: 1986)

Jones, C., 'Sisters of Charity and the Ailing Poor', *Soc. Hist. Med.,* 2/3 (1989), 339–48

Jones, E., and Eyles, J., *An Introduction to Social Geography* (Oxford: 1977; 1979)

Kearns, A. J., 'Active Citizenship and Urban Governance', *Instit. Br. Geog. Trans.,* New Ser. 17 (1992), 20–34

Bibliography

Klein, R., *The Politics of the National Health Service* (1983)

Idem, 'Labour's Health Policy', *Br. Med. J.* 304 (29 Feb. 1992), 517–18

Knight, P., 'Women and Abortion in Victorian and Edwardian England', *Hist. Workshop J.*, 4 (1977), 37–81

Knott, S., *The Electoral Crucible: The Politics of London 1900–1914* (1977)

Koven, S. and Michel, S., 'Womanly Duties: Maternalist Politics and the Origins of Welfare States in France, Germany, Great Britain, and the United States', *Am. Hist. Rev.*, 95/4 (1990), 1076–108

Idem, (eds), *Mothers of a New World: Maternalist Politics and Origins of Welfare States* (1993)

Koven, S., 'Borderlands: Women, Voluntary Action, and Child Welfare in Britain, 1840–1914', in S. Koven and S. Michel (eds), *Mothers of a New World: Maternalist Politics and the Origins of Welfare States* (1993)

Labour Party, *Your Good Health: A White Paper for a Labour Government* (1992)

Idem, *Health 2000: The Health and Wealth of the Nation in the 21st Century* (1994)

Lake, M., 'A Revolution in the Family: The Challenge and Contradictions of Maternal Citizenship in Australia', in S. Koven and S. Michel (eds), *Mothers of a New World: Maternalist Politics and the Origins of Welfare States* (1993)

Langan M. and Schwarz, B., *Crises in the British State, 1880–1930* (1985)

Leat, D., *The Development of Community Care by the Independent Sector* (1993)

Leathard, A., *The Fight for Family Planning: The Development of Family Planning Services in Britain 1921–74* (London and Basingtoke: 1980)

Leavitt, J. W., 'Birthing and Anaesthesia: The Debate over Twilight Sleep', in J. W. Leavitt (ed.), *Women and Health in America* (Wisconsin: 1984)

Idem, '"Down to Death's Door": Women's Perceptions of Childbirth in America', in J. W. Leavitt (ed.), *Women and Health in America* (Wisconsin: 1984)

Idem, *Brought to Bed: Childbearing in America 1750–1950* (Oxford: 1986).

Idem, 'Joseph DeLee and the Practice of Preventive Obstetrics', *Am. J. Publ. Health*, 78/10 (1988), 1353–9

Lechtig, A. *et al.*, 'Effect of Maternal Nutrition on Infant Mortality', in W. H., Moseley, *Nutrition and Human Reproduction* (New York and London: 1977)

Lee, C. H., 'Regional Inequalities in Infant Mortality in Britain, 1861–1971: Patterns and Hypotheses', *Popul. Stud.* 45 (1991), 55–65

Lee, R., 'Uneven Zenith: Towards a Geography of the High Period of Municipal Medicine in England and Wales', *J. Hist. Geog.*, 14/3 (1988) 260–80

Le Grand, J., 'Can We afford the Welfare State?', *Br. Med. J.*, 307 (23 October 1993), 1018– 19

Leventhal J. M., *et al.*, 'Does Breastfeeding Protect Against Infections in

Infants Less than 3 Months of Age?', *Pediatrics,* 78 (5 November 1986), 896–903

Levy, A. B., *East End Story* (*c.*1949)

Lewis, J., 'The Ideology and Politics of Birth Control in Inter-War England', *Women's Studies International Quarterly,* 2 (1979), 33–48

Idem, The Politics of Motherhood: Child and Maternal Welfare in England, 1900–1939 (1980)

Idem, 'The Social History of Social Policy: Infant Welfare in Edwardian England', *J. Soc. Pol.,* 9 (1980), 463–86

Idem, What Price Community Medicine: The Philosophy, Practice and Politics of Public Health Since 1919 (Brighton, 1986)

Idem, (ed.) *Labour and Love: Women's Experience of Home and Family, 1850–1940* (Oxford: 1986)

Idem, 'The Working-Class Wife and Mother and State Intervention, 1870–1918', in J. Lewis (ed.) *Labour and Love. Women's Experience of Home and Family 1850–1914* (Oxford: 1986)

Idem, Women in England 1870–1950 (Brighton: 1984; 1986)

Idem, 'Reconstructing Women's Experience of Home and Family', in J. Lewis (ed.), *Labour and Love: Women's Experience of Home and Family 1850–1940* (Oxford: 1986)

Idem, 'Mothers and Maternity Policies in the Twentieth Century', in J. Garcia, R. Kilpatrick and M. Richards (eds), *The Politics of Maternity Care. Services for Childbearing Women in Twentieth-Century Britain* (Oxford: 1990)

Idem, 'Models of Equality for Women: The Case of State Support for Children in Twentieth Century Britain', in G. Bock and P. Thane (eds), *Maternity and Gender Policies: Women and the Rise of European Welfare States, 1880s–1950s* (1991)

Idem, Women in Social Action in Victorian and Edwardian England (1991)

Lister, R., 'Tracing the Contours of Women's Citizenship', *Policy and Politics,* 21/1 (1993), 3–16

Lodge, M., 'Aspects of Infant Welfare in Coventry 1900–40', in B. Lancaster and T. Mason (eds), *Life and Labour in a Twentieth Century City: The Experience of Coventry* (Coventry: 1986)

Loudon, I. S. L., 'Historical Importance of Outpatients', *Br. Med. J.,* 1 (1978), 974–7

Idem, 'Deaths in Childbed from the 18th Century to 1935', *Med. Hist.,* 30/1 (1986), 1–41

Idem, 'Obstetric Care, Social Class and Maternal Mortality', *Br. Med. J.,* 2 (1986), 606–8

Idem, 'Puerperal Fever, The Streptococcus and The Sulphonamides 1911–1945', *Br. Med. J.,* 2 (1987), 485–90

Idem, 'Maternal Mortality: 1880–1950. Some Regional and International

Bibliography

Comparisons', *Soc. Hist. Med.,* 1/2 (1988), 183–228

Idem, 'On Maternal and Infant Mortality, 1900–1960', *Soc. Hist. Med.,* 4/1 (1991), 29–74

Idem, 'Some Historical Aspects of Toxaemia Pregnancy. A Review', *Br. J. Obstet. & Gynaecol.,* 98 (1991), 853–8

Idem, 'Some International Features of Maternal Mortality, 1880–1950', in V. Fildes, L. Marks, and H. Marland (eds), *Women and Children First. International Maternal and Infant Welfare 1800–1950* (1992)

Idem, Deaths in Childbirth: An International Study of Maternal Care and Maternal Mortality 1800–1950 (Oxford: 1992)

Lovell, J., *Stevedores and Dockers: A Study of Trade Unionism in the Port of London 1870–1914* (1969)

Lowe, R., 'The Second World War and the Foundations of the Welfare State', *Twentieth Cent. Br. Hist.,* 1/1 (1990), 152–82

Macfarlane, A., 'Statistics and Policy Making in the Maternity Services', *Midwifery* (1985), 150–61

Idem, 'Review and Assessment of Models of Care Using Research Information and Data: The Role of Routinely Collected Data', in G. Chamberlain and N. Patel (eds), *The Future of Maternity Services* (1994)

Macfarlane, A. and Mugford, M., *Birth Counts. Statistics of Pregnancy and Childbirth,* 2 Vols (1984)

Macfarlane, A., *et al., Counting the Changes in Childbirth: Trends and Gaps in National Statistics* (Oxford: 1995)

Macnicol, J., *Family Allowances* (1981)

Maggs, C., 'Nurse Recruitment to Four Provincial Hospitals 1881–1921', in C. Davies (ed.), *Rewriting Nursing History* (1980)

Mahler, H., 'The Safe Motherhood Initiative: A Call to Action', *The Lancet* (21 March 1987), 668–70

Mamdani, M. and Ross, D., 'Review Article: Vitamin A Supplementation and Child Survival: Magic Bullet or False Hope?', *Health Policy and Planning,* 4 (1989), 273–94

Manton, J., *Elizabeth Garrett Anderson* (1965; 1987)

Mark-Lawson, J., Savage, M. and Warde, A., 'Gender and Local Politics: Struggles over Welfare Policies, 1918–1919', in *The Lancaster Regionalism Group, Localities, Class and Gender* (1985)

Marks, L., 'The Experience of Jewish Prostitutes and Jewish Women in the East End of London at the Turn of the Century', *The Jewish Quarterly,* 34/2 (126) (1987), 6–10

Idem, '"Dear Old Mother Levy's": The Jewish Maternity Home and Sick Room Helps Society 1895–1939', *Soc. Hist. Med.,* 3/1, (1990), 61–88

Idem, 'Working Wives and Working Mothers: A Comparative Study of Irish and East European Jewish Married Women's Work and Motherhood in East London 1870–1914', in the Polytechnic of North London Irish Studies Centre, *Occasional Papers Series*, No. 2 (1990)

Idem, 'Ethnicity, Religion and Healthcare', *Soc. Hist. Med.*, 4/1 (1991), 123–8

Idem, 'Carers and Servers of the Jewish Community: The Marginalized Heritage of Jewish Women in Britain', in T. Kushner (ed.), *The Jewish Heritage in British History* (1992)

Idem, 'Mothers, Babies and Hospitals: "The London" and The Provision of Maternity Care in East London, 1870–1939', in V. Fildes, L. Marks and H. Marland (eds), *Women and Children First. International Maternal and Infant Welfare 1800–1950* (1992)

Idem, '"The Luckless Waifs and Strays of Humanity": Irish and Jewish Immigrant Unwed Mothers in London 1870–1939', *Twentieth Cent. Br. Hist.*, 3/2 (1992), 113–37

Idem, 'Medical Care for Pauper Mothers and Their Infants: Poor Law Provision and Local Demand in East London, 1870–1929', *Econ. Hist. Rev.*, 46/3 (1993)

Idem, *Model Mothers: Jewish Mothers and Maternity Provision in East London 1870–1939* (Oxford: 1994)

Marland, H., *Medicine and Society in Wakefield and Huddersfield* (Cambridge: 1987)

Idem, 'A Pioneer in Infant Welfare: The Huddersfield Scheme 1903–1920', *Soc. Hist. Med.* (1994)

Marshall, T. H., *Citizenship and Social Class* (1950)

Marwick, A., *The Deluge: British Society and the First World War* (New York: 1965)

Mather, G. 'Serving You Rights', *Marxism Today* (May 1991), 29

Meckel, R. A., *Save the Babies: American Public Health Reform and the Prevention of Infant Mortality, 1850–1929* (1990)

McClaren, A., *Birth Control in Nineteenth Century England* (1978)

McCleary, G. F., *The Development of British Maternity and Child Welfare Services* (1945)

McEwan, M., *Health Visiting* (1950)

Miliband, R., *The State in Capitalist Society* (1973)

Mitchell, B. R., *European Historical Statistics, 1750–1975* (Cambridge: 1980)

Idem, *British Historical Statistics* (Cambridge: 1988)

Mitchell, H., *The Hard Way Up* (1968; 1984)

Mommsen, W. J. (ed.), *The Emergence of the Welfare State in Britain and Germany, 1850– 1950* (1981)

Moore, M. J., 'Social Work and Social Welfare: The Organisation of Philanthropic Resources in Britain, 1900–1914', *J. Br. Stud.*, 16 (1977), 85–104

Morley R., *et al.*, 'Mother's Choice to Provide Breast Milk and the Developmental Outcome', *Archives of Disease in Childhood*, 63 (1988), 1382–5

Moscucci, O., *The Science of Woman: Gynaecology and Gender in England 1800–1929* (Cambridge: 1990), 185–7

Moseley, W. H., *Nutrition and Human Reproduction* (New York and London: 1977)

Mulgan, G. 'Power to the Public', *Marxism Today* (May 1991), 14–19

Munro Kerr, J. M., Johnstone, R. W. and Phillips, M. H. (eds), *Historical Review of British Obstetrics and Gynaecology, 1800–1950* (Edinburgh: 1954)

Murray, R., 'The State After Henry', *Marxism Today* (May 1991), 22–7

Nicholls, D., *The Pluralist State* (1975)

North Kensington Community History Group, *Women Remember* (North Kensington Community History Group, *c.*1980)

Idem, They were Happy Days (North Kensington Community History Group, *c.*1983)

Oakley, A., *The Captured Womb: A History of the Medical Care of Pregnant Women* (Oxford: 1984)

Idem, 'Wisewoman and Medicine Man: Changes in the Management of Childbirth', in J. Mitchell, and A. Oakley (eds), *The Rights and Wrongs of Women* (1976; 1979)

Idem, Women Confined: Towards a Sociology of Childbirth (Oxford: 1980)

Oddy, D., 'Working Class Diets in late Nineteenth Century Britain', *Econ. Hist. Rev.*, 2nd Ser., 23 (1970), 314–23

Pamuk, E. R., 'Social Class Inequality in Infant Mortality in England and Wales from 1921 to 1980', *Eur. J. Popul.*, 4 (1988) 1–21

Peacock, A. and Wiseman, J., *The Growth of Public Expenditure in the UK* (Oxford: 1961)

Pearson, M., Spencer, S. and McKenna, M. 'Patterns of Uptake and Problems presented at Well Woman Clinic in Liverpool', *J. Publ. Health*, 13/1 (1991), 42–7

Pedersen, S., *Family, Dependence, and the Origins of the Welfare State, Britain and France, 1914–1945* (Cambridge: 1993)

Pelling, M. and Smith, R. (eds), *Life, Death and the Elderly: Historical Perspectives* (1991)

Pennybacker, S., '"The Millenium by Return of Post": Reconsidering London Progressivism, 1889–1907', in D. Feldman and G. Stedman Jones (eds), *Metropolis London: Histories and Representations Since 1800* (1989)

Peretz, E. P., 'The Professionalization of Childcare', *Oral Hist.*, 17/1 (1989), 22–8

Idem, 'A Maternity Service for England and Wales: Local Authority Maternity

Bibliography

Care in the Interwar Period in Oxfordshire and Tottenham', in J. Garcia, R. Kilpatrick and M. Richards (eds), *The Politics of Maternity Care* (Oxford: 1990)

Idem, 'Regional Variations in Maternal and Child Welfare Between the Wars: Merthyr Tydfil, Oxfordshire and Tottenham', in D. Foster and P. Swan (eds), *Essays in Regional Local History* (Hull: 1992)

Idem, 'The Costs of Modern Motherhood to Low Income Families in Interwar Britain', in V. Fildes, L. Marks and H. Marland (eds), *Women and Children First. International Maternal and Infant Welfare 1800–1950* (1992)

Idem, 'Infant Welfare in Oxford between the Wars', in R. Whiting (ed.), *Oxford and its People* (Manchester: 1992)

Pfeffer, N., *The Stork and the Syringe: A Political History of Reproductive Medicine* (1993)

Pfeffer N. and Pollock, A., 'Public Opinion and the NHS', *Br. Med. J.,* 307 (27 September 1993), 750–1

Pfeffer N. and Coote, A., *Is Quality Good for You: a Critical Review of Quality Assurance in Welfare Services,* Institute for Public Policy Research, Social Policy Paper No. 5, 1994

Phoenix, A., 'Black Women and Maternity Services', in J. Garcia, R. Kilpatrick and M. Richards (eds), *The Politics of Maternity Care: Services for Childbearing Women in Twentieth-Century Britain* (Oxford: 1990)

Picchio, A., *Social Reproduction: The Political Economy of the Labour Market* (Cambridge: 1992)

Pickstone, J. V., *Medicine and Industrial Society: A History of Hospital Development in Manchester and its Region* (Manchester: 1985)

Porter, D., '"Enemies of the Race": Biologism, Environmentalism, and Public Health in Edwardian England', *Vict. Stud.,* 34/2 (1991), 160–77

Porter, R., *London: A Social History* (1994)

Powell, M., 'Hospital Provision Before the NHS: Territorial Justice or Inverse Care Law', *J. Social Policy,* 21, Part 2 (April 1992), 145–64

Preston, S. H. and Haines, M. R., *Fatal Years: Child Mortality in Nineteenth Century America* (Princeton: 1991)

Prochaska, F. K., *Women and Philanthropy in Nineteenth Century England* (1980)

Idem, 'Body and Soul: Bible Nurses and the Poor in Victorian London', *Hist. Research,* 60/143 (1987), 336–48

Idem, The Voluntary Impulse: Philanthropy in Modern Britain (1988)

Idem, 'A Mother's Country: Mothers' Meetings and Family Welfare in Britain, 1850–1950', *Hist.* (1989), 379–99

Idem, Philanthropy and the Hospitals of London: The King's Fund 1897–1900 (Oxford: 1992)

Ramsay, E., *East London Nursing Society 1868–1968: A History of a Hundred*

331

Bibliography

Years (1968)

Richardson, R., *Death, Dissection and the Destitute* (1988; 1989)

Richardson, R. and Hurwitz, B., 'Joseph Rogers and the Reform of Workhouse Medicine', *Br. Med. J.* (16 December 1989), 1507–10

Rivett, G., *The Development of the London Hospital System* (1986)

Robbins, M., 'Breaking Up the Blocs', *Marxism Today* (May 1991), 30–3

Roberts, E., 'Working-Class Standards of Living in Barrow and Lancaster 1890–1914', in P. Thane (ed.), *Essays in Social History* (Oxford: 1986)

Idem, A Woman's Place: An Oral History of Working-Class Women 1890–1940 (Oxford: 1984; 1986)

Roberts, R., *The Classic Slum* (1971; 1977)

Rose, G., 'Locality, Politics and Culture: Poplar in the 1920s', *Society and Space* 6 (1988), 151–68

Idem, 'The Struggle for Political Democracy: Emancipation, Gender and Geography', *Society and Space: Environment and Planning,* 8/4 (1990), 395–408

Idem, 'Imagining Poplar in the 1920s: Contested Concepts of Community', *J. Hist. Geog.,* 16/4 (1990), 425–37

Rose, L., *The Massacre of the Innocents: Infanticide in Britain, 1800–1939* (1986)

Rose, M., 'Settlement, Removal and the New Poor Law', in D. Fraser (ed.), *The New Poor Law in the Nineteenth Century* (1976)

Rosenfield, A. and Maine, D., 'Maternal Mortality – A Neglected Tragedy: Where is the M in MCH', *The Lancet* (13 July 1985), 83–5

Ross, E., '"Fierce Questions and Taunts": Married Life in Working Class London, 1870– 1914', *Fem. Stud.,* 8/3 (1982), 575–602

Idem, 'Women's Neighbourhood Sharing in London before World War One', *Hist. Workshop J.,* 15 (1983), 4–27

Idem, 'Labour and Love: Rediscovering London's Working-Class Mothers, 1870–1918', in J. Lewis (ed.), *Labour and Love: Women's Experience of Home and Family 1850–1940* (Oxford: 1986)

Idem, Love and Toil: Motherhood in Outcast London, 1870–1918 (Oxford: 1994)

Rowbotham, S., *Hidden from History: 300 Years of Women's Oppression and the Fight Against It* (1973)

Idem, Royal College of Obstetricians and Gynaecologists, Report on a National Health Service (1944)

Ryan Johansson, S., 'Sex and Death in Victorian England', in M. Vicinus (ed.), *A Widening Sphere* (Indiana: 1977)

Ryan, P. A., '"Poplarism" 1894–1930', in P. Thane (ed.), *The Origins of British Social Policy* (1978)

Bibliography

Saint A. (ed.), *Politics and the People of London: the LCC 1889–1965* (1989)

Idem, 'Politics and Relief: East London Unions in the Late Nineteenth and Early Twentieth Centuries', in M. E. Rose (ed.), *The Poor and the City: The English Poor Law in its Urban Context, 1834–1914* (Leiceste:, 1985)

Saunders, P., 'Rethinking Local Politics', in M. Boddy and C. Fudge (eds), *Local Socialism? Labour Councils and New Left Alternatives* (1984)

Savage, M., *The Dynamics of Working-Class Politics: The Labour Movement in 1880–1940* (Cambridge: 1987)

Schasse, C., 'Social Mothers: The Bourgeois Women's Movement and German Welfare-State Formation, 1890–1929', in S. Koven and S. Michel (eds), *Mothers of a New World: Maternalist Politics and the Origins of Welfare States* (1993)

Schofield, R., 'Did Mothers Really Die? Three Centuries of Maternal Mortality in "The World We Have Lost"', in R. Smith, L. Bonfield, and K. Wrightson (eds), *The World We Have Gained* (Oxford: 1987)

Scott, J. W., 'Gender: A Useful Category of Historical Analysis', *Am. Hist. Rev.* (1986), 1053–75

Idem, *Gender and the Politics of History* (New York: 1988)

Searle, G. R., *The Quest for Efficiency 1899–1914* (Oxford: 1971)

Semmel, B., *Imperialism and Social Reform* (1960)

Sheard, S., 'Gagging Public Health Doctors', *Br. Med. J.*, 309 (17 December 1994), 1643

Smith, E. R., 'Jews and Politics in the East End of London, 1918–1939', in D. Cesarani (ed.), *The Making of Anglo-Jewry* (Oxford:, 1990)

Smith, F. B., *The People's Health 1810–1930* (1979)

Smith, R., 'An Unfree NHS and Medical Press in an Unfree Society', *Br. Med. J.*, 309 (17 December 1994), 1644

Smith, S. J., 'Society, Space, and Citizenship: A Human Geography for the "New Times"', *Trans. Inst. Br. Geog.*, 14 (1989), 144–56

Soloway, R., 'Counting the Degenerates: The Statistics of Race Deterioration in Edwardian England', *J. Contemp. Hist.*, 17/1 (1982), 137–64

Idem, *Birth Control and the Population Question in England, 1877–1930* (1982)

Idem, 'Eugenics and Pronatalism in Wartime Britain', in R. Wall and J. Winter (eds), *The Upheaval of War: Family, Work and Welfare in Europe, 1914–1918* (Cambridge: 1988)

Stedman Jones, G., *Outcast London: A Study in the Relationship Between Classes in Victorian Society* (1971; 1984)

Stucke, R. B. (ed.), *Fifty Years History of the Woolwich Labour Party, 1903–53* (1953)

Bibliography

Summers, A., 'A Home from Home – Women's Philanthropic Work in the Nineteenth Century', in Burman, S. (ed.), *Fit Work for Women* (1979)

Idem, Angels and Citizens: British Women as Military Nurses, 1854–1914 (1988)

Idem, 'The Mysterious Demise of Sarah Gamp: The Domiciliary Nurse and her Detractors', *Vict. Stud.,* 32/3 (1989), 365–86

Idem, 'The Costs and Benefits of Caring: Nursing Charities c.1830–1860', in J. Barry and C. Jones, (eds), *Medicine and Charity* (1991)

Sutton, D., 'Liberalism, State Collectivism and Social Relations of Citizenship', in M. Langan and B. Schwarz (eds), *Crises in the British State 1880–1930* (1985)

Szreter, S., 'The Importance of Social Intervention in Britain's Mortality Decline c.1850–1914: A Reinterpretation of the Role of Public Health', *Soc. Hist. Med.,* 1/1 (1988), 1–39

Teitelbaum, M. S., 'Male and Female Components of Perinatal Mortality: International Trends, 1901–63', *Demography,* 8 (1971), 541–8

Tew, M., *A Safer Childbirth: A Critical History of Maternity Care* (1990)

Thane, P., 'Women and the Poor Law in Victorian and Edwardian England', *Hist. Workshop J.,* 6 (1978), 29–51

Idem, (ed.), *The Origins of British Social Policy* (1978)

Idem, The Foundations of the Welfare State (1982)

Idem, 'The Working Class and State "Welfare" in Britain, 1880–1914', *Hist. J.,* 27, 4 (1984), 877–900

Idem, 'Government and Society in England and Wales 1750–1914', in F. M. L. Thompson, (ed.), *Cambridge Social History of Britain,* Vol. 3, 'Social Agencies and Institutions' (Cambridge: 1990)

Idem, 'Genre et Protection Sociale: La Protection Maternalle et Infantile en Grande-Bretagne 1860–1918', *Genèses,* 6 (1991), 73–97

Idem, 'Women in the British Labour Party and the Construction of State Welfare, 1906–45', in S. Koven and S. Michel (eds), *Gender and the Origins of the Welfare States in Western Europe and North America* (1993)

Idem, 'Visions of Gender in the Making of the British Welfare State: The Case of Women in the British Labour Party and Social Policy, 1906–1945', in G. Bock, and P. Thane (eds), *Maternity and Gender Policies: Women and the Rise of the European Welfare States, 1880s–1950s* (1991)

Thompson, B., 'Infant Mortality in Nineteenth-Century Bradford', in R. Woods and J. Woodward (eds), *Urban Diseases and Mortality in 19th Century England* (1984)

Thompson, F. M. L., *Hampstead: Building a Borough, 1650–1964* (Boston: 1974)

Thompson, P., *Socialists, Liberals and Labour: The Struggle for London, 1885–1914* (1967)

Idem, The Edwardians (1975)

Idem, 'Voices from Within', in H. J. Dyos and M. Wolff (eds), *The Victorian City: Images and Reality,* Vol. 1 (1973)..

Idem, Voice of the Past (1978; 2nd edn, 1988)

Thomson, D., 'The Welfare of the Elderly in the Past: A Family or Community Responsibility?', in M. Pelling and R. Smith (eds), *Life, Death and the Elderly: Historical Perspectives* (1991)

Idem, 'Workhouse to Nursing Home: Residential Care of Elderly People in England Since 1840', *Ageing and Society,* 3 (1983), 43–70

Idem, 'The Decline of Social Security: Falling State Support for the Elderly since Early Victorian Times', *Ageing and Society,* 4 (1984), 451–82

Titmuss, R. M., *Birth, Poverty and Wealth: A Study of Infant Mortality* (1943)

Urwin C. and Harland, E., 'From Bodies to Minds in Childcare Literature: Advice to Parents in Inter-War Britain', in R. Cooter (ed.), *In the Name of the Child: Health and Welfare, 1880–1940* (1992)

Usborne, C., '"Pregnancy is the Woman's Active Service". Pronatalism in Germany during the First World War', in R. Wall and J. Winter (eds), *The Upheaval of War: Family, Work and Welfare in Europe, 1914–1918* (Cambridge: 1988)

Idem, The Politics of the Body in Weimar Germany: Women's Reproductive Rights and Duties (1992)

Vallance, E., 'Women in Politics', *East London Record,* 5 (1982), 2–12

Vicinus, M., *Independent Women: Work and Community for Single Women, 1850–1920* (1985)

Vincent A. and Plant, R., *Philosophy, Politics and Citizenship* (Oxford: 1984)

Walker, A., 'Dependent Relativities', *Times Higher Education Supplement* (22 April 1988)

Walkowitz, J., 'Jack the Ripper and the Myth of Male Violence', *Fem. Stud.,* 8/3 (1982), 543–75

Waller, P., *Town, City and Nation* (Oxford: 1983)

Watterson, P., 'The Role of the Environment in the Decline of Infant Mortality: An Analysis of the 1911 Census of England and Wales', *J. Biosoc. Sci.,* 18 (1986), 457–70

Webster, C., 'Health, Welfare and Unemployment During the Depression', *P & P,* 109 (1985), 204–30

Idem, 'Healthy or Hungry Thirties', *Hist. Workshop J.,* 13 (1988), 110–29

Idem, Problems of Healthcare: The British National Health Service Before 1957 (1988)

Idem, 'Conflict and Consensus: Explaining the British Health Service', *Twentieth Cent. Br. Hist.,* 1/1 (1990), 115–51

Bibliography

White, J., *Rothschild Buildings: Life in an East End Tenement Block 1887–1920* (1980)

Idem, The Worst Street in North London: Campbell Bunk, Islington Between the Wars (1986)

Whynes, D. K., 'The Growth of UK Health Expenditure', *Social Policy Administration*, 26/4 (December 1992), 285–95

Williams, K., *From Pauperism to Poverty* (1981)

Williams, N., 'Death in its Season: Class, Environment and the Mortality of Infants in Nineteenth-Century Sheffield', *Soc. Hist. Med.*, 5/1 (1992), 71–94

Williams, R., *Keywords* (1976)

Willmott, P. and Young, M., *Family and Kinship in East London* (1957; 1967)

Winter, J. M., 'Infant Mortality and Maternal Mortality and Public Health in Britain in the 1930s', *J. Eur. Econ. Hist.*, 8 (1979), 439–62

Idem, 'The Decline of Mortality in Britain 1870–1950', in T. Barker, and M. Drake (eds), *Population and Society in Britain 1850–1980* (1982)

Idem, 'Aspects of the Impact of the First World War on Infant Mortality in Britain', *J. Eur. Econ. Hist.,* 11 (1982), 713–38

Idem, 'Unemployment, Nutrition and Infant Mortality in Britain, 1920–50', in J. M. Winter (ed.), *The Working Class in Modern British History* (Cambridge: 1983)

Idem, The Great War and the British People (1986)

Wohl, A. S., *Endangered Lives: Public Health in Victorian Britain* (1983; 1984)

Women's Group on Public Welfare, *Our Towns: A Close-up. A Study Made in 1939–42* (Oxford: 1943)

Woods, R. I., Watterson P. A. and Woodward, J. H., 'The Causes of Rapid Infant Mortality Decline in England and Wales, 1861–1921 Part I', *Popul. Stud.,* 42 (1988), 343–66

Idem, 'The Causes of Rapid Infant Mortality Decline in England and Wales, 1861–1921 Part II', *Popul. Stud.,* 43 (1989), 113–32

Woods, R. and Woodward, J., 'Mortality, Poverty and the Environment', in Woods, R. and Woodward, J. (eds), *Urban Diseases and Mortality in 19th Century England* (1984)

Woodward, J., *To Do The Sick No Harm: A Study of the British Voluntary Hospital System to 1875* (1974)

Wray, J. D., 'Maternal Nutrition, Breastfeeding and Infant Survival', in W. H. Moseley (ed.), *Nutrition and Human Reproduction* (New York and London: 1977)

Wrigley, E. A., *Population and History* (1969; 1973)

Yeo, S. and Yeo, E., 'On the Uses of "Community": From Owenism to the Present', in S. Yeo. (ed.), *New Views of Co-Operation* (1988)

Index

337

Index